PENGUIN BOOKS

BODY WORRY

The Body Worry Team

Remar Sutton is a syndicated columnist, consumer writer, and novelist. His health and fitness journal, "Fit After 40," currently appears in *The Washington Post*. He also serves as a consulting editor to *American Health* magazine.

Sutton is considered one of America's foremost automotive experts, and his best-selling book, *Don't Get Taken Every Time*, is regarded as the definitive guide to the automobile business. A frequent guest on talk shows such as "Donahue," "Nightline," "Today," "Good Morning America," "The Oprah Winfrey Show," "Hour Magazine," National Public Radio's "All Things Considered," and the Cable News Network, Sutton also appears regularly on scores of regional radio shows to talk directly with consumers. His first novel, *Long Lines*, was published in 1988.

Christopher Scott and Mary Abbott Waite make up the research and editorial parts of the team. Scott, a cum laude graduate of Springfield College, holds a master's degree in sports science and served an extensive internship at Dr. Kenneth Cooper's Institute for Aerobics Research in Dallas, Texas. Waite received a Ph.D. in English from Duke University and has worked extensively as a teacher and an editor.

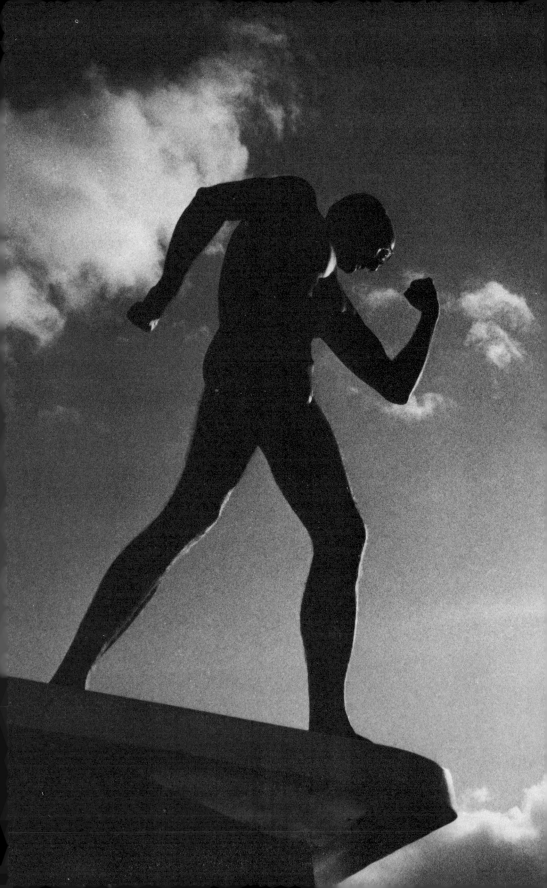

BODY
WORRY

BY REMAR SUTTON

PENGUIN BOOKS

PENGUIN BOOKS

Published by the Penguin Group
Viking Penguin Inc., 40 West 23rd Street,
New York, New York 10010, U.S.A.
Penguin Books Ltd, 27 Wrights Lane, London W8 5TZ, England
Penguin Books Australia Ltd, Ringwood,
Victoria, Australia
Penguin Books Canada Limited, 2801 John Street,
Markham, Ontario, Canada L3R 1B4
Penguin Books (N.Z.) Ltd, 182–190 Wairau Road,
Auckland 10, New Zealand

Penguin Books Ltd, Registered Offices: Harmondsworth,
Middlesex, England

First published in the United States of America by
Viking Penguin Inc. 1987
This revised edition published in Penguin Books 1988
Published simultaneously in Canada

LIBRARY OF CONGRESS CATALOGING IN PUBLICATION DATA
Sutton, Remar.
Body Worry.
Bibliography: p.
Includes index.
1. Health.   2. Physical fitness.   3. Body image.
I. Title.
[RA776.S945   1988]   613.2   87-7282
ISBN 0 14 00.9744 9

Printed in the United States of America by
R. R. Donnelley & Sons Company, Harrisonburg, Virginia
Set in Aster

DEDICATION

To 603 and G.A.P.
To M.A. and M.M.
And to N.L.

ACKNOWLEDGMENTS

Before I started my remake, I knew as much about hunkdom, health and fitness as I know about the moon. And I am not an astronomer.

Hundreds of people, therefore, needed to educate me, if my experience was to be valuable for others. I can't name them all here, but would like particularly to thank these.

Christopher Scott and Dr. Mary Abbott Waite are my two fellow members of the Body Worry Team. Chris Scott's knowledge and research skills in the medical and physiology fields are the reason this book is, I hope, an unusually complete layman's guide. Dr. Waite, my friend, personal editorial adviser, and partner in most endeavors, researched, organized and edited the enormous amounts of information in the narrative and discussion portions of this book. Mary Abbott makes writing a joy for me. *Body Worry* would not be a book without these two people, and I am thankful for them and look forward to working with them on other books.

Margaret Mason, then the Style Plus editor at the *Washington Post*, believed in my year before anyone else in the media found it interesting. The power of that paper, and therefore the impact of her decision, have in many ways changed my life. Since Margaret has retired, Peggy Hackman and the rest of the Style Plus staff have been as helpful to me.

As has Tracy Brown, my editor at Viking Penguin. Tracy has fought many battles for me.

ACKNOWLEDGMENTS

Thomas P. Rosandich, Ph.D., president and founder of the United States Sports Academy, advised me on the structure and make-up of my Body Worry Committee. Tom's enthusiasm for my idea kept my enthusiasm high when others weren't so encouraging. His contacts, and the help of the Academy, were invaluable.

Dr. Kenneth Cooper, president and founder of the Aerobics Center in Dallas, has provided me constant advice, testing and access to his medical and sports associates throughout the year. Dr. Arno Jensen, Pamela Neff, Georgia Kostas, and Kia Vaandrager all worked with the Body Worry Team virtually weekly. Dr. Cooper, Dr. Jensen, and Georgia Kostas, M.P.H., R.D., L.D., director of the Aerobics Center nutrition program, also spent hours reviewing this manuscript, and all improved it. Dr. Jensen, his wife, Joan, and their son, Eric, have been particularly helpful in preparing the revised edition of *Body Worry*. You will see their pictures in the exercise section, too.

Kia Vaandrager, her daughter Kiki, and her husband, Dr. Johan Vaandrager, have gathered more research papers and answered more of Christopher Scott's questions than I think *they* want to know!

Gideon Ariel, Ph.D., LaVon Johnson, Ph.D., and Robert Stauffer, Ph.D., all worked with me, thanks to Tom Rosandich. Gideon Ariel has advised me on my weight lifting goals and techniques, and has also been a valuable source on many matters. Spending a weekend with him is like spending the weekend with a rocket—brilliant! Von Johnson, at that time Chairman of the Department of Fitness Management at the Sports Academy, both recommended Christopher Scott as my physiologist and planned portions of my year's physical regimen. Bob Stauffer, a fellow of the American College of Sports Medicine, introduced me to Dr. Kenneth Cooper. During the entire project, Bob has guided me down the middle road in research, exercise, and hunkdom. The soundness of his advice is very evident in this book.

Dr. Robert Bell, at the very beginning of my planning, encouraged me to make my year a search for health and then hunkdom. I didn't want to listen to him at first, but I owe him thanks for his insistence. Bob's testing, advice, and suggestions on this manuscript were all important to me.

David Heber, M.D., Ph.D., Chief of the Division of Clinical Nutrition at UCLA's School of Medicine, answered many questions for both Chris and me. Dr. Art Leon at the University of Minnesota

ACKNOWLEDGMENTS

shared his considerable epidemiological knowledge with Chris; Michael Pollock, Ph.D., an internationally noted exercise physiologist, talked with us several times from his offices at the University of Florida. Dr. Herbert deVries, a noted authority on exercise and aging, advised us on our comments and opinions on those topics.

Eric Goldstein, Ph.D., shared with us his insights on stress. He is a stress management specialist in Miami. Dr. Frank M. Kamer raised my opinion of plastic surgeons. When I visited his very upscale practice in Beverly Hills, he recommended against surgery for me. How long since a doctor has sent you away?

William T. Jarvis, Ph.D., taught me a lot about quacks. He is President of the National Council Against Health Fraud, and a Professor of Health Education at Loma Linda University. Dick Clark, Clinical Director of the Hyperbaric Center at Richland Memorial Hospital, gave me a first-hand education in hyperbaric medicine, and I am thankful for him.

Kelly Kehlet, R.D., reviewed early drafts of our Godly Eating Plan in the new how-to section. Our thanks for her insights.

David Prowse, both in London and in the Bahamas, has taken a great interest in my year. His advice on weight lifting techniques and strength-building exercises has contributed a lot toward my remake.

Former Mr. Universe Tony Pearson not only helped me with my weight lifting routine, he allowed me the great fantasy of kicking sand vaguely in his direction at muscle beach, as did Champ McGregor and Debra Walker. Mike Christian, Mr. Universe 1985, brought me back to earth when he showed me his routine *and* his right biceps. Do not compare right biceps with him.

Russell Burd, my trainer, has done the most to actually change my body. Russ had the terrible chore of getting me to the gym six days a week, for months on end. His patience and skill as a trainer in working with me made these days nearly pleasurable. Russ and Kim, his wife, are now back in Perkiomenville, Pennsylvania, and I look forward to the day they open their own gym. I would like to work out there.

Until that time, I work out most often with Bill and Marilynn Carle at the Grand Bahama YMCA. Neither Bill nor Marilynn, owners and managers of the gym, has ever laughed at my weight lifting efforts, and that in itself endears them to me. Dr. John Clement, my island doctor, both doctored my weight lifting ills and my spirits. He makes a great neighbor. Doc was even a part of the Body

ACKNOWLEDGMENTS

Worry aerobics class. Lauren Hunt-Manning, now living in Taiwan, ran that class for me, and all of us alumni would like her back: Warren Manning, Gerry Matt, Judy Graham, Bill Nelson, Joan Munnings, Pam Ferguson, Keith Thompson, Sarah Lihou, Kim and Russell Burd, plus Ricky and Doc. Thanks to you all for participating.

John Englander, president of The Underwater Explorer's Society, didn't ever exercise with us, but he did keep my brain working. He has been a good sounding board for me during the year, and also spent many hours reading this manuscript for accuracy. Will and Deni McIntyre *did* exercise with us, and did about everything else with me, too, as they took over 18,000 photographs of me during the months.

Hunkdom and health don't mean much without the right people to share them. My right people include my family: Mom, brother George and his family, Bunny and Buck, Peggy, and all the cousins and friends in Swainsboro and Marietta.

Chris Scott wouldn't have made it through the year without the help of Debbie and Bob Spusta, John Sheetz, Tom Sekeres, Keith Markolf, Michele Coyne, and Jonathan Scott, Chris's identical twin brother. I do not think the world is ready for two.

I wouldn't have made it through the year without all of the people listed in these pages, and thank them all from the top to the bottom of my healthy and semi-hunky body.

Because in many instances I have provided my own interpretation of others' works and thoughts, I, of course, am solely responsible should those interpretations or any fact be in error. Since I'm pretty strong now, though, I wouldn't pick a fight with me. Muscles and health.

CONTENTS

CONTENTS

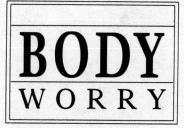

INTRODUCTION TO THE REVISED EDITION

Nearly two years ago I started writing to a group of friends and media contacts around the country, telling them about my grand plans to remake my body—a body much in need of overhaul. Since letter writing runs in my family, I hoped the recipients would enjoy a personal and very informal blow-by-blow account of my trials and triumphs (assuming there would be triumphs) just as I over the years had enjoyed many of their personal experiences via mail.

It perked me up quite a bit, therefore, when Margaret Mason from *The Washington Post* called and asked to run my letters as a bimonthly column. United Feature Syndicate didn't exactly make me feel bad, either, when they asked to run versions of the letters as a weekly column around the country.

Because the letters were so popular, I used portions of them as the basis for many of the narrative sections of *Body Worry*'s first edition. Rewritten and expanded, they remain as the basis for the narrative of this edition, too. But beyond the narrative, *Body Worry* has changed somewhat, become one of those "new and improved" models auto makers always seem to brag about.

Well, as we know, "new and improved" sometimes seem to be in the eye of the maker, not the user, so let me quickly tell you what this book is about and why it can help you if you are honestly concerned about the state of your body. First, put it back if you already exercise regularly, are careful about what you eat, don't abuse drugs (including alcohol and cigarettes), can still fit into your high school clothes, and are happy about your looks. Go buy a book on Tantric Yoga or something. You are obviously a health nut or worse, so go away.

But if you are like most of us—not really interested in physical fitness or dieting or doing things that hurt or giving up things that taste good—please continue to read, because this book will tell you about health and then tell you how to get it with modest changes in your eating habits and doable changes in your activity level. (That last phrase sounds so much better than "exercise.")

Body Worry first answers the questions I think most of us want to ask about health and fitness in general. Since I had never really thought about health and fitness much, and was essentially unschooled in even the basics of those things, I gathered up a committee of experts such as Dr. Kenneth Cooper (the man who coined the word "aerobics") and Dr. William Jarvis (president of the National Council Against Health Fraud) to educate me.

For instance, what is health? What is fitness? Why is fat bad, if it is? Why are seemingly all the things that taste good bad for you? To my surprise, a lot of the simple questions hadn't been answered in layman's terms. They are here. Because health is such a dynamic field, I have updated and expanded all of the first-edition answers, when necessary, and plan to keep updating this book, too.

I had originally intended to report on shortcuts to health and fitness. Since I hate a fat stomach, and had one that qualified for the *Guinness Book of World Records,* I wanted to buy one of those machines that supposedly melt the fat away with electrical currents. And I thought about getting the machine that looks like a barrel-shaped abacus and supposedly just rolls the fat off you.

As you would expect, I found out those things were junk, as were an awful lot of the products, books, and methodologies in health and fitness. The only quick fix out there was the fast injection of money into the pockets of those who take us for suckers. I decided to write about those things, too.

Then I decided to write about the myths and true but unusual realities in health. For instance, I used to think that exercise, when you got around to it, would make up for bad eating habits. You know, walk a mile and work that greasy piece of fried chicken and that biscuit soppy with butter out of your system. Lots of people have died because they believed that myth. Or do you know a man with thin arms and legs but a large pot belly? That person, particularly if he is bald, is statistically much more likely to have a heart attack than a more symmetrically shaped person.[1] And I do hope you notice *my* shape back when this all started.

AND THEN ALONG CAME THE REVISED EDITION

The first edition told you how important the road to health was and how damnable stepping off that road could be, but it didn't really give you a detailed road map to get there yourself.

The revised edition gives you that in a very unusual format. It lets you decide how much you and/or your family are going to change your eating habits, and then tells you exactly how to make those changes without making life miserable. Our approach shows you how to design an eating modification program you can live with for life.

We take the same approach with exercise, based on your particular goals and time limitations. If you, like me, really do hate exercise per se, you'll probably choose the most modest exercise programs, and that's fine. But if you get enthusiastic as changes begin to take place in your health and shape, we will show you how to increase your activities, too.

The exercise and eating portions of *Body Worry* have added over 150 pages to the book, and *work with your goals in mind.*

Finally, *Body Worry* still deals with "surface" things like looks. My own looks—or, more specifically, my insecurities about my looks—have probably ruled my life more than I want to admit. You may feel the same way about yourself, and I think you'll find these parts of the book interesting.

The information we give you in *Body Worry* may not be what you want to hear at times—for instance, flat bellies, contrary to what the television commercials say, are about as hard to come by as cheap books—but it is as accurate and updated as possible, and without hype.

Very little is black and white in health and fitness. Many issues are complicated and controversial. But the work of my committee, dozens of other doctors and scientists, and *Body Worry* physiologist Christopher Scott means the answers you will see here are thoughtful, carefully formed, and backed by much research and cross-checking. In the back of the book you'll find sources for my thoughts, all of them noted in the text.

A *WORD ABOUT PHIL, NORMA, AND THE KIDS*

Please, oh God, I hope you don't have a family like this. As I was writing the discussion portions of this book, this unusual family, how shall I say it? . . . "appeared"—I don't know any way to describe Norma and Phil and Busbo and Blinki other than to say they're real nice folks but probably not the type you would want to sit by at your twenty-fifth high school reunion. They all certainly seemed to be looking over my shoulder as I wrote, however, butting in, adding their questions to mine. I think someone once said great things come from little minds, and am sure you will agree that little nugget applies very well to my friends.

As I said in the beginning, I'm a layperson, and, even after changes in my health and happiness, I still don't read the AMA journal or jogging magazines. I still don't love exercise, either, even after nearly two years of work and dramatic changes in my health brought on by exercise, and I still wish there was a health and fitness pill.

But there isn't. I therefore hope you will find *Body Worry* the least painful entryway to that most mystical world of health, fitness, and good looks. And I think the way to start is with my first letter.

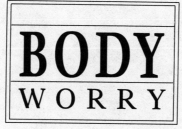

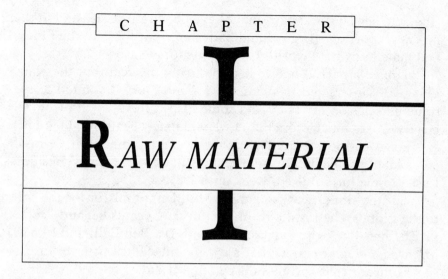

RAW MATERIAL

Week 1

<u>*Grand Bahama Island*</u>

I can look out the window and see the ocean, a calm one, and a shimmering red Bahamian sun breaking through scarlet clouds scattered low along the horizon, like in the movies. A very nice day to start, I think.

I am a forty-five-year-old man without muscles, bald, twenty-seven pounds overweight, no longer involved in much physical activity, somewhat self-conscious about my looks, and even more self-conscious about the thought of trying to improve them within smirking range of those god types who were born fit, don't sweat, and seem to be everywhere I am when vanity prods me to the thought of exercise.

In June 1985, I decided it would be nice to chuck it all and spend a year devoted solely to making myself handsome. By November, even my publisher seemed to be intrigued with the idea. What could you do to a middle-aged body in a year? By December, we had come to terms—a milestone, I might add. It takes a lot of money and discipline to chuck it all, hire a full-time trainer, move to an island, recruit a fancy committee of medical, strength, and fitness experts, build lots of muscles, turn a watermelon belly into a sexy, flat

1

stomach, perhaps add hair, maybe even have a face-lift, and in the process report on the good and bad things out there in the fitness and male hunkiness world. I was game, though.

I planned a partial nod to health during the year, but the plans that really interested me centered around looks. I wanted to see some muscles on my body and some lust in the eyes of a tropical beauty or two much more than I wanted to feel healthier. I felt fine, anyway. Most people are a little overweight and get a little tired and a lot of people used to smoke and still drink regularly. Besides, I used to jog forty miles a week until 1981.

About the time I was packing my full-length mirror for the trip to the islands, the results from my physical exams began to come in. The first doctor to call was a friend, Dr. Bob Bell, and I knew him well enough to know that a cough and slight stutter before he speaks means that bad news is coming. It did.

"Remar, I'm afraid you're not as well as you think." He paused. I remember the pause very well and don't know how to describe its feeling other than lonely. "I'm afraid you have some heart disease."

What was this man talking about? I wanted to be a hunk, not worry about my health. Even before I could try to hide from his words, Dr. Bell emphasized them with specifics. The thallium stress test and first-pass radionuclide angiogram showed that I have mild coronary heart disease: mild left ventricular dysfunction. Reduced left ventricular ejection fraction; drop in the stroke volume; abnormality on the front and back walls of the left ventricle. The possible causes? Probably the result of too little exercise, too many cigarettes, and those extra pounds. Another test showed that I have a small pulmonary dysfunction. The cigarettes I enjoyed for so long, of course. A final test showed that one of my liver functions is abnormal.

None of these unpleasant bits of information, incidentally, would show up during the normal yearly physical you may undergo, even if you have a stress EKG and standard bloodwork. I had three stress EKGs, and they were all normal. I hope that's an unnerving thought for you but I am not complaining here. At least I know what is wrong with me. According to my good adviser Dr. Kenneth Cooper, the man who started America jogging, forty percent of people with coronary heart disease have only one symptom of that disease: death from a heart attack.

Well, if all of this wasn't enough to temporarily still my yearnings for a high lust factor, two other members of my medical team rated me in the high-risk category for heart attack, even though I don't have high blood pressure, exercise more than the majority of people, and haven't been a smoker in over a year. The extra pounds and lack of meaningful exercise and my diet, too, are the culprits in their minds.

Dr. Von Johnson, Chairman of the Department of Fitness Management at the United States Sports Academy, tested my oxygen consumption per kilogram of weight, a measure of cardiovascular fitness. He did not comment on the results, but simply handed me a chart entitled "Risk Category" with my name at the top and a red circle around the fifth line from the bottom, the one labeled "very high."

Finally, Dr. Cooper, who had put me on another treadmill and poked and pried some more, said if I didn't change my ways, I could look forward to bypass surgery, developing angina pectoris, heart attack, or sudden death. Sudden death. I don't know why that sounded worse than death alone, but it did. Does sudden death mean there's no time for regrets? Does it hurt?

I dream a lot when things bother me, and my dream that night was of a very well-built Remar Sutton, dressed to show my muscles, laid out in a coffin.

I still want beauties to swoon when they glimpse the new me. But my year is going to be a more balanced one now. I have to make my insides as healthy as my outside will be hunky, a thought with some urgency in it. I want to understand more about my decline in health, too. In 1983, my hometown doctor rated me as a nearly "ideal" health profile. What happened? Can you lose your health in two years? If you can, that's a damn scary thought for a lot of people.

It's 7:30 A.M. now. Before noon I'll have stretched for thirty minutes, walked for a good distance along a palm-fringed beach lined with half-naked people (most of them overweight), biked, and lifted weights for the first time in my life. By sunset I will have talked to a few of the doctors who are worrying over me more than I like, eaten fresh conch salad, drunk papaya juice, and probably flipped through a copy of a muscle magazine. I'm clipping pictures of sample muscles, sort of a hit list for the new surface me.

Doc Clement, my local doctor, lives across the backyard, even closer to the ocean. He checks on me nearly every day, more out of curiosity than concern, I believe.

I am not at all sure what is going to happen to me this year, but I do know it will not be a boring time. More later.

Muscles and health.

So *what is health, anyway?*

Being without pain mentally or physically, having an engine and supporting parts which don't labor under any unnecessary burdens, and possessing habits which protect you mentally and physically from the attack of disease and age.

What *is fitness?*

A state of training in which your body performs tasks efficiently, without undue fatigue. Because it is a trained response, fitness decreases with inactivity.

Can *you be physically fit—a jock—and not be healthy?*

Physical fitness has to do with your ability to do things. For instance, to run hard and fast or to be strong and flexible. Health has to do with the state of your engine and its supporting systems, as I said earlier. Your health is impacted by the things that come into your body. Food. Liquids. Things in the air. You can change your health, and probably the likelihood of having many diseases, without doing any exercise. Simply changing your intake habits can improve your health. Health is also impacted by heredity. Health and fitness, therefore, don't necessarily go hand in hand. If you have a choice between being physically fit and healthy, choose the latter. Now, with all that said, most people who are physically fit are healthy, and most people who are healthy are physically fit. But don't assume one brings the other.[2]

Does heredity predispose us to physical well-being or the lack of it?

It does in many ways. For instance, many diseases appear to haunt families; aging itself seems to be passed through genes, and lots of people are from long-lived backgrounds. The tendency to heart attacks definitely seems to be genetically passed on.[3]

But those heart attacks may also be related to family eating, smoking, and drinking habits. Those are definitely learned and passed along, too. Recent research indicates that family history of heart disease disappears at times when these poor health patterns are factored out.[4]

If I've inherited bad genes in the health sense, what's the sense in trying?

If you know your particular danger areas in health—for instance, a history of high blood pressure or family tendencies to cancer or heart attack, you can learn to stop damage before it begins in many instances. If you can't stop it, you can modify it. What kills people normally isn't simply a disease itself, for instance, but a disease gone wild.

How much of my shape itself is determined by heredity? (Which is a sneaky way of asking, "Can my wife Norma blame her fat on bad genes?")

The American Medical Association recently reported on the largest study done to date on obesity and identical twins. If it's right, about 80 percent of body composition is determined by heredity.[5] For some people, fat may not be due solely to that extra piece of chocolate or one more six-pack of beer. But a genetic tendency to obesity does not mean any of us is doomed to fat. It may mean we have to control our fat problems differently, and we'll talk about that later.

Speaking of fat, is a little fat all that bad?

Probably not from a health point of view, but the problem is in the definition of "little." Too much fat places a strain on the heart and joints simply from its weight, probably causes increased cholesterol (a fat itself) in our blood, and may lead to "adult onset" diabetes. It also may lead to high blood pressure, arthritis, gall bladder disease, increased blood lipids, increased risk from surgery, impaired heart function, lung problems, and, that most familiar demon of all, psychological distress from looking blimpish.[6]

So how much fat is too much fat?

Five percent above your age group's norm would be considered dangerous.[7] For instance, for me, 16 percent of my weight in fat would be ideal, and 20 percent would be considered normal. When the sickening "before" pictures for this book were taken, my fat level was *30 percent*. In the "after" pictures I'm 15 percent.

How is a body fat percentage determined?

You are composed of bone, lean tissues such as organs and muscles, and fat. Bathroom scales may be good for tracking the changes in your weight, but they can't measure fat itself, obviously. Doctors do that several ways, including underwater weighing and skinfold tests which I'll describe more fully in Chapter 3. But there are a couple of tests you can do at home that are highly accurate. Also, free is nice:

1. Take off your clothes, all of them. Men, grab a pinch of skin on your love handles, and don't be dainty. You will feel the fat, unconnected to your skin. If your pinch is more than an inch thick, you probably need to read on. Women, take a pinch on your hips, legs, or back of the upper arm, where women put on most of their fat. If the results depress you, administer the pinch test to your spouse—if you dare.
2. Stand in front of a mirror and look at yourself. Don't hold it in. Rolls of fat and a memory of a far thinner body when you were younger are good indications of too much *dolce vita*. If your stomach is larger than your chest, you may have a real problem. Did

you know actuarial tables deduct two years of life for every inch a man's stomach is larger than his chest?[8]

Are *you saying even five pounds overweight can be a bad thing?*

Dr. Cooper, president of the Aerobics Research Center, certainly thinks so. On his desk sits a brand-new teaching model of five pounds of fat. How big would you guess the model is? A cupful? The size of a bag of sugar? The model, an exact replica, is eighteen inches long and approximately the height and width of a loaf of bread. From its size most people think it weighs fifteen pounds.

Well, *I may be a little overweight, but I'm in shape. I mean, I cut the grass each week, work around the house, and run like mad at work. Doesn't that count in fitness?*

The only real fitness that counts is fitness that helps your cardiovascular system do the best job your particular system can do. And the cardiovascular system is hard to exercise. Most doctors believe that any conditioning effect requires at least twenty minutes of sustained exercise that substantially raises the level of your heart's work at least three times each week. That's called aerobic exercise, and only takes place when you are working very large muscle groups (such as legs when you jog, or legs and arms when you swim) for long periods of time.[9] Stop-and-go activities don't count aerobically, and simple exercise, such as pushing the lawn mower, doesn't count, either. Any movement more than your normal daily movements is good in building endurance and stamina, but it will not really help your engine and its support systems.

But *I thought you said exercise may not make me live longer.*

It may not, but the *factors associated with the LACK of exercise— overweight, bad intake habits—can definitely kill you.*[10] And exercise will definitely improve the quality of your life, however long that may be. "Quality of life" has nearly become a trite, buzz expression in health and fitness, but is really all that counts. I want to feel good as long as I'm conscious, don't you? And when things go wrong, when that probably inevitable heart attack happens to me, for instance, I want to know that I've made my engine and its support systems as strong as possible to lessen damage. And exercise makes many things strong. Just to give you some hope: the heart, a muscle, responds quickly to it; bones, which grow brittle with age, actually gain more calcium and become strong because of it; soft saggy skin tightens; the lungs provide more oxygen; and the blood actually changes.

But you don't know how I've abused my body, and for how long. Can all this health stuff rebuild burned bridges?

No one can be as bad to his body as I have been. I smoked three packs of cigarettes a day for fifteen years, did the right type of exercise for only two of the past twenty-five years (and overdid it then), and ate foods that would make any sensible person gag or die of fright. I am a "Type A"—high-strung, intense. I could drink Hemingway under the table, and tried to best his types for years. But my insides and outsides have totally changed in a matter of months without radical changes in my life. Too late is only when you're dead.

Well, anyway, let's get on with the story.

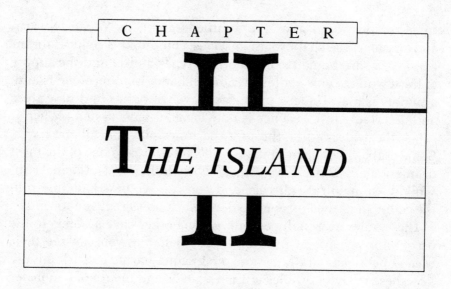

THE ISLAND

Week 2

<u>*Grand Bahama Island*</u>

Grand Bahama Island is located about fifty miles off the coast of Palm Beach, Florida, in the Gulf Stream, in Columbus's path to the New World (*National Geographic* says he stopped in the Bahamas first), and in the path of pirates and bootleggers at various times during the last five hundred years. Back in the early days of the Spanish explorers, the island was occupied by Lucayan Indians, but later the European colonists of Hispaniola and Cuba decided all those heathen Indians needed saving and carted virtually the entire population of our island off to work in their mines and plantations and to find God.

Pirates used to hang around here because the waters are deceptively shallow and booty-laden boats sank as regularly as the tides rise and fall. I don't feel sorry for any of the captains of those booty-laden ships, either, for maps as early as the sixteenth century labeled our waters the *"Gran bajamar,"* the great shallows. Even now treasure finds refuge in those shallows. In 1964, within sight of the Lucayan Beach Hotel, four divers stubbed their flippers on a cache of gold coins and jewels worth over two million dollars.

Former slaves—both freed and escaped—liked the island for the same reason we do now: the weather's great, the ocean is warm and air clear; the shallows themselves, composed of living, vibrant coral reefs, are home to thousands of types of fish, and the supply of fresh water seems endless. Grand Bahama is a limestone island, a porous island. Under our surface layer of palms and pine trees and deserted white beaches is an enormous cave system. When it rains, the waters filter through the limestone and fill the caves. Some of the caves open in the island's interior, and one of the most dramatic ones, Ben's Cave, is part of the Bahamas National Trust. Walk down a spiral staircase and you can see bats hanging from the ceiling and the entrance to deep black holes that run for miles.

These holes eventually end up joining other cave systems in the ocean, and when you fly over Grand Bahama, you can see their ocean openings: dark-blue dots on an aquamarine sea. Island lore says these particular holes are the nostrils and mouth of a monster called Luska. Luska lives under the island. He (or she—the sex of this monster is as of now undetermined) sucks in when hungry, and *watch out*! if you're around that hole. Children have disappeared. Luska blows out, too, making the water boil. Hence, the name Boiling Holes. Scientists say this blowing and sucking has to do with the tides, but I prefer this more likely version.

The bootleggers were aware of these holes, too, and filled their barrels with our pure water just about as regularly as they off-loaded bootleg liquor down on the island's west end. From big, slow boats it was stored in warehouses until sleek mahogany speed-boats picked it up for the night run to the Florida coast. One or two of the warehouses which housed that good Canadian still sit in the village of West End, an exotic community about twenty buildings long, and outside the most run-down, you can occasionally find a man who will tell you Joseph P. Kennedy's yacht used to anchor right offshore a good bit each year. Maybe he liked our fishing.

I use the word "our" in referring to Grand Bahama, because I have vacationed here regularly for the past seven years, and am fond of both the island and its people. My friends here are both native and expatriate, and all of them have seen my weight go up and probably my health go down with the regularity with which I used to drink island rum. Ollie Ferguson, a Bahamian, has always been very diplomatic about my shape. "Well! You're looking, uh, like a fullback these days, Remar." Judy Graham, in her forties and with the energy of a high-tide boiling hole, was just as nice, but got the message over to me, anyway. "Do you need help in zipping your wet suit?" she said once as we prepared to scuba dive.

When I decided to remake myself, therefore, the site for the effort was a given. All I needed was a house, which I found near the beach, and a plan, which God knows everyone wants to give me. Also I need more energy, a thought which fills me after about one hour of my normal day.

After stretching and jogging, I bike five miles to the YMCA with my trainer. Right out of an ad for Soloflex, Russell Burd is a young gymnast from Perkiomenville, Pennsylvania. Put my brain in his body and I'll be happy. Russ spent two months meeting with the doctors who are planning the new me, and moved here to the island with his equally dramatic fiancée, Kim, to implement my Master Body Plan. Quiet, calm, and patient, Russ doesn't make me feel like a fool when I do foolish things. On our first bike trip to the gym, for instance, we stopped by a sporting goods shop to buy some gym shorts. Against the back wall of the store was a set of chrome hand weights. I thought they looked handsome, even serious, and quickly pointed them out to Russ as I reached for a credit card. "Boy, I really like these," I said as I waved to the brawny Bahamian behind the counter, "Let's get them for the house." Russ gave a fleeting glance to the Bahamian. The man had not seen or heard me, thankfully. "We call those 'La Femme Spa' weights, Remar," Russ said quietly. Shiny weights are not in vogue in serious gyms, I've since learned. My hands now touch only the most rusted ones.

Our weight room is filled with them, too. The Grand Bahama YMCA, a modest place, leases the gym to Bill and Marilynn Carle, both Bahamian weight lifting champions. Marilynn recently won the Miss Southeastern United States title, too. With a waist about like my arm, arms like my waist, and a pair of legs only a giant rabbit could emulate, she isn't the type of woman I would pick a fight with; she is very feminine and bright, though, qualities that surprised me. Bill, her husband, is an equally humbling sight for neophytes. Arms like the trunk of an old oak.

Each day, the faithful and the hopeful gather here. But in the mornings, when we usually arrive, only the enormously well-developed seem to occupy the large white-walled, blue-carpeted room. Bill is usually putting Marilynn through her workout in the front part, his voice deep and loud, pushing, taunting her. Other voices mix with his, drifting from behind the partition which divides the gym. One of those voices invariably belongs to the l985 World Games posing champion. Henry Charlton is referred to as a "big boy" in the parlance of lifting circles, though he is relatively small-statured. He has developed a posing routine which is now his ticket to weight lifting competitions all over the world. It's akin to watching the movement of a person under a strobe light, and in London last year it brought down the house. As Henry began to twitch, the audience "went crazy, hooting and hollering," he says calmly. At the memory, he flexes involuntarily and watches his muscles jump in one of the thirty mirrors which line the walls. Except for the glass section which allows lesser mortals standing in the hall to watch, mirrors line the walls.

My first view of the gym was from the hall, too, and the sight of all that rust and sweating muscle and the sound of all that power vibrating the glass partition poured insecurities and fears on me like a lumberjack pours syrup on hotcakes. Though I am six-one, my self-image has always pretty much been that of a nonmuscular, rather frail-looking, nonathletic, recently fat wimp, and at that terrible moment, my image seemed like reality. My bike was wrong, too. Lollipop red with shiny new chrome accents, it was the La Femme Spa of gym bikes, pretty in the midst of black, fenderless, and, yes, rusted bikes.

I had never walked into a weight room before with the intent of lifting weights or consciously looking at muscles, never been embarrassed by a bicycle, and certainly never prayed as fervently that I wouldn't be noticed as I did that first day. An unanswered prayer. The big boys looked at me. I fully expected to see Henry Charlton, the posing champ, lose his composure at the sight and roll from the bench in uncontrollable laughter. He gave me the most inconsequential nod instead, the reaction of the others, too. I was to learn that serious lifters don't go out of their way to greet novice lifters, but they don't laugh at them, either, a respectful pecking order on both sides. Henry said nothing of consequence to me until the second week, incidentally, but when he spoke, I listened and wanted dearly to believe: "Legs you got, and you're gonna have a good chest, too," he said, his eyes seemingly ignoring the twenty-odd pounds of fat on my belly. Henry is a man of vision, maybe a man of blurred vision, but I think he sees real well.

We are in the weight room for about two hours each day, but our actual lifting time is no more than ninety minutes. On Mondays and Thursdays we work only shoulders and back. Tuesdays and Fridays are for arms, and Wednesdays are for legs. It will take a few weeks, Bill Carle says, for my body to adjust to the type of straining and pain weight lifting brings, but both sensations are bearable and at times pleasant. So far. Some of the pain, such as that brought on by leg lifts, is high-pitched and vicious in its intensity and slightly delayed, a flood hitting you an instant after the last push. The relief which follows the pain puts the relief which accompanies a desperately needed leak to shame.

It will be worth it, however, if the muscles come. I obviously can't see them yet. All of me is hidden under fat. The experts say I already have some under there which will begin to show within the month. My new muscles will supposedly begin to show within three or four months. Since I've been waiting all my life, that doesn't seem too long.

Eating and Weight Loss. I have been putting on my fat quietly for about five years, drops of sand steadily piling. The insidiousness of the change made it even worse, of course, for I was never bothered by the gains. Except when I changed closets each season. In 1981, my winter thirty-threes seemed tight. In 1982, spring thirty-fours just wouldn't fasten. Thirty-sixes felt nice in 1983, tight in 1984, and caused a hernia and a move up to thirty-eights in the spring of 1985.

I attributed the tightness to heat shrinkage in my closets at first (they just didn't make clothes like they used to) but finally faced a version of reality in June 1985. June was the month I first thought about redoing myself and I instantly took the thought as an excuse to worry even less about my weight and shape. I needed fat. My thirty-eight-inch stomach didn't seem big enough to deserve its own book yet, and, more importantly, I theorized that muscle was simply rearranged fat. A little weight lifting would in essence tie a string around the two ends of a blob of fat, thereby shaping it, much like a balloon filled with water can be shaped with a knot or two. Ergo . . . more fat meant more muscle.

My theory, fortunately, didn't carry much weight with the doctors who advise me. My excess twenty-seven pounds of free-flowing, greasy-smelling fat, just like the fat I hope you pull from a chicken before cooking, had already jeopardized my health, a jeopardy multiplying geometrically, not arithmetically, with each new pound.

I therefore undertook my new eating patterns with the utmost seriousness. Nothing less than pure would touch my lips. For two days, even the juice we drank was extracted seconds before we drank it with our new ninety-dollar juicer. Liquefied apple, banana, plum, peach, and sapodilla fruit was delicious and supposedly teeming with living vitamins and other terribly healthy organisms; each four-ounce drink took only a minute to make, too. Unfortunately, we figured each four-ounce drink cost about three dollars in fruit, and it took twenty minutes to clean the juicer each time we wanted a four-ounce-three-dollar drink, something I tired of quickly, so I traded the juicer to a fisherman friend for thirty lobster tails (about a hundred and twenty dollars' worth), started buying juice at the grocery store, feel just as healthy, and eat a lot better.

In addition to lobster, fish, and lots of chicken, our diet consists of many vegetables lightly steamed or raw and lots of fruit. We eat pasta at least twice a week, steak probably once a week, and wheat pancakes smothered in a heated sauce of fresh orange juice, crushed bananas, and cinnamon on Sunday. Conch salad, low in fat and calories, is in the fridge at all times for snacking. Every single thing I eat or drink is logged in our computer with a code which identifies the item, quantity, and time consumed. I attribute my weight loss solely to the fact that it's a damn lot of trouble to write down everything you eat or drink, so I eat and drink less. Try it sometime.

My island friends are tremendously supportive of all my efforts, both exercise- and food-wise. They honk and cheer when passing me as I jog or bike. If I'm asked to dinner, all sinful things are kept hidden away as securely as bottles of booze from an alcoholic. I accidently found a chocolate cake in one friend's closet, though, and did take one bite. I tried to make the hole look rat-ish.

R*emar, you spend more time being good than I'll probably ever spend. I want to know if a little exercise—all I'll ever do—is better than no exercise at all.*

Cardiovascular fitness requires an absolute minimum of twenty sustained minutes three times a week. Period. But if you absolutely refuse to think about cardiovascular/aerobic fitness, do something anyway.

Recent research on physical activity and longevity suggests that an active lifestyle will help you keep what you've got and may keep you living longer (more on that later).[1] Any activity or exercise is an improvement over sitting still. A long walk three times a week will at least build stamina. Walking up one flight of stairs at work is better than riding, and you never know who you'll meet on that stairwell. But your engine and its supporting systems won't adapt and strengthen themselves if you don't push them long enough to make them change for the better. This threshold, sorry to say, is twenty minutes three times a week.[2]

But remember, particularly if you've been a couch potato, that consistency is the key. You cannot safely go without exercise for even a few days and then try to make up for your sins by overdoing. A lot of people injure themselves, even die of heart attacks, doing that. So if you've laid off for a week or a lifetime, start moderately and work up.

O*kay. Let's say I'm overweight, depressed, high in cholesterol, and thinking about living a long time. Specifically, what can exercise do in each of these areas?*

Life span. A very interesting study of Harvard alumni indicates that persons with active lifestyles *do* live longer than those of us who seek the tranquillity of minimal movement.[3] Exercise is part of an active lifestyle. Painting the house is an active lifestyle. Pulling a Tom Sawyer is not.

Changing your lifestyle, something my year was all about, isn't as hard as you think, either. And do remember that feeling better is more important than living longer.

Lowering cholesterol. Cholesterols are chemical compounds in the blood. Most doctors believe high levels of the wrong types definitely increase the incidence of heart disease, most particularly the development of atherosclerosis (a narrowing of the arteries). Exercise can increase your good cholesterols.

Losing weight. Run a marathon, 26.2 miles, and you won't even lose a pound of fat. Why not? A marathoner burns only about 2,400 calories during the race,[4] and a pound of body weight has 3,500 calories. The six- and seven-pound weight losses many marathoners experience is caused primarily by temporary fluid loss. So if you're close to thirty pounds overweight like I was, you would need to run over a thousand miles to lose your fat. I'd rather be fat. But exercise helps you lose weight in more ways than the simple burning of calories. As we'll see later, exercise can lower your appetite, make your body more efficient in burning fat, and simply make you look healthier. Looking better makes diet changes more worthwhile.

I don't want to exercise because all those muscles will turn to fat when I get bored and quit.

Both men and women use this as an excuse, but big muscles don't have to come with exercise, even though they can, nor can muscle turn to fat. Big muscles do atrophy when they're not used and lose their tone. Athletes who decrease their exercise programs without decreasing their caloric intake do get fat, too. Too much fuel for too little work. That's exactly what happens to lazy amateurs, too, who use weight lifting as an excuse to overeat and then blame the fat on flabby muscle. It can't happen—fat is fat.

Do diets really work?

No. Diets for most people mean being *deprived*, and no one other than the occasional weird monk can deprive himself for all of his conscious life. That's why serious weight-loss researchers say that being overweight is not the *problem* with anyone—it is the *symptom* of the problem.[5] As with most problems, treating the symptom solves nothing, and usually just creates more problems. Lasting weight loss happens only when your long-term consumption of calories is balanced with your long-term consumption of food.

Do you mean to say all those diet books in our kitchen that promise quick weight loss aren't going to bring sveltedom?

Any diet that cuts calories will bring about weight loss. Any diet that dramatically cuts back your caloric intake will bring dramatic weight loss. But diets that promise weight losses of more than two pounds a week can be dangerous and are certainly taking off more than fat. For example, rapid loss usually takes water with it and virtually always takes muscle tissue with it. Because muscle tissue burns calories much more actively than fat, any loss of muscle will make it harder for you to lose weight the next diet book around.[6] Some of the dangers posed by too-rapid weight loss include dehydration, nausea, dizziness, and impaired kidney function.

Why are there so many diet books?

Because people like to make money.

But, if it's in a bookstore and promoted like mad on television, and associated with or written by some doctor, doesn't it have to be legitimate?

There are no moral or legal restraints in the diet business. Anyone can think up a new diet, and virtually any publishing house will publish it if it's radical or new-sounding enough. Money is the motivation, not good information.

Even the best-sellers?

Some of them, the quack diets, kill people. Virtually all of the fad diets will leave you discouraged and even more overweight. Most diet books are like a math book that says four plus four equals nine. Most of us don't understand the math of weight loss and we therefore don't see the obvious mistakes.

The only way to get svelte again is this: you must slightly modify your eating habits for the rest of your life. An article in the *Journal of Addictive Behavior* says it best: successful weight loss only happened when people *"recognized their own responsibility for their body size. They felt a strong need to take charge of their own weight loss plan"* [emphasis added].[7] Real weight loss, like real health changes, only take place with lifestyle changes. Those changes do not have to be radical.

So *how do we recognize a fad diet?*

They promise dramatic results; their authors have discovered a "secret"; they present one-food solutions; they claim persecution from medical and scientific authorities; they misrepresent basic information; they use scare tactics.[8]

An average man will burn nearly 2,500 calories in a day if he simply sits in a chair. Burning calories isn't magic and dieting doesn't require a quack's book.

What *is a calorie, incidentally?*

It's an amount of food energy measured in heat. One calorie is the amount of energy it takes to raise the temperature of one liter of water one degree Celsius. If you eat a 900-calorie meal, for example, you've just eaten enough energy to raise the temperature of 900 liters of water one degree. This is a handy way to calculate how much food we eat because we are engines burning food to release energy to keep us alive.

How *do researchers actually know how many calories are in something?*

They burn it. The item, such as a chocolate fudge sundae with crushed nuts, fresh cream, and a cherry on top, is actually ignited in something called a "Bomb Calorimeter." The heat released by that tragedy is measured.

How *many extra calories do I have to eat to gain a pound of weight?*

Approximately 3,500. And, logically enough, fat has a lot of calories itself. More than twice as many as carbohydrates and proteins per measure. So it doesn't matter whether you're a connoisseur of greasy pork barbecue or well-aged, well-marbled prime beef; the more fat you eat, the faster you grow fat. To say nothing about what you do to your arteries, but more about that later.

How *do I really know how much food to eat to keep my weight stable?*

Doctors can measure this with complex tests, but if your clothes seem tighter each year, as mine did, you're eating too much.

So *what weight should anyone want to be? Isn't fat inevitable with age?*

"Creeping fat" is real. As we grow older, our lean body mass—the muscle, essentially—is replaced somewhat by fat. But you can dramatically retard that process. Exercise and good eating patterns can make you nearly as lean as an eighteen-year-old swimmer. It will take away that softness in your flesh.

Do *you really mean I should look like I used to in high school?*

The healthy state for any body is lean. If you were lean in high school, in shape in high school, there's absolutely no physiological reason you can't be that way now and forever. If you've never been lean and in shape, like me, you can still be that way.

Let's *get back to exercise, then. No living person is going to see the real state of my body other than my spouse. (Thank God love is blind.) Can I start all this changing and exercising alone? Do I need a gym?*

You don't have to have a gym or a partner, but it helps. Partners can monitor each other's effort and simply be there to help and to share the misery. Gyms of some sort can actually be fun, once you realize other people are as bad off as you may be. Gyms provide lots of toys, too, and supposedly provide good supervision. But many are in business only to sell memberships, and their tactics make the car business pale in comparison, and I should know.

How *can I choose the right gym?*

They're all different, so don't choose one quickly, don't fall prey to a pressure sell, and don't fall simply for high-tech looks. First, decide what your goal is: aerobic fitness, social contact, or muscle work. Serious weight lifting gyms, for instance, aren't good places to meet a date for the night. When you do meet someone there, they can break your arm if you cross them. Second, visit the gym during the time you'll normally be working out there. If the gym is too crowded for your particular activity, choose another one.

If you decide to go to a real gym, the lingo there can be pretty foreign; here are few terms to roll off your tongue casually, if you're game:

• *Z-bar* (also called a curl bar) It weighs about twenty pounds, and is angled in the middle to relieve pressure from the wrists.

• *Nickels* Five-pound weights.

• *Dimes (biscuits)* Ten-pound weights.

• *Quarters* Twenty-five-pound weights.

• *Ripped* What I'm going to look like at the end of this year: having well-defined muscles.

• *Pumped* Muscles filled with blood from hard exercise.

• *Bodybuilder* A lifter interested primarily in esthetic changes.

• *Power Lifter or Olympic Lifter* A lifter interested primarily in strength changes.

• **Big Boy**   Larger, stronger, or better proportioned than the average person. I'm going to be one of these guys, too.

• **Pencil Neck**   Opposite of a big boy, and a term I'm trying to forget.

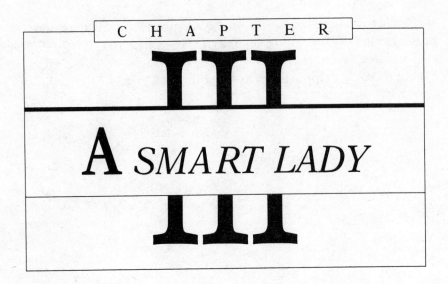

CHAPTER

III

A SMART LADY

III

Week 4
Grand Bahama Island
One month of my remake is over and I'm still alive after 204 bicycling miles, fifteen days of jog-walking, my first injury, and no
booze (do you know how scary that thought was at first?). I'm also
seventeen pounds lighter and six inches smaller around the waist.
I lifted weight six days a week, too. How much total weight do you
think a nonmuscular first-time lifter can lift his first month? Would
10,000 pounds impress you? 75,000 pounds? Neither should. For
you are reading about a man who lifted 385,000 pounds.

The greatest thrill of the month? When Kathy, a friend's very
beautiful, blond, and athletic steady, said, "My God, Remar, you
look good." I think she said it with an exclamation point, but I'm
trying to be conservative here. I don't think I detected the least bit
of swoon or a *soupçon* of lust in this perceptive lady's words or
demeanor, unfortunately, but there was a lot of surprise there, and
I'm real patient.

Just a few minutes ago, something nearly as exciting happened.
After finishing my thirty-minute, twenty-two-position stretching
routine, I, on impulse, decided to try a push-up. I did three. With

perfect form. Though that may not sound impressive for a man who in one month lifted 385,000 pounds, the accomplishment was as sweet to me as the small piece of chocolate pie we had for dessert Sunday, the day we pretty much forget our normal eating routine, for I have never been able to do push-ups.

Many of the small gains mean a lot to me. One month ago standing up quickly and walking to the beach path, only fifty feet away, tired me; scared me, too, since the reality of heart disease had entered my consciousness. I jog-walk two miles now, jogging until I'm breathing hard, then walking until my breathing calms, then jogging again. The first day, I shuffled along for twenty seconds before stopping. This morning, I went five minutes, passing an old lady and a slow-moving dog.

I had one real scare in the gym, or rather I scared the hell out of Russ once. I was doing curls with a forty-pound Z-bar, my third set. After twenty repetitions, my form became sloppy. On the twenty-first repetition, rather than keeping my back straight and my knees slightly bent (which keeps the weight on the legs), I stood straight, then shifted my back to one side. That instantly pulled my back and I turned white, started to drop the bar, and nearly fell backward. Russ, who stands facing me during exercises like this, caught the bar, but was positive I was having a heart attack. The look on his face even scared me.

Funny pains do affect me a little more, now that I think about it. When I'm walk-jogging, I am at times conscious of my heartbeat. When it occasionally skips a beat, as all hearts do, I wonder if the skipping will become more frequent and then become pain and then really become a heart attack. The first time it skipped, I thought of my grandparents. I used to look forward to my summer stays with them because they, like all good grandparents, let my brother and me get away with things. Grandmom let me drive their white 1950 Ford station wagon, handsome wood paneling down the side, the day they bought it. As a ten-year-old driver, my skills weren't too good, and when I backed into the corner of the garage, she did not yell. Granddad didn't yell, either, he simply said I needed more driving lessons and took me out himself. I remember driving by some summer friends of mine, and holding my head high enough, it seemed, to touch a good homemade kite in the Swainsboro sky.

But on my fifteenth birthday my grandad did yell, a sound that still haunts me over thirty years later. On that morning, my grandparents had arrived in Marietta, Georgia, with a new pet for my brother and me, a 300-pound sow quickly nicknamed Petunia the Pig. The pig was to join our growing menagerie of country pets—dogs named Rumpus and Mickey, horses named Trigger (of course), Toni, and Red, and a large gray field rabbit named Humphries. Grandfather worked hard to unload and pen our new pet, trained on command to roll over on her back and "oink," and seemed tickled with his gift.

I was asleep that night when I heard the first yelling, a gasping for air when the heart attack struck him. I had never been that scared before, because I had never seen a person facing death, and did not know that anything could hurt that much. Do you know what really bothered me about that night? There was nothing I could do, there was nothing my grandmother could do but watch the pain. Though my grandfather survived that attack, it was the first time I had ever thought seriously about heart attack. His death from a second attack was one of the few other times I thought about heart disease until this year.

Here on the island, when I become a little discouraged and a lot worn-out from all the work it's taking to remake myself, I think about that night, and the feelings of mortality it brought me. Living is not just a gift. It is earned, too.

And, God knows, I am earning it. My first month's gains in both strength and endurance were more than even my most wishful supporters had thought possible; my looks are improving, and none of my clothes fit me any more (the first time in years that problem has made me smile). And, most important of all, I feel so damn good about myself. Do you know how nice that feels?

I*f it's earned, when does the work begin to pay off?*

Changes on the inside. Even if you spent a lifetime abusing your insides with bad food, smoking, and a sedentary and/or sinful lifestyle, you can make things better relatively quickly. Cardiovascular changes begin to take place in three to five weeks, cholesterol and other blood-related factors in as little as three to eight weeks, depending upon the individual.[1]

Strength and stamina. Changes here can take place quickly, within a week or two, if you are consistent in your exercise program. Anything more than your current activity level will promote change in these areas.

Muscle growth.   Muscles grow very slowly. Change is measured in pieces of inches. If you're a man over forty, be happy with an inch on your arm in a year. But an inch on your arm combined with several inches off your belly makes for a dramatically different shape. I refer you to the handsome devil on the cover of this book. Woman can have bigger muscles if they want to, but they don't have to.

Weight loss.   The slower you lose it, as I said, the longer it will be off. Eliminate 200 calories a day, for instance (drink two diet drinks rather than regular drinks), and cut out enough calories to lose twenty pounds, probably permanently, in a year.

T*hat's all very interesting, but what is the very first thing I will notice if I begin to exercise?*

A dramatic improvement in energy. Most people notice that within days, along with improvements in their sleeping. But some of the long-term changes are as interesting. Did you know consistent, sustained exercise will eventually increase the number of blood vessels throughout your body? Increase the pumping power of the heart? Make the burning of fat, not that you have much, a much more productive process?[2]

P*hil says he hates exercise, period. Does it ever become fun?*

People who really don't like exercise probably are not ever going to begin giggling about it. But attitudes do change somewhat. Tell him to pick the exercise he likes the most (or hates the least) and stick with it for a few months. In time, it will become habit, just like taking out the garbage.

Okay, muscles may not come easy but you seem able to lose weight easily and that makes a big difference. But not at my house. I always quit dieting and quit exercising because the changes seem to stop. I know I'm weak-willed, but am I also running into physiological plateaus?

I have a feeling you and Phil run into a lot of things, including plateaus. Weight loss may stop, according to one current theory, because of a protective survival mechanism dating back to caveman days when we humans stored fat like other animals for use in times of famine. This "setpoint" theory says that when weight loss such as that caused by fasting or near fasting threatens the body's encoded minimum fat requirements, it lowers metabolism, cutting back on the calories normally needed for proper function.[3] In other words, the body simply stops burning as many calories, and you hit a plateau. Of course, Phil's problem is that midnight snack of chocolate cake you don't know about. He hides it in your wig box, the one that held your platinum beehive for the senior prom, remember?

You will reach plateaus in your strength and/or muscle-building programs, too. Your body simply adapts to your new level of activity. Increase the level again or change the activities themselves to keep your progress going.

What about fasting as the answer? Will it help me lose weight faster, clean out my body, or do something spiritual to my mind?

Fasting can obviously bring rapid weight loss, but it's virtually never permanent, can cause traumatic loss of lean tissues such as muscle, and eventually harm even organs. It should be undertaken under the care of a doctor only, and most doctors recommend it only for extremely obese persons as a last-ditch effort before surgical intervention.[4] People out there have died from it, too. So, even if it'll clean your body and mind (which it probably won't), don't undertake it lightly.

Well, *what if I just eat only one big meal a day?*

What you'll probably do is interfere with your body's metabolism if you do this often. The one-meal-a-day diet can also lead to an increased appetite, and a poor blood-fat profile because your system cannot efficiently handle the rapid intake of a large amount of fat.[5] Spreading your calories over the day is the best way to eat.

Shortcuts—fasting or one big meal—don't work.

You *had a bunch of tests before beginning your program. But most people aren't going to exercise as radically as you do. Is a physical really necessary before beginning exercise? What can it show?*

I didn't really think my physicals were necessary from a safety point of view, and I was very wrong—remember my heart disease. A physical is good even if you are healthy, simply to give doctors measuring points for later changes in your health. But any time you undertake a change in the stress patterns on your body and heart, a physical should be a must. (In Chapter 17, I pass along some guidelines for getting the right one.) Since I was planning a pretty rigorous year, I wanted to know precisely how overweight I was, what my endurance levels were, and how healthy my engine and its systems really were.

Norma *wanted to know how much fat was on her body, too, before she let any doctor see her naked. She took the home pinch and mirror tests you mentioned in Chapter 1, and thinks you're a dolt. How can we get a second opinion?*

Second opinions are always a good thing, and here are some precise methods used by professionals.[6] Norma probably won't like them, either.

1. Underwater weighing is probably the most accurate way. You're dunked in a water tank. Since fat floats and lean tissue sinks, your weight out of water and in (used in the proper formula) gives a good indication of your total fat. You can't, incidentally,

put your bathroom scales in the tub for this one, since other lab tests are required for accuracy. Fitness clinics and some health clubs have special weighing rooms, though they are not numerous. Your best bet of finding a place near you is to check with the physical education department of a local college or university or with any preventive or sports medicine clinics.

2. Another popular but probably not as accurate method is the skinfold measurement. Skin calipers measure the amount of fat in predetermined areas.[7] Most health clubs and fitness centers can do this for you, but the results can vary widely, based on the experience of the user.

3. The bioelectrical impedance analyzer is another way.[8] It sends a small unfelt current through your body and measures the greater resistance of current through fat. Analyzers are new and are looked down upon by some doctors and clinics, as are all things new, as being inferior. I don't know who will win that argument, but these machines are probably a lot better than nothing.

You've said you're glad you had all those fancy tests because they showed heart disease. Everybody from my doctor to you to the margarine commercial on TV tries to scare the hell out of us with the words. But nobody explains. Just what is coronary heart disease?

A narrowing process in your coronary arteries, three major arteries attached to the walls of your heart. Arteries carry oxygen-loaded blood from your heart to feed your organs and other cells. Block the coronary arteries and you strangle the heart.

Coronary heart disease kills nearly half the people who die of any cardiovascular disease. It is particularly scary because of its first symptom in 40 percent of us: immediate death. It is also one of the few very deadly diseases for which the risk factors respond quickly to changes in our health patterns, good or bad.[9]

How can I tell if I am a high-risk candidate for coronary heart disease?

If you smoke, have the wrong cholesterol levels, or have high blood pressure, your chances of dying from it are greater. If you, like me, claim a couple of these things, your chances of dying from it are a lot greater. If you claim them all, your risk of death increases geometrically.

Other things you can control probably contribute to coronary heart disease, too: the lack of meaningful exercise, high body fat, diabetes, tension, and stress. And finally, your age, personal history, and heredity will have some impact.[10]

What tests can tell me if I have coronary heart disease?

Doctors don't entirely agree on what tests tell them. But the ones presented here are the best indicators to date of the presence of CHD, and if they err, they do so on the conservative side. By that I mean the side of heart disease. The side which might make you make some changes in your lifestyle.

One test usually indicates a need for the other here, too. If the first seems perfectly okay, the others may not be necessary. Remember, however, that my regular stress tests, the tests you'll find at health clubs and most clinics, indicated no problems, but my extra tests indicated a problem—even though I had no symptoms of heart disease.

EKG Stress Testing. You are probably familiar with this test. Electrodes, up to fifteen, are attached to your chest. All simply pick up the heart's electrical activity, the activity which makes the heart beat. As you move on the treadmill, the electrodes pick up any changes in your heart's electrical activity as you place it under stress. For instance, missed beats, extra beats. Electrical changes can indicate problems in getting oxygen to your heart.

How accurate is an EKG?

Dr. Henry Solomon, a cardiologist from Cornell and author of *The Exercise Myth*, argues that "stress tests are not sensitive enough, specific enough, or reproducible enough for anyone to be sure they're telling you anything at all."[11] At times, he states, they show heart disease when none is present. At times they don't show disease when it's definitely there.

But the problem with EKG stress testing may lie not with the test but with the test administrators. Because many factors are associated with heart disease, not just the presence of an EKG irregularity, physicians monitoring the test need to look at many aspects of a person's physiological response to exercise: heart rate, blood pressure, time of the onset of changes in electrical patterns, and the shape of those patterns; the duration of the electrical wave changes and the like.[12]

Women under forty-five have a statistically higher rate of incorrect EKG test results. Skillful administrators can compensate for this with careful laboratory procedures and especially complete evaluation of your medical history.[13]

Evaluation of EKGs isn't as clear-cut as math, but in the hands of a skilled administrator, many people believe this test can save your life if you have heart disease.

Stress tests have also become a gimmick. Health clubs perform them. Stress clinics open up weekly. Physicians with an extra room buy stress treadmills as an easy income-producer. My barber's even thinking about installing a few. Some of these people may be administering meaningful tests, but most are not.

Should I go have a test?

If you are over forty-five, have a family history of coronary heart disease, or are in one of the three high-risk groups, the American Heart Association and the American College of Sports Medicine and many other reasonably nonbiased scientific types consider you a "candidate" for an exercise stress test.[14] This very cute word is their way of dancing around a yes-or-no answer.

So what are the real risks to you if you do?

If you pick a quack administrator, you will waste your money and time; if a test shows you have heart disease and you don't, it will scare the hell out of you, probably make you turn to clean and godly living (which is good), and definitely make you see a heart specialist (which isn't bad after forty anyway), but you will have wasted about a thousand dollars in total. If the test shows you don't have heart disease and you do, that can obviously be a problem. To minimize this risk, you must go to a competent testing center or individual.

If the test correctly shows you have heart disease, and if you take the right corrective measures, it could save your life.

However—you could die from one, too. But the odds here are astronomically in your favor. At the Cooper Clinic in Dallas sixty-five thousand maximal stress tests have been administered with no fatalities.[15] In a study in Indianapolis, twelve thousand tests have been administered with no fatalities.[16] When the rare death has occurred, it has usually been among high-risk persons.[17] It's absolutely imperative, therefore, that your test (if it's a "maximal" test, where you go until exhaustion) be administered by very experienced personnel and that you be absolutely honest in giving your personal history before the test.

Does a correctly administered stress test do anything other than check for heart disease?

The other things it can show are very important. For instance, it can indicate your physical work capacity—what levels you are capable of working up to at a particular point in time. How much exercise can you tolerate? Don't start a meaningful exercise program without knowing that, especially if you're over forty-five. A stress test is also a good base-line measurement for later changes in your health. Four years from now it might let a doctor see changes in your heart's electrical patterns which could indicate heart disease or other irregularities.

How do you know a good testing place from a bad one?

Generally speaking, go to a place that specializes in cardiovascular testing. Your local fitness spa probably doesn't fit in that category. Remember, interpretation is the key to a meaningful test. A person who administers many stress tests might understand their implications better. Your regular family physician probably doesn't administer them regularly, either, though he may have a treadmill machine.

Also before making an appointment ask the administrators these obvious things: (1) The EKG machine should have at least seven leads, or terminals, fastened to your body. Does it? (2) The attendant should monitor your blood pressure at frequent intervals. Will he or she? (3) A physician should definitely be within walking range. Does this center have such an on-staff physician? Some testing centers don't have on-staff physicians, and therefore can't take you to your maximal workout range, where most trouble would probably show up.

What if the test does show a problem?

If the test shows anything, it will probably indicate you simply need other tests. Obviously a good doctor should do the choosing, but you should know the types of tests available.

The **Tomographic Thallium Stress Test** "often provides the earliest information about reduced blood flow to the heart, the cause of most heart attacks," says Dr. Bob Bell, my nuclear medicine adviser. First, you run on a treadmill, then thallium, a radioactive material, is injected into your bloodstream. Images are then taken on film which show blood flow in the heart.

The **Stress Radionuclide Angiogram** determines how the heart works as a pump. You sit on a bicycle with your chest against a camera. Radioactive technetium is injected into your bloodstream, and moving pictures of your heart pumping under stress are made. Quantitative data is also collected—for instance, the volume of blood pumped, the speed of the blood in and out of the heart.

An **Echocardiogram** uses sound waves to determine heart anatomy and function. It is a noninvasive test now being used to evaluate the motion of heart valves and heart walls. Although it is used primarily to depict anatomy, future improvements will probably provide more functional information. (At present this is not used primarily for coronary artery disease detection.)

A **Cardiac Catheterization** is the most accurate test, but it is usually the last resort because it is also the most dangerous. One out of a thousand people die from this test, also called a coronary angiogram, so you don't want to undertake it casually.[18] A catheterization places a catheter, a long, thin, flexible tube, in an artery, and literally pushes it through the body to the heart. A dye is injected into the catheter. The dye lights up the coronary arteries, which give an indication of blood flow in the coronary arteries. This test is very accurate. It tells which arteries are blocked, how much they are blocked, and also can help a good physician determine a course of action.

Catherizations require hospitalization and a very experienced staff, and may cost several thousand dollars. Before undertaking one, you should definitely ask for a second opinion.

I'*ve had my blood pressure taken a hundred times, but those numbers are a mystery. What does it all mean?*

Your blood system is obviously a closed system; therefore, the blood exerts pressure at all times on the vessels. Your "blood pressure" is determined by measuring in millimeters of mercury (just like a barometer) the pressure applied to all the interior walls of your arteries. The systolic number, the one on top, is the pressure the vessels are under when the heart pumps. The diastolic, the bottom number, is the pressure when the heart is at rest, between beats.

So *what is high blood pressure, then, and how bad is it?*

When your systolic and diastolic pressure measurements move up out of statistically normal ranges, you have "high blood pressure" or hypertension. And why is it bad? When your blood pressure is within normal ranges, the pressure itself does no damage to the arteries. However, when that pressure is high enough, over a period of time, it can damage the artery walls and make them less elastic. Arteries must have elasticity to help move your blood properly. High blood pressure also places a strain on the heart. The increased pressure forces the heart to work harder and can eventually lead to congestive heart failure, a general deterioration of the heart's pumping capacity.[19]

Are *there any physical symptoms for high blood pressure?*

There are none specifically, but certain types of people are more likely to have it: those with a family history of it, black males, people who are overweight, and people under stress and tension, perhaps.[20]

Will a blood pressure check in my drugstore tell me anything?

If these instruments aren't calibrated regularly, they can be inaccurate. But it's better than nothing. If it does indicate your pressure is a little high, have it checked again professionally. Don't use this "curbside" check as an excuse to delay a doctor's checkup.

Everyone I know seems to have a little high blood pressure. Everyone seems to put off doing something about it, too, and I don't see them having strokes and heart attacks from it. So what's the big deal?

Please don't be casual about this stuff. Some people I've loved very much are dead from it, and each year, more people develop cardiovascular disease, particularly strokes, from it than from anything. Dying is one thing, but being paralyzed and conscious enough to live to regret your carelessness is another.

Okay, how can it be treated?

Many degrees of high blood pressure can be safely and reasonably quickly treated with changes in your eating habits, changes in your weight, and changes in your exercise patterns.[21] If you have high blood pressure, don't put this book down and go jogging, but do see a doctor who understands the importance of exercise. If you're already on medication, for God's sake, don't stop taking it simply because you start exercising. Let your doctor make that decision.

In my wilder days, doctors constantly told me my blood pressure was high. My reaction was to drink a little more and worry a little more. When I began to exercise, my personal blood pressure problem went away, and did not return even when I took on my barrel shape.

What if I already have heart disease? Can clean and godly living and exercise reduce, arrest, or reverse it?

Evidence exists that shows all of these can at times happen. Stopping or retarding the progression of this killer is an obtainable goal perhaps for the first time for many of us.[22]

Isn't your risk of dying much greater during exercise?

According to a very respected epidemiologist, Dr. Steve Blair, there is a slight, short-term increased risk of sudden death during exercise. But sedentary people are at greater risk overall than people who exercise. In fact, more people die from a heart attack in bed than while exercising.[23] And a recent study reported the risk of death in cardiac rehabilitation programs as only one death in 800,000 hours of exercise.[24] Go do something.

But in time will exercise make me live longer or not?

Some people, such as Dr. Henry Solomon, like to say there is absolutely no proof exercise increases life span, and they've sold an awful lot of books saying that, too. Technically they may be "right" because how could any study, for instance, ever prove a person had lived longer because of anything? Direct evidence here is impossible.

But the evidence is overwhelming that sedentary living increases the risk of CHD;[25] the evidence is building that physically active people have lower mortality rates in general;[26] the evidence is specific and convincing that aerobic exercise can improve the work of the heart and its supporting systems.[27] Cumulative evidence points to longer life for those who exercise correctly.

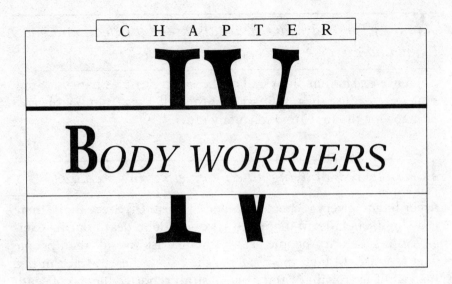

C H A P T E R

IV

BODY WORRIERS

Week 6
<u>*Grand Bahama Island*</u>
George Plimpton called me today, elated and relieved at the rapidly declining state of my stomach. "Why, you're a virtual wisp these days!" he proclaimed.

George was elated because he's a good friend who cares for my health; relieved because, almost single-handedly, he was responsible for creating the last four inches of my former belly. As I tried to sell my idea for a book on redoing my body, George encouraged further deterioration for the sake of the book. "How's the belly today, Bub?" he'd say. "Are we gaining some more weight?" He was concerned about my drinking habits. "Drink cheap scotch, doubles, lots of them," he advised on one call. He took an interest in my exercise program (don't have one) and my sleeping habits (late to bed was recommended).

Plimpton is a participatory journalist of some note, so I, of course, wanted to trust his judgment in these matters as a true chocolate lover wants to trust a chocolate diet plan. Except for George's heart theory. "You know, I was thinking," he said in August, "a little stroke would be nice. Nothing debilitating, you understand." We both laughed.

We both laughed even when it appeared my publisher was having second thoughts. ("You mean we're belly-up, great Bub?") But the next week, when we met in Florida for a strategy session, when George saw my forty-three inches of freshly wrought flesh, he did not laugh. *"Good Lord,"* he said, "Poor Bubba, what have I done?" Earned an unusual title as the first member of my Body Worry committee, that's what—Chairman of the Debauch.

Normally, I don't think much of committees. They seem to either be for things we already agree on ("Keep America Beautiful"), or things we'll never agree on anyway (tax reform), or things we need to meet on to see if we agree or disagree. On the surface, my committee is no different. Let's face it, my body is a mess—it doesn't take a committee to decide that—and none of my members will ever entirely agree on what it takes to make me whole. *All*, nevertheless, are convinced that two, maybe three, tax-deductible visits here to my tropical island will make everything right.

Similarities to other bodies aside, my group has a real purpose: I want my health back. I want muscles. I want to be able to touch my toes again, and know that whatever exercise I do is the right exercise. I want someone like Kathy to keep telling me I'm looking more handsome these days. And more than anything, I want answers to questions. There the committee excels. Though my experts may not all agree, their opinions in their particular fields are as good as you can get.

Dr. Kenneth Cooper, for instance, doesn't really care about any of my muscles except for my heart. A quiet, slender man with a Texas-dry sense of humor and a great sense of mission when it comes to God, aerobics, and preventive medicine, Dr. Cooper does two things that especially impress me. Though he has sold more books than there are committees and is an international celebrity in the sports and medicine fields, he still practices medicine regularly. Would you be giving proctoscopic exams to middle-aged men when you could be giving autographs and interviews?

Dr. Cooper also admits when he's wrong. Years ago, Cooper believed that exercise alone could overcome poor diet and bad habits such as smoking. He was wrong: runners and sports addicts who ate fatty foods and smoked developed heart disease and died just like the rest of us who do those things. Cooper tells the story often, and I think of it when temptation sends me to the fried food portion of menus.

Cooper is balding, a sign of great intelligence. Some say he is too evangelical when it comes to aerobic fitness. But that's okay. In the past six weeks, over 100,000 Americans have died from some disease of the heart and blood vessels, much of it preventable.[1] That's more than twice the population of Grand Bahama Island. I think of the number during the hard part of my jogs, the first part.

Remember how far I could jog when I began? Less than thirty seconds the first day, about five minutes on the fifteenth day. On the twentieth jogging day, I jogged down Royal Palm past the sea streets—Sea Fan, Sea Horse, Sea Shell, etc.—to the ocean at Silver Point Jetty and then back to my street, twenty minutes without stopping. I was very smug after that, even called Dr. Cooper to casually drop the news, for twenty minutes of jogging three times a week is all the aerobic exercise most people need to remain healthy.

The smugness stuck to me as tightly as the barbed spines of a sea urchin until about eleven-thirty the next morning when I watched Ruth Goldfarb cross the finish line at the Bahamas Princess 10K Race (6.2 miles). Ruth isn't even five feet tall, isn't fast, either, but she still finished in good time. She is eighty-three.

I told Gideon Ariel, another member of my committee, about Ruth, and he immediately asked me if she also did strength training, an expected question from him. Many believe Gideon is the preeminent authority on strength in America. Gideon jogs, swims, and works out every day. He doesn't lift weights in the normal sense but uses instead his own innovative setup, a computer-driven, piston-powered, four-color gizmo which beeps at you, makes you stronger, burps when you try to cheat, and makes weight training infinitely more interesting. The machines are called Ariels and are considered the most advanced around.

Aside from being a strength expert and equipment designing wiz, Gideon is known as the Godfather of Biomechanics, the science that combines the study of physics with the study of human anatomy and movement. Boxers (Muhammad Ali), horses (Spectacular Bid), the U.S. Olympic Committee, and just about everything in between, including bald and plump writers, have been to Gideon's Coto Research Institute to profit from his understanding of the things the eye can't comprehend.

Rosy-cheeked, Gideon looks like a grown-up but well-developed cherub; his smile is mischievous in a comfortable way, and his thoughts move about as fast as the spin of the discus thrower he used to be. He likes to invent things, tinker with things. He is trying hard to make me an athlete and to make me constantly stronger.

Though I test on his machines in Miami, Gideon's strength training routine for me essentially involves free weights, since my gym
on the island doesn't have an Ariel machine. Free weights are *great*—
but while there are only two Ariel machines to remember (they do
just about everything), free weights are like an iron jigsaw puzzle.
Our gym set has hundreds of pieces.

At first, I didn't even try to keep things straight or understand
the importance of the clipped phrases which make up gym dialect.
I used instead a drawn-out but logical-sounding approach when I
needed something: "Pardon me, but could you hand me that short,
crooked bar over there and two of those medium-sized weights?"
People looked at me as if I were from the moon.

As I calmed, the sentences shortened. Today I worked out next
to Henry Charlton, the World Games posing champion, and I said
it like this, "Hey, man, hand me that Z-bar and some quarters, will
ya?" Henry didn't blink an eye as he reached for the bar, but before
handing me the twenty-five-pound "quarters," he looked me up and
down, then picked up some thirty-fives. "You look like you're ready
to pump some heavy iron now," he said.

I'm thinking about adding Henry to my committee.

R*emar, you say raising my heart rate is the thing that counts
in fitness. If that's the case, why won't watching a porno
movie make me aerobically fit? Or smoking?*

Aerobic activity requires the movement of large amounts of oxygen
in the blood and the absorption of that oxygen by tissues. The
absorption of large amounts of oxygen requires the work of large
muscle masses, such as your legs. Simply increasing your heartbeat
won't increase the absorption of oxygen in areas other than your
heart. The ability to pump volumes of oxygenated blood is the key
to developing cardiovascular fitness.[2]

I*s all exercise aerobic exercise?*

Our bodies have essentially two ways to derive energy from its fuels:
aerobic metabolism and anaerobic metabolism. Aerobic metabolism refers to a production of energy requiring oxygen, much like
a fire requires oxygen to burn. Anaerobic metabolism is a process

that releases energy to the body without the presence of oxygen.

These two types of metabolism happen at specific times. Aerobic metabolism is a slow-reacting process. It doesn't react instantly to an immediate increase in energy requirements, such as a sudden sprint in the rain from the car to the store, when your individual cells suddenly gasp for breath. At that point, sugar in the cells begins to break down and form lactic acid, releasing energy—anaerobic metabolism.[3]

Lactic acid is a by-product of metabolism. During intense activity, the acid builds up in our cells. When lactic acid production is greater than the body's ability to remove it, your blood and muscles become acidic. Your muscles don't work as well in this acidic state, and you fatigue quickly.

Anaerobic exercise, generally speaking, is a more traumatic exercise for your body. Just like drag car racing wears engines more than everyday driving. Most people can't continue exercising at an anaerobic pace, either. Instead your engine and its supports systems need long-term, lower-intensity demands on them to provide the most cardiovascular benefits. For safety and practical reasons, anaerobic exercise isn't appropriate for most people.

What are the aerobic exercises?

Running, jogging, brisk walking, rowing, swimming, race-walking, cross-country skiing, biking, and any other movement that uses large muscle groups continuously and for sustained periods of time.

Are some aerobic exercises more efficient than others?

Some aerobic exercises provide your body a better total workout by working more muscle. For instance, cross-country skiing. But twenty minutes of aerobic work at the right level is twenty minutes, regardless of the sport or machine. You can't cheat the twenty minutes, that's the point.

So *are you saying walking briskly is as good as running at a fast pace?*

Yes. Especially if you're out of shape. If your goals, for instance, are weight loss and stamina increase, low-intensity, long-duration exercises are particularly good. Fat really doesn't even burn itself up much faster during exercise until you cross the twenty-minute barrier.[4]

Norma *wants me to go to an aerobics class and jump up and down like Richard Simmons. Aren't the men who do that a little "funny"?*

Constant movement of your major muscle groups like this is aerobically like running a race, and a lot more fun at times, as you'll find out later when you read about our island class. Go with Norma.

How *safe is aerobic dancing?*

A lot of people do injure themselves with regular aerobic dancing, mostly injuries related to the pounding of your feet and the movement of your back. If you're really out of shape, find a place that teaches low-impact (or soft) aerobics. Low-impact aerobics are designed to provide the same cardiovascular benefits with minimized trauma. You keep one foot on the ground to reduce the impact, but still get your heart rate up through exaggerated movements such as high steps, lunges, and vigorous arm motion.

Whichever you chose, high- or low-impact, do start out in a class that fits your fitness and ability level.

If *I'm out of shape, can I build endurance and strength at home before I put my act on the road?*

Push-ups, even partial ones with your knees on the floor, will definitely help build your strength. Running in place or stepping up and down on something like a box can quickly build your stamina.

Things you can do at home can do as much for you as most machines and clubs (and cost you a lot less, too), but gyms and the like can provide you company, which is good for misery, as we know.

I'll *do the aerobics if it's good for me, I guess, but weight training appeals to me more. What can it do for me?*

For most of my life, I've wanted to be comfortable in weight rooms but was sure people like Bill and Marilynn Carle, god-type bodies, would laugh at me if I went there.

For most of my life, I also thought weight lifting was for the narcissistic or worse—guys and women who put the size of muscles above their health. Part of that, I think, is true: serious weight lifters at times jeopardize their health for their looks.

But weight training (the term generally used for people who aren't competing) has health values, physically and mentally, if you are a person who undertakes it with some sense of proportion. Weight training (or any good resistance training) is the only thing that will take the softness from your flesh. Jogging, for instance, will not create a washboard stomach. Aerobics won't take the softness from your arms. The right weight program will, and, more importantly, it will make you feel so good about your body if you stick with it. Change comes so very slowly here, but that in itself makes the change meaningful. After what I've been through to have a flat stomach, no fat will ever live there again.

Well, *if I weight train, can I skip aerobic exercising altogether?*

You can't skip it at all, for weight lifting is not aerobic, regardless of what some weight lifting advocates say. When aerobic gains are made as a result of lifting, they're nearly inconsequential.

"Circuit training," a type of weight training involving moderately heavy weight and many repetitions with little or no rest between exercises, is pushed by many gyms as a way to be aerobically fit and get the benefits of lifting at the same time. Most studies show improvement in aerobic capacity doesn't happen significantly, though.[5] Separate your activities. Or, perhaps, do something aerobic such as running in place or cycling between lifting exercises—Rambo-level training!

Won't weight lifting give me high blood pressure? Maybe damage my heart or something?

Lifting does little to improve the heart's function, but it doesn't hinder it, either. It definitely doesn't cause high blood pressure, but it raises your blood pressure when you're doing it, which isn't bad if you're healthy and normally pressured, but can be very bad if you already have high blood pressure.[6]

Some cardiac rehabilitation centers, incidentally, are beginning to use light to moderate weight training for rehabilitation in very supervised settings.[7] If you have any type of heart problems or high blood pressure, talk to an experienced doctor before undertaking a program.

Won't weight lifting make me less flexible?

No. A lot of flexibility can be hereditary, but most physiologists believe the proper weight training can increase your range of motion.[8] I personally am bored with too much stretching.

Should I start out lifting with free weights or with machines?

Free weights require more balancing skills than machines, since the weight isn't guided by anything but your skills. Machine weights usually move along some form of controlled track. It's hard to drop them on yourself unless your klutz factor is very high. Machines also give you a faster workout, because changing weights is usually done with a pin rather than actually moving and rearranging weights.

Manufacturers of machines will also tell you their products are more efficient in building muscles and strength because they vary the resistance to make you work harder where you're stronger. The pitch is appealing, but no one has proved it's true.

I learned how to lift with free weights, so my opinion may be biased (disagree with me and I'll punch you out), but I like free weights better. Lifting a hundred pounds on a machine just isn't as satisfying as attacking that hundred pounds by yourself. Doing a bench press with a free weight also uses more muscles than doing a press on a machine: a machine press essentially uses up and down muscles. A free press uses up and down muscles plus front and back and left and right muscles because you must balance the weight. Got that? There's a lot of healthy tension with free weights.

Phil is fat; I simply have "weak flesh." Will a weight training program help me?

Flesh on your arm or leg or neck sags from several things, including the effects of gravity, the aging process itself, and, most important, from the loss of muscle tone. Muscle tone really means muscle is always in a state of partial contraction. Quit using a muscle, and it loses that tone. Start using a muscle again, and lots of the sagging will eventually go away.

I want muscles. Norma wants tone. Do we do different things?

It takes strength, and therefore more tissue, to be able to lift steadily increasing amounts of weights. It takes endurance, and therefore more stored fuel, to keep lifting a weight for a large number of repetitions. To build or keep your muscle balance (tone) follow a weight lifting program which emphasizes moderate weight and large numbers of repetitions. To become a hunk, build your weight program around steadily increasing resistance. Tone, incidentally, obviously comes with increased muscle size also, but muscle size isn't a necessity for tone.

Can weight training do anything to protect me from heart disease?

Weight training can make you look good, strengthen your bones, obviously strengthen and enlarge certain muscles, improve your mental attitude, give you more energy reserves for such fun things as cutting the grass or going to the market but . . . weight training's beneficial impact on your engine and its support systems is minimal.[9] Don't substitute weight work for cardiovascular work.

What about the kids? When should they start lifting?

Let your kids learn about weight lifting as you learn about it. Making them comfortable and interested in this healthy sport is great. But, according to Christopher Scott, don't let your children become serious lifters until their bodies are nearly full grown, middle to late adolescence. On no account should children or early adolescents engage in strength contests because heavy strains can affect proper bone growth.[10]

Our weight lifting section will help everyone in the family start a sensible lifting program, and for inspiration let me tell you here about a couple who lift together and whom I met on a trip to California. Bryant Cushing, fifty-nine, and his wife Carole, forty-nine, have been lifting for six years. They are not jocks. Carole said she tried jogging but hated it and tried roller-skating but couldn't come to a stop. They started lifting as a lark and quickly found they liked it. Carole doesn't look muscular; she looks tight. The same goes for Bryant. He, incidentally, has had a quintuple heart bypass operation. He is also a believer in stress tests. Bryant was feeling just fine, but a maximal stress treadmill test uncovered his heart disease and probably saved his life. These two say a lot of their friends think they are crazy—"They call us Mr. and Mrs. Schwarzenegger"—but they don't care. "We have more energy than all of them," Carole told me as she pressed sixty pounds over her head.

C H A P T E R V

TROUBLE

Week 8

<u>*Grand Bahama Island*</u>

I am approaching slim and healthy with great speed, it seems, but some cracks are beginning to appear in my smile.

My right shoulder (specifically, the rotator cuff) isn't taking well to weight lifting; that's the first problem. I haven't been able to work it at all for a week. And then an acquaintance, I think without meaning to, belittled both my progress and my effort. And then the real world came to visit my island and hasn't left yet. My phone rings too much, my budget isn't working, and my typewriter won't talk to me.

But my shoulder scares me the most. Right now, I worry about it more than my health, a stupid thing to say but the truth, for it is part of the very beginning of my story. I have wanted muscular shoulders and arms—really wanted a whole new body—longer than I want to admit. The thought was never overpowering, but it nagged.

The nagging started with a patch I had my mother sew on a shirt when I was in the first grade. It was a large red "S" purchased at Dupree's Five and Ten. I collected Superman trinkets and comic books avidly until that patch. I don't think it was the beauty of muscles which attracted me to the Man of Steel, but rather the fact that he was strong and invulnerable to bullies; I had felt frail and, worse, had recently drawn the attention of a bully named Lawton.

Lawton didn't beat me up much, but he threatened to all the time, occasionally using his right center knuckle to raise a frog on my arm and constantly standing too close to me, reminding me that he could invade my territory at will. If a very young person can feel adult impotence, I felt it then.

The feeling was especially strong the first day I wore my Superman "S." I ran to the small wooded area where Lawton and his friends held their secret meetings, hoping that they would accept me, knowing that belonging to the group would protect me. But the boys were not impressed with my shirt. Lawton laughed first, and then he punched me once in the stomach, at the very bottom of the "S." I buried the shirt that day and gave my comics and trinkets to a kid much smaller than I.

After that I decided that muscles and strength were not as important as personality. I smiled a lot. Boy, could a smile and a few well-chosen words make things happen. By the third grade I was a glib, friendly, very gregarious young boy, and by the end of that year I had been elected to my first class office. Vice-president of Mrs. Dasher's homeroom may not be very important to the outside world, but to me it was a heady, powerful moment. My body said very few negative things to me for several years.

Ah, but puberty arrived on a dark horse, or more precisely, in the person of Lawton again. Lawton (to this day I think out of spite) asked my first great love, Felicia, to attend the seventh grade dance with him. When I had asked her, Felicia had unconsciously glanced up and down my body and begged off. She looked at Lawton's body, too, slowly, then said yes. When neither of them acknowledged me, my arms felt especially frail.

Looking back, I think that incident was pretty much an epiphany for me in the negative sense. I first went to a doctor who told me that I had not been born with the right body for large muscles. I tried to accept those life-changing words right then (the doctor's office, his words, even the color of his tie under the white jacket are as vivid to me now as the pain in my shoulder). I began several lifelong habits. I learned to dress to be comfortable with my arms and shoulders. Long-sleeved shirts rolled up just right gave an impression that muscles might be hiding under the folds. Short-sleeved shirts, when they had to be worn, couldn't have elastic in the cuffs.

I avoided sports which required me to perform in front of others and became a water skier and scuba diver and, on one, uh, hair-raising occasion, a sky diver—things which were a little exotic and conversationally interesting.

But I never, never could really put away my dream of shoulders and arms. Last year, when those who know muscles said I really could have honest-to-God muscles, my heart skipped a beat, like the flutters brought on by my crush on Felicia thirty years ago. Last week, when one of my doctors said matter-of-factly my dream could end with too many shoulder injuries, it skipped again, an unpleasant lurch which seemed prolonged and dangerous.

Now, intellectually, I know the shape of my body isn't important. I am happy my life has been guided more by the meatiness of the mind than the shallowness of muscle tissues. I know how very trite it is to be bothered by surface things. And, hurt shoulder or not, I'm living an exotic year. But I'm still very capable of a trite and shallow thought or two. As I sat glumly nursing my shoulder after visiting the doctor, a friend tried to perk me up by admiring the many pluses in my life. To his kindness, I snapped, "And I suppose you're going to tell me I have a nice personality, too."

The following day things got worse. An acquaintance who'd recently returned to Grand Bahama stopped me outside UNEXSO, the Underwater Explorers Society, with a "My God, Remar, you look awful! Stringy." The word took me back years. She continued, "You know, you should take up weight lifting." This to a man who had lifted over half a million pounds in the last two months. I had a fleeting image of what it would be like to trip her accidentally into the sharp spikes of the giant century plant by the front door, but simply nodded. "Yes, that would be a good idea. Nice to have you back," I lied as I walked on, rubbing my hurt shoulder.

It's a mile from UNEXSO to my house, a pleasant walk even when things aren't going well, past tennis courts, three oceanside hotels separated by large open spaces, and dozens of large mushroom-shaped banyan trees.

I stopped under the banyan before the Holiday Inn and purchased a Styrofoam cup of conch salad from the small native stand there. The tree virtually surrounds the stand, roots touching its roof and sides, attaching there in places, but Bertha, the proprietress, doesn't seem concerned about the creeping roots. Good island psychiatrist that she is, Bertha sensed my mood. "Give it away," she said when I told her about my slight depression. I blinked. She was right. If exercise even when it brings a little injury is good and if diet even when it makes you look "stringy" is healthy, decent people like me should share their blessings. Right then, under the banyan tree, I decided to form my own exercise class.

I called Lauren Hunt-Manning. Laurie and her husband are both instructors at UNEXSO; she is also a certified aerobics fitness specialist. During the past ten years, the Mannings have lived, exercised, and scuba dived from the Great Barrier Reef of Australia to the Taiwan Straits, the Gulf of Siam, the island of Barbados, New Guinea, and finally back to Grand Bahama. Laurie is slightly built, a wisp, and blond. For a while there, she dyed a small shock of her hair pink. Coupled with her smile, the effect was fun and indicative of independence rather than punk.

Laurie looked me straight in the eyes without blinking when I asked her to form an aerobics class at my house. She spoke quickly, "Why do you want a class, Remar?"

"Well, I thought it would be good for my book, you know," I said, "understanding the dynamics of exercise physiology and all that."

She smiled, and continued as if her words were part of my sentence, "You mean the principle of misery loves company, eh?" Bingo.

We met for the first time last night, a get-acquainted session. Five other scuba instructors have joined, all under thirty. Three ladies over forty have joined, too. None of them appear overweight to me, but all say they feel that way. Doc Clement has agreed to participate and serve as our official medical attendant. Dr. Clement's wife seems to be very glad he's participating, too. "She's been pushing me to do something about this," he says as he smiles broadly and rubs his stomach. Doc is tall, chisel-chinned, and enormously jolly in a clipped, British way. In my opinion, he has way too much hair for a man over forty, but he will not share it.

Everyone in the group says they want to slim down and firm up; everyone says they want more energy. Those under thirty seem to want more energy to party. Those of us over forty want more energy to function. The men, at first, were hesitant to discuss specific body goals, but when I told the group about my desire for muscles enough to bring swoons from the opposite sex, all of the men in unison said, "Yeah, *that's it*." Keith, considerably overweight, was the most honest and most touching. "I want to feel better about myself," he said quietly.

The men are also a little nervous about the thought of aerobic dancing itself, of doing those "funny Richard Simmons movements" I mentioned earlier. I laughed when he said it, for Laurie had already shown me how much work those funny movements really are.

I also told them about my cousin Wayne's friends at the Daniels Creek Hunting Club, down in the pine woods of South Georgia. Dressed in beat-up boots and beat-up clothes, driving a truck even more beat-up, and probably fortified with some good whiskey, lots of beer, and a chew or two of tobacco, the boys arrive at their leased 6,000 acres at about five in the morning during hunting season.

The guys spend about five hours there, usually bag some game, then drive back to downtown Swainsboro (population 8,000 on Saturdays) just in time for their aerobic dancing class. Kenny Loggins provides the beat and a black man leads the class.

Now, if Chuck Yeager or my cousin's friends had been the first people to adopt and promote aerobic dancing, probably a lot more men would be doing it now. It *is* fun, especially with people who are as rotten at dance as I am, and God knows it is work. I lasted about four minutes of the first forty-minute class before finding an excuse to make a very long phone call. But Simmons is the person many men associate with aerobic dancing, and, unfortunately, he doesn't fit the physical image we dream of having, the Yeager image. He's short, fuzzy-haired, and wildly enthusiastic. Before you raise an objection to aerobic dancing as an unmanly pursuit, however, I suggest you try it nonstop for even ten minutes. You won't be able to raise your hand to swat a fly.

Our class meets three times a week for an hour. My living room, with furniture pushed against the walls, serves as our stretching and limbering-up room. I, like most of the men, am as limber as a rock. After about twenty minutes of warm-up movements to music, we move to my backyard and dance among the palm trees, to fast music. Laurie demonstrates the motions, but I can't follow them too well yet. I try, but everything comes out like some funny version of the Twist.

But my cousin and his friends would not laugh at me, especially Gary Curry. Gary belongs to *two* hunting clubs, a big deal in South Georgia, and is a darn good shot, too, a bigger deal. But he's most proud of the sixty pounds of fat and twenty points of blood pressure Richard Simmons's funny movements have taken from him. On second thought, Gary Curry really does have the last laugh, doesn't he?

Meanwhile, my injured shoulder still continues to slow the weight lifting. If it hasn't improved in another week, the shoulder doctor is sending me to the States to a specialist. If it's better, I'll be working shoulders that day in the gym. The difference between "stringy" and "hunky" in inches is very small—perhaps three more inches on the biceps and a couple of inches over the shoulder. I am beginning to realize how far those distances may be.

Too bad about your shoulder, Remar, but you know what they say: "No pain, no gain."

I think Cher is explosively good-looking, so when I first heard her say, "No pain, no gain," about the time I started to redo myself, I didn't doubt the wisdom of her words. Nothing bad could be uttered by a body that charged with sex. I, however, don't like pain and was, therefore, happy to learn that Cher was wrong. Real pain doesn't and shouldn't come with proper exercise.

Stress, on the other hand, is what exercise is about. The proper stress causes beneficial change. Sometimes after the proper stress, you will feel soreness, too, usually from the buildup of fluids or tissue damage in an area.[1] Soreness happens when your body isn't used to stress, and generally isn't bad for you. Pain on the other hand—an instant feeling that something isn't right—should not happen. If it does, slow down or stop exercising, depending on the severity of the pain. If it continues, seek medical help.

The healthy soreness you feel a day or two after first jogging or weight lifting will go away quickly as your body adjusts to the new stresses you're putting on it. Incidentally, static stretching (when you hold a position) and repeating the exercise that made you sore (believe it or not) will decrease soreness, at times significantly.

No body has ever needed muscles like my body needs muscles. If I work out twice as hard, will I results come as fast?

I used to think that. For a while, I worked out much more than any of my doctors or weight coaches recommended. That's when my real injuries started, too.

Think of weight training—really, any exercise—as a prescription from your doctor. It generally isn't safe to take twice the dosage. Exercise twice as much and your injuries will increase nearly geometrically and, more importantly, your improvements may come slower. My strength and muscle gains have been much more dramatic since I started cutting back on my lifting.

That's the best news I can give you, too. No one has to devote his life to exercise and no one has to spend literally hours each day to accomplish the things I've accomplished.

Will stretching exercises have me touching my toes in no time or at least touching my knees?

Flexibility does not come easily. I told you I stretched at least thirty minutes a day and made only minimal gains in that area. The only thing that touches my toes is my feet. That depressed me until I was told that flexibility by itself probably doesn't do anything for your health. I now stretch about five minutes a day, since stretching muscles may lessen the chance of injury.

What about warm-up and cool-down?

Especially if you are over forty or out of shape, warm-up is very important. Start hard exercise without it and you can bring changes in your EKG and maybe worse. Warm-up also reduces injury, lets your oxygen-carrying cells and enzymes work more efficiently, and generally increases blood flow to the muscles you are working.[2] My five-minute stretching, for instance, is a part of my warm-up.

Cool-down is just as important, regardless of your age. After exercise, large amounts of blood build up in the muscles you've been working. The muscles then actually help return the blood to the heart by squeezing the veins. A sudden stop in exercise can cause the blood to pool in the veins, which may reduce blood flow to the brain, which can make you faint or worse.

Both warm-up and cool-down should be for at least five minutes, and should contain a gradual buildup or build down of activity: walking to jogging, then jogging to walking, for instance.

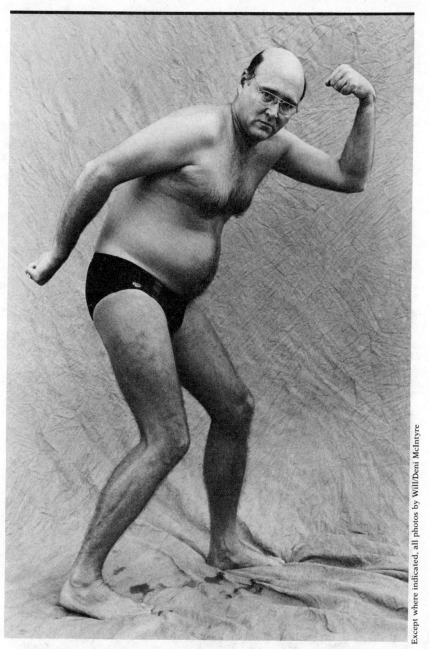

This is the story of a 201-pound man, and let's start it with honesty: My shape on January 1 elicited very few swoons.

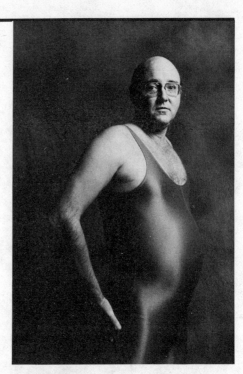

I wore this to hide reality.
It didn't work.

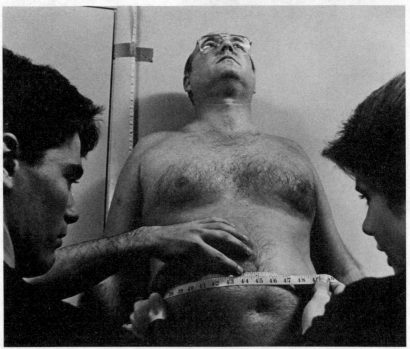

My trainer Russell Burd and my photographer and friend Deni McIntyre confront the belly of the beast: forty-three inches on January 13.

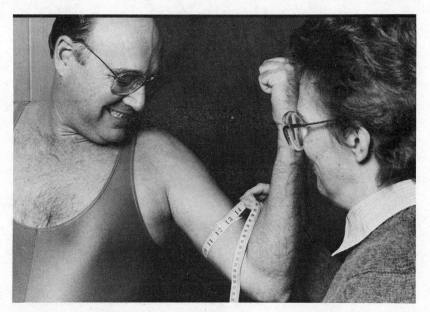

Mary Abbott Waite is my best friend and my editor, a nice combination. She's trying not to laugh as I attempt a flex. How do you like my double chin? January 13.

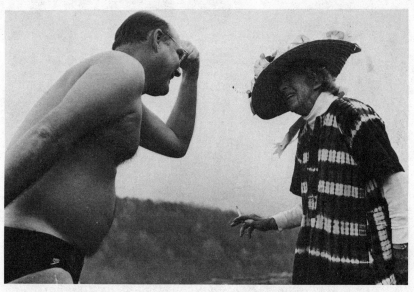

I am standing on a friend's fieldstone patio. She's smoking, and I'm freezing, since it's thirty-eight degrees. In her eighties, my friend has her own theories about health, and I think she's wondering about mine.

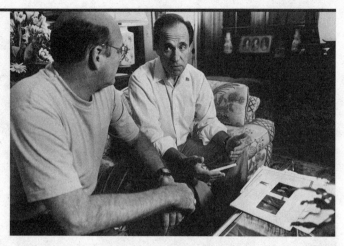

The pictures on the coffee table are color shots of my heart beating. During this meeting, Bob Bell, my nuclear physician, is telling me for the first time about my heart problem.

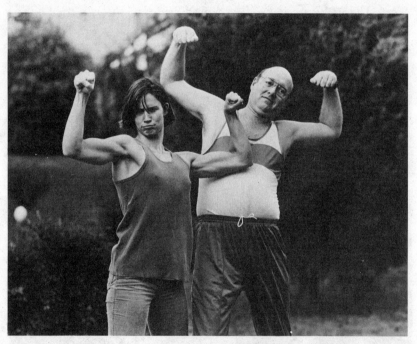

Jenny Bell, M.D., one of Bob's daughters, joins me in a pose-off. At this point, there's no contest. My jowls are bigger than my biceps.

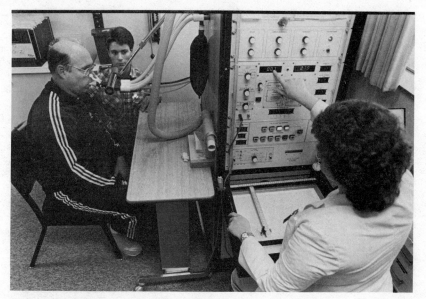

This machine, a spirometer, told me that 15 percent of my lung capacity was gone—probably due to smoking.

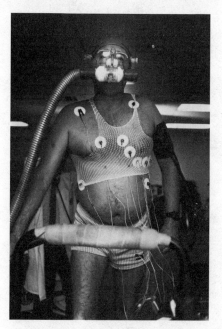

I am trying out for a Godzilla role. The handsome mask directly measures oxygen consumption as I work out on the treadmill.

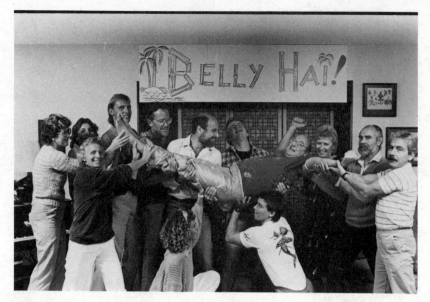

Members of my aerobic dancing class and a couple of other friends practice lifting maximum weight. John Englander, president of UNEXSO, is the bearded but bald fellow. Doc Clement is to his left. Kathy, the first beautiful woman to sense my emerging hunkiness, is two over from Doc. Kathy is very smart.

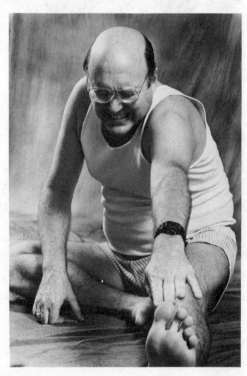

In mid-January, I can barely reach past my knee; my weight still hovers around 200 pounds.

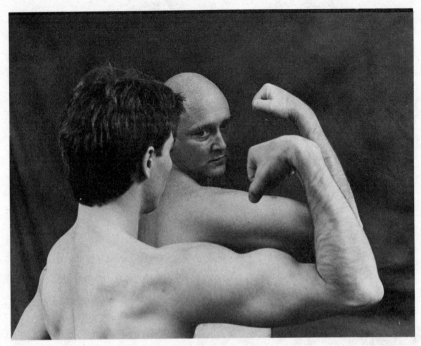

I like Russell Burd, my trainer, but I don't like his bicep. He also has far too much hair.

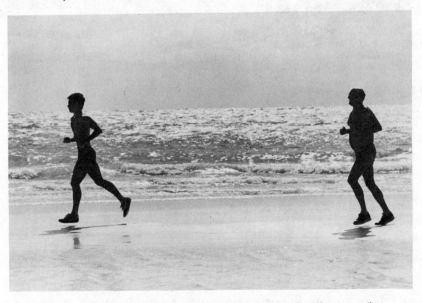

Sunrise on Grand Bahama Island, my home for the remake. Jogging at sunrise is really breathtaking for me, especially during these first weeks.

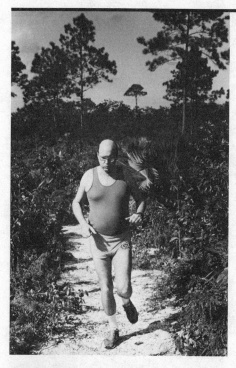

I jogged a lot at the Lucayan National Park. Did you know that caves and tunnels there run miles out into the sea, where they're called Blue Holes?

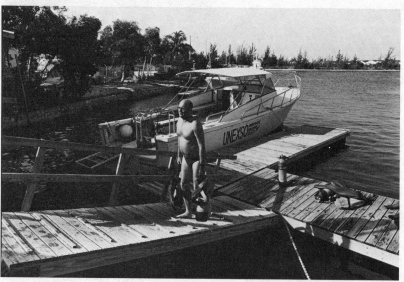

UNEXSO has been my main island hangout for years. Here, I'm exercising by hauling up empty scuba tanks. The people who usually hauled scuba tanks endorsed my exercise. They were disappointed when this mode of exercise didn't last more than fifteen minutes.

If *I'm going to do all this work, do I need to stock up on Gatorade and the like to really quench my thirst?*

When you exercise, your body heats up and begins to sweat, depleting your water supply and passing off certain minerals such as salt and potassium. The manufacturers of commercial thirst preparations, looking for an honest way to make a healthy buck, decided to duplicate the ingredients of sweat under the logical assumption that a drink which duplicates sweat does good things.

Unfortunately, all commercial thirst quenchers have something sweat doesn't, unless you're weird: sugar. Sugar definitely isn't good for quenching thirst, either. It actually impairs the passage of water from the stomach to the body, eventually to your individual cells.[3]

Thirst quenchers also contain calcium, potassium, and magnesium in the equally logical assumption that, since these items are depleted to some degree during exercise, we should replace them. Depletion doesn't happen very quickly, though. And a normal diet adequately replaces them. A study of participants in a grueling twenty-day road race showed even these hardy folks didn't need any mineral supplementation.[4]

So what does this tell you commercial thirst quenchers actually replenish? People's pockets, of course. And what's the very best, most healthy drink before and during exercise? Cool water. Faster than commercial preparations, and even faster than warm water, it enters your system quickly and efficiently.[5] The only thing it doesn't do is stimulate further drinking. The commercial thirst quenchers do and in that sense can be good. If you forget to drink, you might want to use them watered down. But remember to use sugared drinks only during exercise, not before.

You may also have caught wind of a new product on the market called "glucose polymers." These things are supposed to increase endurance time and delay fatigue by preventing the body's store of glucose from running out.[6] If you don't run marathons or compete in triathlons, don't waste your money. Glucose is a carbohudrate. Your stores of carbohydrates aren't depleted easily during exercise. Marathon runners and other weird types usually reach that depletion point, but real Americans don't.

At least thirty minutes before beginning a sustained exercise program, drink two to two-and-a-half cups of water, and try to drink a cup or two every fifteen minutes during your exercise. You must not trust your thirst reaction to tell you when to drink during exercise. The sensation of thirst doesn't really keep up with your body's need for water.[7]

Well, *how about a candy bar or something else with a little sugar in it for an energy lift as I exercise?*

When you are fatigued, your body is telling you it needs fuel, energy. What you're physically feeling is the effects in the brain of depleted blood sugar. I used to think M & M's were the perfect energy pick-me-up, which still seems logical to me, and I still do love them as a snack, but they, like all high-sugar-based candies, don't really give you a productive energy boost. After you eat one of those sugary, tasty treats, the level of blood glucose raises quickly in the body. Your brain and nervous system use glucose specifically as a fuel, and are very sensitive to these changes in the glucose levels. They don't like it, and your brain tries to compensate for the extra glucose by having your pancreas secrete extra insulin. Insulin, in effect, tells the body's cells to soak up the extra glucose.

When you take in large amounts of high-sugar things—and large here can be one candy bar—the overproduction of insulin results in drastically lowered blood sugar. Lowered blood sugar, of course, is what makes you feel fatigued.

For most of us, this rebound effect of eating high-sugar sweets doesn't do anything but make us feel weaker and fatter, but for some people it brings on depression of the central nervous system. Excessively high blood sugar can also cause cell dehydration.

Fructose, on the other hand, the sugar found in fruits, has a much more stable effect on blood glucose. It doesn't seem to cause the overproduction of insulin which causes the problem.[8] So, occasionally nibble on a good candy bar just for the hell of it, but plan on getting your energy from fruits.

Are you saying that refined sugar in itself is bad?

Refined sugar isn't bad in itself, but the calories it provides aren't very productive. Except in the fat-building area, where they're very productive.

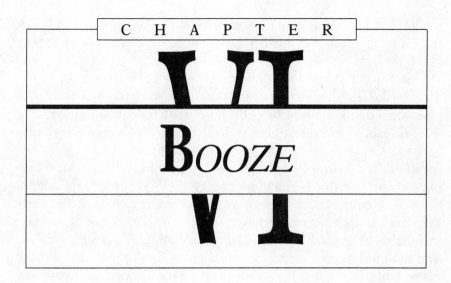

CHAPTER VI

BOOZE

Week 10

Marietta, Georgia

For two and a half months, since I moved to Grand Bahama, my life has been controlled and sheltered. Gluttony and sloth, former friends, haven't seen much of me. Insecurity, an acquaintance, has been pretty much kept at bay, too. I've been safe, others shoring me up and keeping me from all temptation.

Leaving the island without my trainer last night, in the company of strangers who cared only about their hangovers and sunburns, was therefore wonderfully tempting and a little nerve-racking. Airplanes serve *real* food. Junk food. No one told me to avoid butter, or select baked chicken over greasy, tasty stew, and not a soul acted like the dessert was anything but healthy. Even the coffee wanted to seduce me. For two and a half months I have avoided my usual six cups, drinking hot apple juice or bubbling cranberry juice instead. The doctors didn't make me do that, either. Hot juices just sounded a lot healthier and more exotic and they did fill my craving for something hot in the mornings or after a meal.

Until the plane. I decided moderation was just as good as abstinence when it comes to dessert and coffee and consumed them without guilt. Small sins are so nice.

The cart with liquor bottles rattling away rolled by for the last time and my eyes followed it for a moment until I realized how much it tempted me.

I have quietly enjoyed wine and whiskey for over twenty years. I say it like that for no one has accused me of being a drunkard or a problem drinker, and even I didn't realize how much I depended on reasonably moderate amounts of alcohol to help me handle things. Insecurities, worries, pressures, rapid changes in plans, great opportunities, exciting things and terrifying things, boredom, thinking too much, fatigue—I had an encyclopedia of reasons for a glass of wine or beer. The amounts were modest at first, too. But over the years, more and more things seemed to bother me or at least seemed to be a good reason to have another and a stronger drink. And though I never drank alone during the daylight of any of those years, I did like a drink at night to help me sleep. The before-bed drink became the one I really needed. It, of course, only put me to sleep for a few hours and then woke me up.

Now, as I write this, the words look an awful lot like those of an alcoholic, and they scare me as much as my memories of the times I needed *that drink*. They also embarrass me in a way: I may not elicit swoons yet, but I'm quite proud of most of me and don't really like to admit that alcohol was necessary for me to be more comfortable with myself.

"Was" is the operative word here, I hope. I stopped drinking the first night of my remake. Though I was nervous and didn't sleep well for a night or two, I now sleep like I used to sleep back when my biggest worry was going out to feed my horse on a cold morning.

Much more important, I like myself better. People have always seen me as an outgoing, relaxed person with others, especially strangers. Their perception has always been wrong. My heartbeat picks up when I'm alone in an unknown situation. I worry if people will like me and worry if my looks fit the situation and worry about my worry breaking through my well-tended façade. I really thought booze helped me through those moments, too. It probably did loosen my tongue but, on more objective reflection, it brought me a quiet dread of others rather than tranquillity.

I realized that at my first no-booze party two months ago. Though I was nervous at the thought of handling myself without my high-octane friend (still am at times), the gathering was enjoyable and surprisingly nonthreatening. Not a goblin chased me. Even more important, my mood swings don't have peaks and valleys these days. I have spent an awful lot of the past twenty years terrified of things that never happened or happened with no great consequence, and excited about things that would elicit a yawn from most. I thought a drink or two would help me through those moments. When I realized they caused many of them and exacerbated all of them, I felt a nicer high than any drink can bring.

A lot of that old agitation was chemically created, my doctors tell me. The brain acts like a sponge in the presence of alcohol. Though I took my last drink two and a half months ago, portions of it were still having a fun time with my brain cells a month later. I don't want to think about all of the important decisions I've made and foolish things I've done over the past twenty years with the assistance of tipsy gray matter.

But I do like to contemplate this quote from my first blood analysis since the Reformation: in two and a half months, my "triglycerides have dropped precipitously from 355 mg/dl to 174 and the GGT, a liver enzyme study most commonly related to the abuse of alcohol, has dropped from 117 to 51. It is almost back to normal." A liver to elicit swoons.

Heaven, incidentally, did not arrive with abstinence. I still worry about things (like my shoulder, which is better but not well enough for serious lifting), still am nervous at times around others, still have occasional grumpiness and depression. Not a weakness or problem left me permanently, but they all did lose ground to equanimity.

I don't plan to check out an ax from the Carry Nation Club, either. I don't think drinking per se is bad, and still think the cool bite of a beer when you're hot and thirsty is delightful. I don't even think an occasional convivial high with friends is more than a small, pleasurable sin. But in this year of rebuilding my health and my body, I am more aware than ever of the need to exercise a few gray matter muscles, too. When I drink again, I don't think it will be for the same effect.

I thought about that as the drink cart continued down the airplane aisle. It didn't seem as filled with magic elixirs as it used to. And though I don't like the idea of facing a world of weight lifting, temptations, and pleasures without some support, I am becoming very comfortable facing it without liquid support.

I *have a beer at lunch, a glass of that fancy Gallo wine with Norma's Chef-Boy-Ar-Dee special, and a beer with my Alka-Seltzer before bed. What does that say about me?*

That you are classified a heavy drinker by the National Institute on Alcohol Abuse and Alcoholism and most other research organizations. The institute defines light drinking as under four per week, and moderate as four to thirteen per week.[1] You're talking about *twenty-one drinks per week.*

Exactly how much booze is "one drink"?

One and a half ounces of eighty-proof liquor, one five-ounce glass of wine, or one twelve-ounce beer.[2] But most people's idea of "one drink" is more than that. Many researchers say that home drinks mixed without the use of a jigger usually contain two to three ounces of booze and most wine glasses hold more than the five ounces of wine which constitutes "one drink." Some surveys also show that many restaurants and bars may also pour more than one-and-a-half-ounce drinks.[3]

I *drink four or five "drinks" a day, but I never feel tipsy. Does this mean I'm doing okay?*

Generally speaking, each "drink" takes about two hours for your body to burn it up, and nothing—not coffee or food or raw eggs or cold showers or pure oxygen or "hair of the dog"—can speed your particular body's burning process. If you drink one drink every two hours, your body can pretty much burn off the alcohol as you drink it. If you down two drinks quickly, you begin to overload your system, and that's when you begin to get drunk.[4]

You could theoretically drink four or five drinks, therefore, and never be drunk. But that's not the way we drink. Two drinks with lunch at one, consumed over an hour, put your body in a slightly alcoholic state. It sobers up at five, when you drink two more, and remain under their influence until nine, when your nightcap takes over. Your body, particularly your liver, has been in overtime for about ten hours. A regular pattern like this, not uncommon, can cause health problems.

But *I don't feel drunk. So what's wrong?*

As professional drinkers (like I used to be) know, experience covers many sins. Our bodies adjust to the alcoholic state, developing a higher tolerance, requiring more alcohol for that "high." But that doesn't mean we have any lower blood alcohol levels than the amateurs.

Now *I feel a little depressed. Won't a drink or two give me a lift?*

For most people a cocktail or beer will give you a feeling of relaxation and euphoria at first, why most of us originally like drinking. But alcohol is definitely a depressant. Oddly enough, the first thing it depresses is our inhibitions. That's why Norma took off her bra at your Christmas party last year and you took off what I won't mention for modesty's sake.

Norma *and I are kind of heroic around the belly. Does that mean we get drunk slower than runty types?*

How fast you get drunk depends on your weight, the speed of the drinking, how much food and what type of food is in your stomach, and the type of beverage you're mixing your booze with. If you are muscular rather than fat, you can handle booze easier, too.[5] But don't think that eating a large meal before a drinking bout prevents you from getting drunk. It simply postpones the drunken state.

Protein, such as milk, incidentally, does a real good job of slowing down alcohol absorption. But that is still "slow down," not "prevent."

When *does alcohol consumption begin to affect my liver? Are there any symptoms?*

Alcohol, unlike most major sources of calories, can't be stored anywhere in the body for use as future fuel. The body therefore tries to burn it immediately, putting it in the fuel chain before any other fuel. Other fuels, such as fatty acids, have to wait before the body can burn them, and fatty acids in particular seem to favor the liver as a waiting place. This infiltration of the liver by fat is the first abnormality of the liver associated with alcohol overconsumption, the first step in a progression of conditions which culminates in cirrhosis.[6] A blood test which measures your liver's levels of two enzymes called SGPT and SGOT can tell you if you're there yet. I was. But in less than three months away from the bottle, my liver was virtually back to normal.

What is cirrhosis, and will it clear up if I'm good?

Cirrhosis of the liver is a progressive disease in which some liver cells are replaced by fibrous, connective tissue. The more cells affected, the more poorly the liver functions, until finally it can't function at all. At that point, you die. Damage from cirrhosis is not reversible, though it may be arrested or slowed.

What about all that publicity about a drink or two being good for your heart?

Please don't lift a sentence or two from this and say it's gospel, for the "drink or two a day is good for you" debate isn't settled yet. But several studies did indicate that moderate drinkers had significantly lower risk of fatal heart attack than either heavy drinkers or nondrinkers. The researchers speculated (didn't state as a fact) that this protection might arise from the seeming ability of alcohol to raise the level of high-density lipoproteins (HDLs) in the blood.[7] A high level of HDLs, as we'll see later, seems to indicate a lower likelihood of coronary heart disease. High levels of HDLs, as we'll also see, are associated also with people who exercise regularly. For example, *Consumer Reports* summarized the findings of one study by saying: "Sedentary men who drank moderately had HDL levels similar to those of moderate drinkers who jogged regularly. When the men who jogged abstained from alcohol for three weeks, their HDL levels remained relatively unchanged. HDL levels in the sedentary men fell significantly, however, when they abstained from drinking."[8]

Now, needless to say, I liked hearing about this study. It seemed to indicate that a slug-type person who didn't exercise or drink could be as well-off cardiovascular-wise as a jock simply by hitting the bottle a little. My type of exercise. Reality is never that nice, though. Like most things in health, these findings are filled with ifs:[9]

1. Many of the most popular studies comparing rates of heart disease and mortality for drinkers and nondrinkers did not separate lifelong abstainers from those who had given up drink, something usually done for health reasons. In the studies where these types were separated, people who had never drunk (lifelong abstainers) and moderate drinkers usually had about the same risk of heart attack. *Ex-drinkers*, incidentally, had a death rate four times the expected rate.
2. Some studies do correct for never-drinkers/past-drinkers and still show that the moderate drinkers come out slightly ahead. These studies may fail to correct for cigarette smoking. When corrections for smoking take place, never drinkers and moderate drinkers have about the same rate of heart problems.
3. Some researchers say many teetotalers may be type A people, the driven folks already at higher risk of heart attack.
4. Changes in HDLs. Remember that HDLs, high-density lipoprotein, in high numbers, do seem to lower the risk of heart disease. Very moderate amounts of alcohol do seem to raise HDL levels, too. But HDL is not one substance. It's made up of components called subfractions. Very hard research is now showing that HDL_2 is the factor protecting against heart disease. HDL_3, another subfraction, seems to be the HDL raised by alcohol consumption.
5. These studies had to do with heart disease only. Many other conditions, such as high blood pressure or high body fat, can take the wind out of your sails, and these things can be prevented or helped with the proper exercise.

S*o can Norma and I forget the dancercise classes at the Moose Lodge or not?*

If you've read this carefully, you probably feel like I do and like most of the heart experts at this stage in the research. A drink or two isn't going to hurt me, but it's not going to make me healthier, either. Didn't you really know it couldn't be that easy?

But *will that drink or two add to our girths?*

Drinks are filled with those evil "empty calories"—calories which don't do anything but put on weight. But an occasional drink is no worse for your diet than an occasional piece of chocolate cake. If you plan to drink, at least cut down their calorie content. Make your wine 25 percent water and you'll hardly notice the difference. Make your hard drinks with one bottle cap rather than a big pour. Buy mini-cans of beer. So much of drinking is psychological, you'll be surprised how these tricks will help you.

I*'ve been drinking a six-pack a day for years. Am I running any risks?*

Regular heavy drinkers increase their risks of developing a number of health problems. A recently released study, for example, found the risk of stroke to be four times higher.[10] Heavy drinking is also associated with increased risk of cancers of the mouth, throat, stomach, liver, pancreas, and colon; increased risk of heart disease; increased risk of high blood pressure; and increased risk of stomach and intestinal orders.[11] In fact, the National Institute on Alcohol and Alcoholism stated: "Chronic alcohol consumption leads to ubiquitous toxic effects in the body, with medical consequences ranging from slight functional impairment to life-threatening disease states."[12] Recent studies also suggest that, for women, even moderate drinking (as few as three drinks a week) is associated with an increased risk of breast cancer.[13] You decide about the six-pack.

How *do you know if someone you know is drinking too much?*

If you and others quietly wonder if someone is drinking too much, they probably are. They may not be an alcoholic by definition, but that doesn't mean they don't need help. Alcohol can begin to control things much faster than most of us (including me) want to recognize. For instance, if reading all this makes you nervous enough to want a drink, you have a reason to be nervous.

Nervous? Who me? I'll just have a little nip or two to make me sleep better.

One one-and-a-half-ounce drink consumed leisurely before going to bed probably won't bother you much.[14] But if you, like me, really need a stiff one to fall asleep, you're probably looking at several problems. First, you're likely to wake up a lot to go to the bathroom or to take a drink of water. Most people find that wake-up period like the morning, and find it hard to go back to sleep. Second, needing a drink to "relax" you at any time is a very scary sign of alcohol dependency. And finally, if that drink is gulped, and is a strong one, you're placing extra burdens on your liver.

I don't want to think how many years that drink was important to me, but do know how nice it feels to be able to go to sleep without it.

Some people can be heavy drinkers for their whole lives and probably not have addictive problems associated with their drinking (though most will have health problems). Others become alcoholic quickly. If you see someone you care for developing alcoholic problems or habits (such as keeping booze too readily available at all times or constantly looking for an excuse to have a drink), ask others who care for the person if they, too, are a little worried. If you all agree there's a problem, go to the person's spouse or closest friend and talk honestly about the problems you are seeing. Real alcoholics, virtually all of them, will die prematurely unless someone helps them.

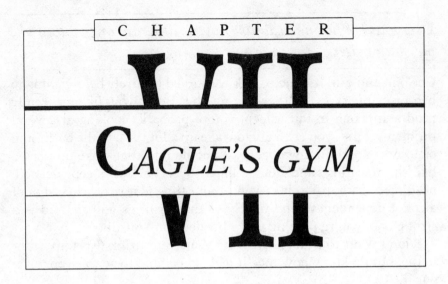

Week 11

Marietta, Georgia

Today I lifted weights by myself in a strange gym, my first workout without the prodding and emotional support of my trainer and other gym members who know me. Sounds like a trite accomplishment, doesn't it, like walking down the street? Though I survived with my dignity reasonably intact, it was more like walking through a field of sand spurs with spring feet.

First I had to choose a gym. Though I'm in my hometown, I didn't have the slightest idea how to find a comfortable place. I left the first fancy fitness center when the "hostess" tried to sell me their own brand of cologne before selling me a day membership. I couldn't get through the lobby of the second place. A large group of "Samba Saturday" class members were dancing through there on the way to a seminar entitled "Human Sexuality and Aerobics." Next I drove to a couple of "serious gyms," so-called because everyone in them looks so *intent* and chiseled. The gyms themselves looked like something from an old Brando movie. A person could get beat up in a place like those. I drove on.

Discouraged, I stopped at the Ace Hardware close to my mother's home to collect another bedding tray of bright red salvia for her.

Here, chance in the person of a very friendly guy named Jimmy Beasley solved my problem. Jimmy is as serious about weight lifting as he is friendly. Since he had both the body and the personality I admired, I asked where he worked out. Cagle's. That would be the gym for me.

"Friendly" may fit Jimmy perfectly, but when I pulled up in front of Cagle's, I wasn't sure the adjective fit his gym. A low, gray building with one shuttered window squatted in a small gravel lot. The single door faced the world from behind mirrored glass. A big, deep-red Harley-Davidson motorcycle leaned rather arrogantly by the door, its fat wheels digging ruts in the gravel.

Two deserted shanty houses right out of *The Grapes of Wrath* sat across the narrow paved alley. A large, red and white sign on the more run-down of the derelict structures said *THIS PROPERTY NOT FOR SALE OR LEASE BY OWNER*, a nearly laughable sign if you don't know the neighborhood. The gym and the houses are a minute's fast walk from the Cobb County Courthouse and are the last pieces of property not yet gobbled up by law firms whose partners like to walk to work.

I was in my mother's car, a silver Lincoln about the size of my insecurities at that moment. It didn't make the right statement, something which hit me as a truck holding two massive, barrel-shaped, and nonsmiling men parked on my left. You don't just sit in a silver Lincoln in front of a serious gym as barrel-shaped and nonsmiling people look at you, especially if your only companion is a tray of pretty flowers, unless you're doing something. I quickly shifted the tray of salvia, shuffled through my mother's mail and slipped a magazine from its wrapper as the two barrel types walked by my window. We saw the cover at the same time, *Gourmet*. I could have been playing with dolls. I thought briefly of explaining: "Flowers? Hell, I *stomp* gardens, myself." Instead I just forced the car door open and headed to the gym. It was a very long walk.

I think fast when I'm nervous. As the gym door shut behind me, I planned the response which I thought would make me sound calm when greeted, stuck my hand out to the guy standing behind the counter, and without waiting for the question blurted, "I'm fine."

Charlie Thompson, the owner of Cagle's, endeared himself to me by making my gaffe seem normal. "Glad to hear it; I am, too."

As he spoke, the reception area came into focus. An old Spanish-style Naugahyde sofa with the corners gnawed off leaned against the right office wall. Two high school boys sprawled on it, paying more attention to Charlie's two towheaded sons running across the green outdoor carpet than to me. An older man in a Gucci sweatshirt walked from the dressing area and playfully kicked one boy's feet as he walked by, stepping over the other set. Charlie's wife knelt on the floor by several battered black filing cabinets and waved to another young man as she called to her sons. Trophies, some on their sides, some dusty, were everywhere, conveying a pleasant nonchalance about winning.

The place and the people who drifted in and out had the feeling of our old cabin at Lake Sinclair, where the furniture was theft-proof (who would want it?) but perfect and comfortable for our needs, and the company was nonstop and happy.

Charlie Thompson, thirty-three, as wholesome-looking as a glass of milk, has been in the gym business, what he always wanted to do, since he graduated from the University of Georgia nine years ago. He refers to Cagle's as a "heavy weight" gym rather than a health club or fitness center. Charlie looks like a bodybuilder, one of those guys who spend their time sculpting their bodies and are judged in competition on the symmetry of their muscles, on their beauty. In my gym in the Bahamas, virtually everyone is a body-builder (me, too). Charlie's background, though, is in power lifting. It's similar to the Olympic weight events you've watched on television in that power lifters are judged solely on their ability to move weight. Those who move the most win.

But power lifting events are different from Olympic events. In the squat, the contestant rests the weights behind his neck on the shoulders and tries to squat then stand up. In the dead lift, the contestant squats, grabs the bar, and tries to lift the most weight from the floor while keeping his arms straight. In the bench press, the contestant reclines on a bench and attempts to press the greatest weight to his chest and then return it to the starting position.

Since power lifters win with strength, not shape, they aren't afraid of fat, and many of them own a good bit of it. Charlie Thompson even says fat adds leverage and cushioning. I don't doubt him, either. Cagle's Gym took first place in eight out of eleven events at the 1986 Georgia Power Lifting Championships. A weight lifting sport that accepts the rotund. Maybe I missed my calling.

I felt real comfortable after talking with Charlie, and entered the weight room rather eagerly, feeling nervous only when I caught the eyes of the two barrel types. They watched me as I walked to a bench, sat a bar on the rack above it, and slid weights on each end. I tried to do all of this very professionally. I lay on the bench. Normally at this point, my trainer would hand me the bar, but my trainer was in the Bahamas. I would have to lift the bar and all that weight from the rack by myself, something I had never done before. A very unnerving thought. Could I lift the weight? I placed my hands carefully on the bar for maximum torque, closed my eyes, prayed the prayer of the insecure, "Oh God, don't let me make a fool of myself," and heaved mightily.

Terror gives great strength. The bar nearly flew from my hands, and a weight from the left side sailed through the air, thumping at the feet of the burly types. The older one, who had glared the most at my mother's *Gourmet*, walked to me. "Hey, buddy, how 'bout someone to spot you?" he said with a grin on his face. "You look kinda eager."

I did not argue with his offer or his observation. But I did explain about the plants and that magazine. You can't have those power lifters thinking we bodybuilders are too effete.

Well, *I would never get caught with flowers, but tell me more about the differences between power lifting, Olympic lifting, strength training, and weight lifting.*

Power lifters compete in three events: the squat, bench press, and dead lift. In the squat, a barbell is placed on the lifter's upper back. The lifter then squats down until his upper thighs are parallel with the ground and then stands up. The winner can stand up with the most. The men's record, set by heavyweight Mat Demio, is 1,010 pounds; the women's is 578 pounds, set by Lorraine Costanzo. Squats, incidentally, aren't graceful, but they're great for building your legs and your buttocks.

Everyone knows the bench press—you're on your back, you lift the bar from a rack, lower it to the chest, and push it back up— but did you know that the record presses are 705 pounds by Ted Arcidi and 331 pounds by Bev Francis? The bench press is a great exercise for replacing flabby breasts with muscle. Women love chests rebuilt with this exercise. Trust me.

The dead lift involves bending down and lifting a barbell off the floor. The records are 903 pounds by Doyle Kennady and 539 pounds by Ruthie Shafer. Dead lifts are primarily a leg exercise, but also strengthen the back.

The three power lifting events are part of almost everyone's weight training, but power lifters simply concentrate on them more.

Olympic lifting, the event you watch in the Olympics, has only two lifts: the clean and jerk, and the snatch. And it's a very fast sport, involving dramatic movement. The clean and jerk starts with the bar on the floor. With a few weights on it. Like 500 pounds for the heavy weight champion. The lifter squats down, grabs the bar and in one lightning-fast upward jerk stands up and pulls that 500-pound bar to his chest, where he may pause for a moment. From there, the lifter literally throws the bar up and goes under it, pushing the weight over his head, where he must control it. It's a damn exciting thing to watch, but a damn scary thing to try.

The snatch also starts with the bar on the ground, but instead of pausing with the bar on the chest, the lifter immediately pushes it over his head. The snatch is probably the most difficult and dangerous maneuver any lifter wants to attempt.

Strength trainers and weight lifters are terms used interchangeably by some to describe people who lift weights, but don't call a power or Olympic lifter either name, or they'll turn you into a pancake. Everyone likes specific terms. So don't forget that bodybuilders care more about their looks than their strength or techniques, and power and Olympic lifters care more about their strength than their looks.

P*hysiologically, what are the mechanisms of getting bigger and stronger? Do my muscle cells grow, or what?*

First, increasing your actual muscle measurements is referred to in two ways: hypertrophy is an increase in the size of the muscle cell itself; hyperplasia is an increase in the number of your muscle cells. Scientists don't know for sure which way human muscles grow, but most agree that hypertrophy (increasing the size of your cells) plays a major role in muscle growth.[1]

Norma is afraid she'll get bigger as her muscles grow stronger. Do women have to worry about that?

Strength depends on the size of your muscle cells and the ability of your body to recruit them. Women (and older men, incidentally) grow stronger from cell recruitment more than they do from increases in the size of muscle cells. It is therefore much harder for them to be really muscular. Women also don't have male hormones, which affect muscle size, too. Do not worry.[2]

What is muscle, anyway?

About 75 percent water, 20 percent protein, and 5 percent minerals, salts, and fuels such as glycogen (a stored sugar). The increase in any of these components will cause increase in muscle size.

What about that theory that you build muscle by "ripping apart" the old muscle tissue?

That sounds real macho, but isn't really right. Muscle tissue *is* a very dynamic tissue. It is always breaking down and being built back up. But this doesn't happen in stages. For instance, the muscle isn't static and then put in a state of frenzy if you lift weights, it is constantly rebuilding itself.

When you weight train, you increase the buildup phase and *decrease* the breakdown phase, according to most theories, although some muscle breakdown does occur and can lead to soreness.[3] This process gives you an increase in the amount of muscle protein actually available to contract your muscle. This contraction, incidentally, is a muscle's sole responsibility. An uncontracted muscle is an unhappy one. It atrophies.

People seem to toss a lot of fancy adjectives around describing strength-building exercises. What's the difference in isometric, isotonic, and isokinetic exercising?

Isometric exercises involve an application of force, but no movement. Pushing like Samson against the sides of a door frame is a good example. Isometrics will definitely build strength, but only at the specific angle in which you are working a muscle. Charles Atlas, incidentally, became a rich and famous man when he introduced isometrics to America's wimps. You didn't kick sand in his face. Isometrics were also popularized by women's magazines as "toning" exercises. Many people, including Atlas, have believed isometric exercises are an excellent way to build muscle. Even football teams have used them for that. Although it works, muscle building the isometric way takes an awful lot longer than muscle building with weights or machines.

Isotonic exercises involve uniform tension but varying speed. Free weights are isotonic exercises. The weight you are handling does not increase or decrease while you lift, but the speed of your movement will be determined by your strength at different points in your range of movement. There are, incidentally, types of isotonic exercise in which the weight does vary, but these are still classified as isotonic exercise because weight and a varying speed are still involved. These "variable resistance machines," which include Nautilus and some Universal machines, vary the weight according to your strong and weak points, a nice selling feature. People like me who prefer free weights are suspicious of most machines. All of the isotonic exercising methods, including free weights, enable you to work a whole range of motion. They can improve both strength and flexibility in the muscles you are working.

Isokinetic exercise machines, the newest thing in strength and weight training, have the ability to control the speed of the muscle contraction. Regardless of how strong or weak you are, you can't change the speed of your motion. That may not seem very important to you or your muscle, but it is. These machines will only give you as much resistance as you give it. If you can only lift a hundred pounds, it resists a hundred pounds' worth, etc. Because we have different strengths at different places throughout a movement, these machines can work us the hardest at our weakest point and our strongest point.

Nautilus and some other variable resistance machines have tried to duplicate this strength-to-resistance ratio mechanically. To do so, they averaged a group of lifters' strengths at different positions in a particular movement and built their machines to provide different resistances to the different strength levels. Their machines will give you a very good workout. But you must adjust your own strength patterns to these machines, they won't adjust to you. Iso-kinetic machines will adjust to you.

For professional athletes, isokinetic machines also provide some very special capabilities. The important movement in most athletic events occurs at very fast speeds. A pitcher's arm may be moving at almost a hundred miles per hour when he throws a fastball, for instance. But most strength and power exercises happen at much slower speeds. Isokinetic machines can allow a person to build his strength and power at the speed his body parts move during an actual activity.[4] They can actually control the speed of the muscle contraction, something that's never happened before.

Dr. Gideon Ariel, my biomechanics and strength coach, definitely does have the neatest isokinetic machines out there. They are very expensive (the two machines you'd need to do most things cost over $20,000), but do the work of many machines. You'll find them at some preventive medicine and physical rehabilitation centers, and at the more advanced human performance centers (health clubs)—no self-respecting place with one of these machines would call itself a gym, would it?

Can I use steroids to speed my progress along?

Whether you are male or female, they'll definitely speed your search, but may kill you along the way. Steroids have anabolic and androgenic qualities. Anabolic refers to the ability of a steroid to convert food into living matter, such as muscle tissue. Androgenic refers to steroid's ability to make the taker more masculine. Side effects include impaired liver function, liver tumors, actual structural changes in the liver itself, lowered HDL cholesterols (the good guys), altered testicular function in men (a nice way of saying your manhood could shrink away to nothing), acne, baldness, and dramatic and negative changes in your behavior patterns. In women, steroids can also bring potentially irreverisble masculinization (body and facial hair, voice changes). Your menstrual cycle can be changed too.[5]

Did *you think about using steroids?*

I did, and I would have used them if they had appeared even reasonably safe. But several months of research and a particular fondness for my manhood convinced me to pass on them. Steroids may speed up hunkdom, but hard work eventually brings you the same result.

What's *the difference in strength and power and endurance and tone? Norma's been reading all this over my shoulder, and she's gonna become a drug-free power lifter, she says.*

Strength is the application of force. It's usually measured by a single repetition, a bench press or leg press. You break strength records when you lift more this week in one repetition than you did last week. Ever had someone take your hand and crush it once in a Texas handshake? That's strength.

Power requires timed movement. Technically, it is your strength multiplied by your speed. If you punch out someone lustfully eyeing Norma, that's power. Be sure the person you punch out isn't more powerful. That's smart.

Endurance is the application of force over a period of time. It's measured by your ability to resist fatigue as you lift the same weight repetitively. When you run from the person you tried to punch out but missed, that's endurance. When he catches you, that's fear.

Tone, as we mentioned earlier, is defined as muscle always in a partial state of contraction. You achieve tone with either strength training or endurance training. Most people's muscles are also in a partial state of contraction when they feel absolute terror, what you'll feel right before the guy who caught you punches you out and doesn't miss.

All of these bad things won't happen to you if you exercise and eat apples and especially if you think before picking on someone bigger than you.

I *worry about "brittle bones," and gulp diet drinks fortified with calcium like Phil gulps beers to beat the blues. Do men have the same worry about brittle bones? Does weight lifting help? Do all those calcium supplements help?*

Although women are more affected by osteoporosis, men's bones can become brittle, too, though usually it happens later in life. But anyone can definitely strengthen his or her bones by lifting weights. The proper lifting program actually increases the mineral content of your bones, the things that make them strong.[6] The best weight program for this is probably high repetitions of low weights.[7] Some people think "circuit training" (remember, that's weight exercises sort of done on the run to get your heart rate up) is very good for this. Start any program under someone's supervision, though. Weight-bearing activity, such as walking or jogging, is also good for strengthening bones.[8]

Making sure you have plenty of calcium in your diet is also important; low-fat milk products, leafy green vegetables, and canned salmon or sardines with bones are good sources. *But* studies show that when osteoporosis is present, it may be too late to begin increasing calcium intake. Start enjoying calcium-loaded foods early in life.[9]

P*hil read in the* It's-Startling-But-the-Gospel-Truth News *that all those little weights will really make his workouts more efficient. Now he's wearing hand weights, ankle weights, and a weighted vest, even to bed. He rolled over and flattened my right arm last night. Are those things worth it?*

Wearing them to bed only makes you kinky, not stronger. But mini-weights, used properly, can increase your aerobic fitness, burn more calories, and increase your strength.[10] Most people don't use them right, though. Because a half-pound weight looks awfully petite, they buy five-pound ones, then attempt to exercise at their normal pace and intensity, or greater. These people are real popular with doctors. Even a half-pound weight drastically increases the stress on the joint and muscles in the area being worked. Ankle weights, for instance, place considerable strain on the knee joint.

If you want to use light weights, start out below your normal pace. Start with very small weights and work up gradually.

Norma's pressing me, but I don't want to buy anything until I think this thing's for sure. Do I really have to have equipment?

You don't have to buy out the store to start, but you will need a few things.

Shoes.   You need a pair for your particular activity, but you don't need twenty pairs for twenty different things. Did you know there are hundreds of sport shoes on the market now? An active person would need a nubile servant just to keep up with all the shoes the manufacturers recommend.

Clothing.   If you want to make a fashion statement, fine, but real men and women don't think about what they wear when they work out. Or at least it looks like they don't think about it. Do wear layers to peel off, though, since exercise heats you up quickly. Of course, many athletes, for instance bikers, take clothing very seriously because it can mean the microsecond difference between winning and losing.[11] But that's not really important for us ordinary types.

Gloves for weight lifting.   I list this separately, because you've got to have gloves if you lift—that is, if you're lifting at a real gym versus a spa and if you want to save your hands from a lot of blisters. Weight lifting actually generates enough friction heat to be uncomfortable. But when you get your gloves, for God's sake, don't take them new to the gym. New gloves are a dead giveaway you are a pro or a wimp, nothing in between. Do what I did: rub 'em in the dirt, throw 'em in a gutter, and stomp on 'em a while. This won't add muscles to your frame, but it will make you look more like a great weight lifter who went to seed and is now coming back.

Well, I'll never wear a wimpy glove. But what about the real equipment out there, bikes and treadmills and the like? Do I need any of that stuff?

The only reason to buy equipment is to make your time devoted to exercise either less boring or more efficient. Many devices can help you accomplish both objectives, depending upon your goals. "But," advises Christopher Scott, my exercise physiologist, "never buy on impulse. Try before you buy and pick something you enjoy. If, for instance, you don't like biking outdoors, you'll probably hate stationary cycling. Finally, be prepared to spend some money—most good equipment is expensive." The following notes may help you begin to think about what equipment, if any, is right for you.

Exercise bikes.   They can bore you to death if you don't have something to do while pedaling, but bikes are a practical way to get your aerobic exercise without going outside. Get one that's portable enough to put in front of a television, if possible. Also get one that holds a carrot out in front of you: one that helps you keep your pedaling goal-oriented. For instance, some bikes have a needle which must be kept in one position to maintain your level of activity. Don't buy a bike without something like it.

Some bikes have handle bars that move and add a degree of strength training to your workout; some have TV screens or little maps which let you pretend you're biking through the woods. Some even have motors which move the pedals and, believe it or not, these monsters can give you the hardest workout of all, if they provide a way to gauge your work level. One good bike requires you to keep a needle in the center of a gauge, which requires about as much effort as running up the Empire State Building. What's important is to try whatever bike you seem to like for a while before buying it, and to avoid flimsy bikes sold by mail order or late-night television.

Rowing machines.   Rowing machines are great: they are nonimpact, use a lot of muscles, and require a lot of work. But they also require a lot of back work. If you have a bad back, don't think about one of these machines without talking with a sports medicine specialist first. Rowing machines take up a little more room than bikes. Most machines have a sliding seat and two piston "oars." Rowing power comes from the legs, really, so make sure the seat and the rails it moves along not only comfortably support you, but support you in your full range of motion along the track. Some new machines on the market duplicate rowing amazingly well by attaching a wooden grip with a length of cable which usually runs around a flywheel in front of the machine. The thing looks a lot like a spinning wheel, but is probably the best type of rowing machine you can buy.

Treadmills. They come in electric and manual models and aren't cheap ($500 to $5,000); but if you really plan to be a hard-core jogger, these things can give you relief from traffic and bad weather. If you look at a manual one, definitely try running on it for at least ten minutes. If you can't run that long without dropping dead, ask the salesperson to demonstrate a running effort. Manual machines vary dramatically in quality, and the bad ones are virtually impossible to run on.

Electric treadmills vary in price with their features but not necessarily with their quality. To find a good one, check out what makes local health clubs use.

Generally speaking, don't waste your money on these things until you're really sure you like jogging over other activities.

Cross-country-ski machines. Did you know the highest recorded cardiovascular level reached by any human being was achieved by a cross-country skier?[12] The machines which duplicate this motion are similar to rowing machines in that they use lots of muscles, but they work you standing up rather than sitting. Because they vary so dramatically in quality, try one for a good long time before buying it, or check out the types of machines available in local clubs.

Jump ropes. I think they were invented by the devil. I tried a jump rope the first day of my remake, and threw my back out on the count of three. Jump ropes do, however, provide fantastic aerobic exercise, take up no room, and work your entire body. But jumping rope also puts lots of strain on your ankles, back, and just about everything else. Jumping can very easily hurt you if you're really out of shape. Don't choose it as a first aerobic exercise, and go slowly when you do choose it.

Minitrampolines. Great for the professionally coordinated and fit, but dangerous for the klutz. You work out by jogging in place on them; bouncers with poor balance usually fall and crack their crowns.

Late-night television specials in general.   Don't buy any exercise equipment without trying it and looking at it closely. That rule applies doubly to the junk peddled on television. As you know, Norma bought one of those "Tummy Wheels" from late-night TV. It's stored under the bed with your "Slide and Slimaway" machine. Most of these gadgets are poorly designed and constructed. Though they may provide some exercise, jumping up and down like a jack-in-the-box provides as much. Don't waste your money. Chris Scott has even invented something as dandy: Gyro Pasties. "The Faster They Twirl, the Fitter the Girl" is his suggested slogan. Chris, a real whiz in advertising, will probably be hired by the people who sell you body wraps.

Weight training equipment.   Whether you want to build endurance, tone up, or become muscular, you can use the same equipment, machines or free weights. Strength and bigger muscles come from lifting progressively heavier weights. Endurance—the ability to do something again and again—comes from lifting a relatively lighter weight for more repetitions. In essence, you are training the body to resist fatigue.

A*re free weights or machines better for the newly serious lifter?*

Free weight or machine, people seem to like what they first lift with, but both have their uses in a balanced program. Free weights definitely teach you balance, and probably work more muscles since the weights are moving three-dimensionally, constantly requiring a tension in all directions. Free weights also look real macho. You don't see machines used in Olympic competitions, and you constantly hear free-weight lifters complaining that "five hundred pounds on a machine doesn't feel like five hundred pounds on a bar." I say that a lot myself around nonlifters. Free weights also instill the essence of weight training: lift anything heavier than normal, and your body responds. When you become used to the movement of dumbbells, you can as easily lift a rock or a heavy log or a chair or, much later, Norma, and receive the same workout. Machines make you dependent.

Machines are safer, however, especially for the newly serious lifter, and machines certainly more easily work some muscle groups such as your lats (latissimus dorsi in formal terms—they give your back a V-shape). In addition, machines let you work out without a partner most of the time. A serious free-weight session always requires two people.

What about those funny spring-type machines I see on TV?

As we said, don't buy something without trying it, and, generally speaking, don't buy machines which provide their resistance with springs. Springs lose their resiliency.

Do you honestly think I'm going to start something like weight lifting at my age? Do you really think I believe my body can change? I mean, you've had all day and tropical beaches and beauties to keep you going. What can a person in the real world accomplish?

I want to tell you about Arno Jensen, a member of my Body Worry Committee, but before doing that, go to the pictures and look at Arno's body.

Wouldn't you like to look like that at fifty-seven? Would you believe he started lifting weights when he was fifty? For those seven years Arno has literally been reversing the most inevitable sign of aging, too. Statistically, everyone loses lean body mass as they age, everyone has more fat. Textbooks accept that fact the way you accept sunrises. But Arno Jensen's lean body mass has *increased* every year for the past seven years. He moves with the grace of a cheetah. He eats 4,000 calories a day. Young women swoon.

He doesn't work out full-time, either, and he didn't even think about being in shape until he was forty. Arnie was a general practitioner then. One night he jumped from bed at 3 A.M. to rush to a maternity patient, made it to the emergency room of the hospital, but had to stop before entering the room because of chest pains. Probably indigestion, he thought. A few hours later he tried to run around the block, and could barely walk around. He started an aerobics program that day.

Arnie's routine includes fifty push-ups every morning, at least thirty minutes on an exercise bicycle virtually every day, and an hour and a half of weight lifting four days a week.

Whenever I wonder what I'm working for, hunkwise and health-wise, I look at pictures of this man.

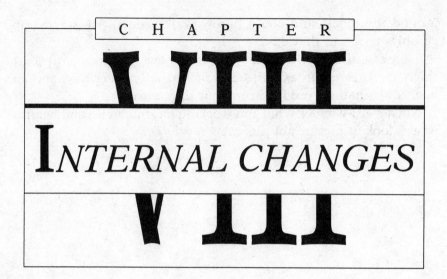

CHAPTER

VIII

INTERNAL CHANGES

Week 14

<u>*The Cooper Clinic, Dallas, Texas*</u>

I hate physical examinations: nakedness, prodding, touching, questions. Everything assaults dignity and pries into places and thoughts that beg to be left alone. Physicals take away our ability to ignore the aging process and to pretend about our health. I, for instance, never felt that any of my bad habits were really catching up with me and secretly believed that there was always time to change things. I was stubborn in those beliefs and steadfast in my ability to ignore any words from my doctors that sounded the least bit threatening to my fantasies of immortality.

You will remember, however, that at the beginning of my remake three and a half months ago, several doctors found the words to get my attention: mild coronary heart disease. Small pulmonary dysfunction. Some abnormal liver function. High risk for heart attack.

I remind you of this because today Dr. Cooper gave me my first complete health evaluation since I took up clean and godly living. And it, in a way, makes the poking and prying worthwhile. In three and a half months my insides have changed. Most of the liquids and tissues and pumping and purifying and growing and dying

80

things have responded quickly to the changes in my consumption and exercise patterns.

I say most because I completely killed some things such as a portion of my lung capacity, and I may have done away with some working liver cells (though I have plenty), and I may not earn back the full function of my heart (though I don't know that yet, either).

But look at what has changed:

My body fat has dropped from 29.7 percent of my total weight to 16.97 percent, a drop of thirty-three pounds of blubber. Aside from the esthetic nicety here, the loss of body fat dramatically cuts down my risk of further heart disease and a dozen other diseases.

My triglycerides have dropped nearly *50* percent. Generally speaking, high triglycerides mean high fat in the blood, which increases the risk of artherosclerosis (more about this in a moment).

My cardiac risk category based on oxygen consumption per kilogram of weight has dropped from very high to low.

My GGT, the liver enzyme which is a nice fingerprint of the steady drinker, dropped more than 50 percent.

My treadmill stress test gave me the most satisfying opinion because I could really savor my progress there immediately. The treadmill gauges many things: aerobic capacity, muscle strength, endurance, cardiovascular fitness, and determination. I added the last category. Three and a half months ago, I collapsed after walking fifteen minutes and achieving a maximum heart rate of 171 beats per minute. Today I walked twenty-three minutes and quit when my heartbeat reached 174. Though that 50 percent improvement may not seem like that much time in minutes, it is. Treadmills increase in angle when you walk on them—the longer you walk, the harder you work. My improvement over the months moved me from a "fair" to an "excellent" aerobic category and literally won me a gold star from Dr. Cooper. The star is made of foil and probably cost a mil, but I value it immensely.

As I write this, I am sitting in the main waiting room of the Cooper Clinic building itself. Cooper opened this place in 1971, then added an aerobics research center and a very fancy gymnasium and guest lodge. The whole place looks like the campus of a very prosperous small college—stately buildings, old trees, joggers, and sports cars everywhere.

Being examined here isn't actually more comfortable physically (they poke you in more places than a regular doctor does, I think), but it all does feel rather cushy. If, for instance, they served more than water or barium for breakfast and if all the victims, uh, patients, around you had on clothes rather than bathrobes, the setting could be for one of those Texas soap operas.

That's the way it should appear, I guess, since an exam here isn't cheap in the dollar sense. A really complete physical exam like mine, including an upper and lower gastrointestinal series (which has to be the most unpleasant thing next to death itself), costs as of this writing about $1,000, plus travel and lodging.

But as with most of the good preventive medicine/diagnostic clinics around the country (there are quite a few, most for profit), the Cooper Clinic is more thorough than you might want to imagine.

Dr. Cooper took my history.

The blood department analyzed my blood.

A psychologist administered a psychological test. (I "stick to a task until mastery.")

A respiratory specialist evaluated my lung function. (Smoking caused a 15 percent loss.)

An audiologist checked my hearing. ("Outstanding at all frequencies.")

A dentist checked my mouth. (No cavities!)

A technician stripped me naked and weighed me underwater.

Dr. Cooper and Dr. Arno Jensen examined virtually every inch of my exterior and interior.

Finally, Georgia Kostas, the clinic's director of nutrition, met with me to plan my diet more carefully.

After all that, no one can pretend or ignore the realities of his health. And for that reason alone I like these clinics. A good physical can save your life.

I hope the man walking down the hall a little self-consciously in his bathrobe and tennis shoes remembers that, for I know what they are going to do to him in the room on the right. The fellow received his visit to the clinic as a perk for a year's work well done, and though I can't help but wonder if he's planning to slack off a little from now on, I hope he knows how lucky he is.

I do. As you can tell, I am proud of my interior gains because what's inside gives me life. But, after three and a half months, I'm different on the outside, too. Excuse me while I go stand in front of a mirror.

Pardon me, handsome, but getting fit doesn't seem to work all the time. Like Jim Fixx. He had one of those slender, Soloflex-type bodies and he ran farther than I can think—the picture of fitness. But he died from a heart attack—while running. Why didn't all that exercise keep him alive?

Jim Fixx was probably the most famous runner in America. When he died at fifty-two of a massive heart attack, thousands of people probably quit jogging from fear of a heart attack and thousands more never started an exercise program because Jim Fixx's death seemed to prove to them that exercise doesn't keep you living longer.

Dr. Cooper knew Fixx well. Several times when the famous runner visited the clinic, Cooper tried to convince Fixx to take a stress treadmill test. Fixx always seemed too busy. Cooper didn't know, of course, that Fixx's father had died at a young age from a massive heart attack. "If we had known that," Cooper says, "we might have finally convinced Jim to have a stress test. And that test would have very likely shown a major problem. Jim Fixx died primarily of a lack of blood flow to the heart caused by blockage in his coronary arteries, an easy thing to detect with proper testing, and a correctable problem most of the time." Dr. Cooper's book *Running Without Fear* will give you an excellent look at Jim Fixx and his health problems.[1]

But aren't there risk factors none of us can do things about?

As I mentioned earlier, we can't literally change our true genetic predispositions to certain things like high blood pressure, high cholesterol levels, or for some of us even the amount of fat on our bodies. But knowing you are in a genetically risky position in any area is the most important reason to fight. If you are from a family of people who die from heart attacks, for instance, you obviously should be concerned about any tests that might show if you have heart disease, and obviously should not do things that already increase your riskier position. If you have genetically high cholesterol, and ignore that as you eat each day, you are simply increasing an already higher probability of trouble.

But remember—for many of us, what appears to be genetic predisposition may not be. If your grandfather's eating, smoking, and drinking habits are the same as yours now, that heart attack he died of may come to you compliments of those habits, not genes.

Norma and I have spent too many years eating the things we like and living the way we like to really change. We've eaten fried for thirty years, smoked for twenty, carried around our bellies for ten, and we really don't feel that bad. And even though I'm on high blood pressure medicine, our doc has never acted like we're going to die any minute. Aren't you being a health nut about all of this?

If you have high blood pressure, eat a lot of fatty foods and therefore have high cholesterol, smoke, and are overweight, you don't need to waste your money to find out if you have heart disease. You do. *Ninety percent of the time* coronary heart disease can be predicted simply by your personal history. And a personal history of excess pounds, cholesterol, smoking, and high blood pressure indicates heart disease.[2] You may not know it yet—they don't call heart disease a silent killer for nothing—but it is definitely there.

Blood pressure you talked about already, but what is cholesterol, anyway? And if it's so bad, why is it so bad?

Cholesterol isn't bad, normally. It's a vital chemical substance both manufactured in our bodies and found in animal tissue we eat. It is not really a fat itself, but the body reacts to it as if it were a fat. Cholesterol is manufactured primarily in the liver, but is so important to the functioning of our body that it is a part of and also manufactured by virtually all of our cells at one time or the other.[3]

Cholesterol, for instance, is the main ingredient in bile. Bile, produced in the liver, breaks all fats down into smaller pieces, making it easier for the body to absorb it. These broken-down fats are stored as fuel reserves, used right away as fuel, and used as insulation and protection of our organs. Cholesterol also makes up a portion of our sex hormones.

When some cells need a little more cholesterol, it is sent there in the blood. Cholesterol, since it acts pretty much like a fat, is not water soluble. If it were released directly in the blood, it would clog it in much the same way that fat poured down your sink will clog the sink. So, to enable the blood to transport the cholesterol, the liver gives each fat and cholesterol package "anti-stick" properties. These packages are called lipoproteins. There are two types of lipoproteins, HDLs, or high-density lipoproteins, and LDLs, or low-density lipoproteins.

HDLs *return* excess cholesterol to the liver for breakdown and disposal. Your body is normally able to regulate the ratio of LDLs and HDLs available to carry cholesterol. But we complicate their work, especially when we eat animal fats. Eating *some* fats is important. For instance, about 20 percent of our diets should be plant fats and about 10 percent animal fats.[4] When we eat too many saturated (animal) fats, however, our bodies begin to manufacture even more cholesterol at the cellular level.[5] For that cholesterol to travel around, more HDLs and LDLs are produced by the liver.

LDLs, the elements which take cholesterols to our cells, for some reason seem to be attracted to our arteries. And here the real tragedies begin.

Arteries, which take blood away from the heart, are flexible when they're functioning correctly. This flexibility actually helps move blood along, a process called elastic recoil. Arteries have essentially three layers. The inner layer, when it's healthy, is smooth. It is also very thin (the thickness of one cell) and fragile. The middle layer is composed of muscle tissue. This layer of muscle normally controls blood flow by contracting the artery when blood flow needs to be decreased and enlarging the artery when blood flow needs to be increased. The elasticity of arteries makes this possible. The outer layer of the artery simply covers the muscular layer.

When LDLs and HDLs are in balance (for a man, 3.5 LDLs to 1 HDL), cholesterol travels through our arteries with little impact on the health of the arteries themselves. But when diseases and chemical imbalances in the blood occur, the interior lining of the vessels become damaged. For instance, smoking, high blood pressure, diabetes, and high fats in the blood (like those in the animal fats you eat) virtually always damage vessels.

The most common damage to that fragile inner lining of vessels is a simple rupture. Much like a hernia, the next layer of tissue protrudes. In this case, the thin layer of muscle. As with any injury, the body reacts to this by sending platelets to the damaged area to attempt a repair. The platelets congregate around the damaged area, causing the beginning of a traffic jam in very fast-moving blood. For some reason yet unknown, the platelets seem to actually draw more muscle tissue through the rupture point, causing an even larger traffic jam.

Floating through the blood, normally without causing any real problems, are the artery-loving LDL cholesterols. As these cholesterols approach the rupture points, they become caught in the traffic jam and attach themselves to the damaged area. The more LDLs in your blood, the more damage. This area is now called a "plaque," and begins to block the flow of blood.

This entire process of damage and plaque formation is called atherosclerosis.[6]

Atherosclerosis? *Is that the same as* arterio*sclerosis?*

Atherosclerosis is the buildup of fat-laden plaques which eventually block arteries. *Arterio*sclerosis, hardening of the arteries, is the replacement of the muscle layer and elastic tissue in the artery with fibrous tissue and certain plaques.

What *are the effects of atherosclerosis?*

In the arteries surrounding the heart, atherosclerosis is simply referred to as coronary heart disease (CHD), usually a progressive disease. Because of the blockage, blood flow decreases to the heart. The muscle literally begins to suffocate. Chest pains can be an indication of that suffocation. Its ultimate progression is a myocardial infarction, death of an area of the heart. Forty percent of the time, the only symptom of this disease is death. Myocardial infarctions cause over 50 percent of the total deaths from diseases of the heart and vessel systems.[7]

If the arteries supplying the brain have atherosclerosis, strokes may result. A portion of the brain literally dies. Strokes usually paralyze, but they also kill approximately 8 percent of all people who die from diseases of the heart and vessel systems.[8] Atherosclerosis is also a cause of senility. Atherosclerosis in other areas of the body, like the legs, for instance, causes the same types of blockages and, in their final progression, kill tissues in those areas.

Can *atherosclerosis be treated?*

There are drugs for the treatment of high cholesterol, but as of now, there are no drugs to actually remove plaques.[9] Many quacks will tell you otherwise, but don't waste your money on a cure without talking with your doctor.

Though drugs aren't available, there are a couple of avenues open to you, which we present here. But remember: there is no treatment as sage or as effective as prevention.

Subcutaneous transluminal angioplasty. A catheter is introduced into the artery and pushed to the injured site. A small "balloon" is inflated to compress the plaques and create a larger opening. Though this is a relatively new procedure, it seems to work very well for many people.[10]

Bypass surgery. The injured area is literally bypassed using a saphenous vein (one near the surface) from some other part of your body, usually the leg. Bypass surgery is effective in most cases, but is a more complicated surgery than angioplasty.

How *important are cholesterols to all this?*

Excess cholesterols cause enormous damage to the arteries. These cholesterols are delivered there by LDLs. When our blood contains large numbers of LDLs—for instance, when we eat too much animal fat—we directly contribute to this process and potentially to all of the terrors mentioned above.

Fighting all this damage are your HDLs. Remember, they *remove* cholesterol from cells and return it to the liver for disposal. Large numbers of HDLs in your blood are a very good, perhaps lifesaving thing.

How *do you lower LDLs?*

Eat less animal fat and more fats from plants. For instance, corn oil, safflower oil, or olive oil—the "polyunsaturates" and "monosaturates." Recent findings indicate that fish oil may be among the most beneficial oils. Certain fibers such as oats, apples, and beans are also helpful.[11] Check out the tips in the eating section, and always listen to your mama when she tells you to eat your oatmeal.

How *ow do you raise HDLs?*

The one scientifically proven way is aerobic activity.[12]

A*re you telling me I can really lower my risk of all these diseases?*

Without question. Remember the things that begin to damage your arteries and rob them of their elasticity even before cholesterols begin to damage them: high blood pressure, smoking, diabetes, fats in your blood. All of these risk factors can be either reduced or controlled by medication, diet, and exercise.

W*hy is it even important that my arteries have elasticity?*

Elastic arteries actually do help move blood through our systems. At the moment the heart beats, vessels near the heart expand to accommodate the increased pressure. As the increased pressure begins to move through the system, the vessel contracts behind this pressure point, helping to push the blood along. The pressure wave, incidentally, is your pulse.

If you should have a heart attack, and if your peripheral arterial system is healthy and elastic, your peripheral vascular system, made up of arteries, veins, and capillaries, may help circulate enough blood to help you lead a more normal life than you might expect with a severely damaged heart. Dr. Robert Bell, one of my advisers, states that he has "seen people whose massive heart attacks have damaged so much of their heart that one might expect they could hardly walk. And yet many of them are able to jog quite well. A relatively healthy peripheral vascular system and good leg muscles probably provide these people with enough assistance to their circulation to allow them to lead nearly normal lives." Research in this area is ongoing, but the results so far make me want to keep my arteries happy and flexible.

Flexible arteries also are less susceptible to wall damage. Remember that blood pumps through your body with constantly changing pressures. Inflexible arteries can rupture easily.

Where do strokes fit in all this? And exactly what is one?

A "stroke" is a general term indicating acutely decreased blood flow to the brain. There are several types:

Aneurysms are weak spots in blood vessels in the brain which burst.

A Thrombosis is a stationary clot which eventually grows large enough to block a blood vessel. Thromboses occur anywhere in your vessel system, but in the brain they often lead to a stroke.

A Cerebral Embolus is a clot which blocks an artery supplying blood to the brain. Emboli often originate as thrombi in other parts of the body (heart and coronary arteries) and migrate to the brain.

Strokes are associated with high blood pressure, high cholesterol levels, and hereditary factors. Many of these risk factors can be managed so the risk of stroke is greatly reduced.[13]

If I cut down on my fats, how quickly will my blood change?

Tests generally measure the two major blood fats, triglycerides and cholesterol. Triglyceride levels in the blood change rapidly, within hours. That's why you are asked to fast for twelve hours before having a blood sample drawn.

Overall cholesterol levels take longer, but most research says modify your diet correctly and expect changes within three to eight weeks.[14]

Are you telling me to quit eating steak? Rare roast beef with that wonderful layer of fat around it? A nice tenderloin smothered in mushrooms and onions?

You probably need to be aware of the foods you eat and modify your eating habits, but that does not require giving up all the things you love. First, be conscious of the problem foods. Because satu-rated fats are found in all animal products, when you eat meat, eat lean cuts. Eat more chicken, very low in fat *if you skin the chicken*. Eat lots of fish, lowest in fat, and that fat seems to be very good for you.

Carbohydrates are found in fruits, vegetables, grains, and cereals. Eat lots of carbohydrates before you fill up on meats. A smart eating habit is to consider carbohydrates as your main course and meat as a side dish. Believe it or not, that isn't a hard habit to acquire, either.

Norma *says I'm a "Type A" personality. I nearly punched her, 'cause I'm not. It just drives me crazy if everthing isn't perfect every second. What the hell's she talking about, and don't be slow with the answer.*

In 1974, Doctors Friedman and Rosenman introduced a concept of heart disease risk as it relates to behavior patterns. Their book *Type A Behavior and Your Heart* separated people into two categories: the "Type A" person who possesses "free-floating hostility" is al-ways on edge, is always ruled by time, and the "Type B" person who isn't ruffled by the lack of perfection or punctuality. Since then, other research seems to back up their theories pretty much. "Type A" people do seem to suffer more heart attacks; tension and stress do elevate blood pressure and cause changes in the blood hormone and lipid levels.[15] While some scientists argue that the separation of all behavior patterns into two distinct categories is an oversimplification, all agree your emotional profile directly af-fects your health.

So *what do I do if I'm an "A"? I already have my secretary remind me every day at 12:10 to relax.*

Very few of us are going to change our emotional compositions any time soon, but we can learn to modify our emotional reactions to things. Exercise definitely can help smooth out your ruffles and give you real thinking time. Simple intake changes can help, too. Less coffee or booze directly affects the depth of your reactions. Though it sounds corny, positive thinking can help, too. Did you know many studies show that simply deciding a particular thing isn't going to bother you, isn't worth anger or frustration, can actually lower your blood pressure?[16] (More on that later.) Because "Type A's" are essentially very competitive in the way they attack problems or opportunities, you might want to pick a sport which requires you to function without competition with others for a while.

*W*ill *anyone respectable give me their absolute guarantee that all these changes in eating and exercise and all that stuff will make me live longer?*

Healthy living can produce a longer, more productive life. Studies have recently been completed which followed people who were able to lower cholesterol levels significantly and to modify their smoking and other health habits. People in these groups had a much lower death rate from coronary heart disease.[17]

Other things point to that conclusion, too. Diseased parts of your body, whatever the part, don't function like healthy ones. Partially functioning organs such as your heart or liver or lungs obviously place more stress on you than fully functioning ones. Genetics obviously plays a big role in each individual's normal life span—but, regardless of your particular genetic life span, your health habits can lengthen or shorten the number of days you have to live.

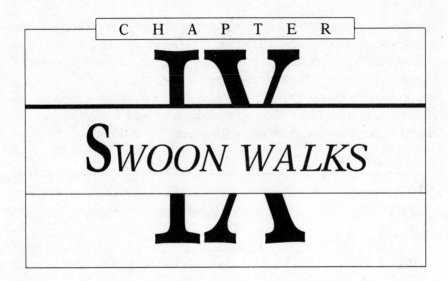

CHAPTER

IX

SWOON WALKS

Week 15
Grand Bahama Island

When I look at the pictures of me taken just a few days ago, I am reminded of the first time I painted something on my own, my brother George's new bike. I painted it red, including the chrome. I was eight and not the best painter, and the finished product didn't seem to impress others (Brother cried and Father spanked), but, to me, it seemed beautiful.

The most obvious change is the fat change. In just under four months, thirty-three pounds of fat have retreated, taking with them nine inches of waist. I say "retreated" because fat cells don't go away. They collapse like a balloon and wait for their next opportunity to attack. Fat cells are hungry, ambitious, strong, impatient, and very, very proud. They don't like retreating and jump at the first opportunity to attack again, gaining more territory with less effort the next time around, too, one of the reasons many people lose weight then gain it back quickly while still eating less. This may not be a scientific explanation, but it's just as accurate and a lot more understandable.

My exercise program obviously brought some change, too. In four months, I have weight-lifted 800,000 pounds, biked 500 miles, run 40 hours, and scuba-dived at least twenty times. I ache thinking about it. But, to my horror, my actual muscle growth in weight is virtually nothing. My total lean tissues (organs and muscle) weighed 141 pounds in January and 141.5 pounds two weeks ago. Since organs don't really change weight, that paltry .5 pound was my total muscle gain.

I didn't sleep well the night I found out that simple statistic. My hopes for this year—encouraged by a lot of weight-training experts' predictions—included at least fifteen pounds of new muscle, I assumed with requisite blonds attached. But at .5 pound per three and a half months, my total gains for the year would be less than 2 pounds. A wimpish-sounding gain.

I went back and looked at my notes from a meeting with Robert Stauffer. Bob is Director of Research at West Point's Physical Education Department, and a member of the faculty of the American College of Sports Medicine. He's also a member of the Board of Visitors at the United States Sports Academy, where we meet from time to time. Bob isn't an official member of my Body Worry Committee, but he is a friend. He is also one of the few people who, from the beginning of my year, tried to realistically quantify the changes that might take place in my body. He never felt my muscles would be enormous in a year. But he did feel I would look dramatically different.

"Remar," he had said, "if you want to have a good appearance and if you want to have that Soloflex look I keep hearing about all the time, you don't necessarily want to have high bulk. What you want is good, sound definition."

Back in January, I hadn't been satisfied with that answer. "But will I have a bicep? Will I ever have real muscles?"

"You can do that. How much you develop will depend on frequency, endurance, and intensity."

I pressed further. "Well, assuming I am motivated, can I have a dramatic change in the shape of my body? And I'm not just talking about losing blubber, either."

"Absolutely. Basically, from cellular physiology, every cell in your body will change. Good-looking bodies don't have to be bulky bodies. The Soloflex look isn't a bulky look." I re-read those comments and decided to call Bob at home that night. After just enough small talk to make it sound like I wasn't worried about a thing, I brought up the thing that was worrying me. "Bob, you know back at the Sports Academy when we were talking about my body shape? That Soloflex look I think I mentioned to you?"

"You mean that Soloflex look you mentioned about ten times?"

"Uh-huh."

"Well, I've decided that I do want that look rather than the bulky look I was kind of toying with."

"Oh, is that right? What brought that on?"

"Just common sense, you know. But there was one thing I was wondering. If I ever do want that bulkier look, can I actually achieve it?"

"Well, maybe. It's just going to take you a lot longer. Didn't I say that around Christmas?"

"Maybe, but I'm forgetful, you know. How much is 'longer'?" I said rather quickly.

"Remar, are you growing slowly or something?"

I was really ashamed to tell him how little muscle had appeared, but I did anyway. He snorted.

"*Remar*. That's an *excellent* growth. Especially considering all that weight you've lost. You're not going to be a Schwarzenegger, but you're not going to be a worm, either. Remember: *definition makes the Soloflex look*, not big muscles."

We chatted on for a few minutes, but my mind fixed on those words. I repeated them to myself silently, like a mantra.

I was feeling better the next morning. Even looking in the mirror was kind of nice. My body did look pretty good, and I decided my frame would look much better with that lean, well-defined look than it would with Arnold's hulking look. Hunkdom meant lean. I rushed through an oatmeal breakfast, looked at my latest pictures once more, and decided this day was going to be just right for a swoon walk, after all.

Swoon walks are simple. I put on the smallest bathing suit my nerves can stand, don a large-brimmed hat, then stroll the mile of beach stretching from the end of my street to the jetty. The hat, angled jauntily above the eyes, allows me to stealthily observe the dozens of ladies along the strand without being noticed. Any look from the gallery accompanied by a smile or any expression approaching come-hitherness counts as a swoon.

Four months ago, I didn't have too much luck out there on the beach. My swoon walk put the lie to the idea that women like minds over bodies. I had enough body for several, but the only female who acknowledged me was about four, thought I was her daddy, realized her mistake, kicked sand in my direction, then ran away. Two months ago, things weren't much better. A mean, stevedorish woman eyed me for a few seconds, then went back to her book on karate. It's real hard being rejected for a book on breaking bricks, especially since the lady herself pretty much resembled one.

My third attempt needed to be more successful, particularly since the "Today" show wanted to film it. Bob Berkowitz, "Today's" men's correspondent, smiled at me each time he mentioned that possibility. Bob is a rather debonair and handsome fellow. He had already laughed long and hard at my expense earlier in the day when, with the cameras rolling, I had fallen from my bike in the most inelegant way. The cameraman had laughed, too, but not enough to prevent the show from using the footage, I feared. Lying entangled with the pedals, I had thought for a moment of using reverse psychology on the guys ("Boy, any good producer would *die* for that footage!") but dropped the idea when I remembered that briar patches were invented by the Fourth Estate. Redemption would have to come on the swoon walk.

And to the surprise of Bob Berkowitz and the crew, it did, in triplicate, in the form of the Smith sisters of New Jersey and their mother. Attractive, perceptive, obviously appreciative of a well-turned swoon walk and the man behind it, the Smith sisters and their mother "ravished me with their eyes," as someone in a juicy pulp story might characterize the feeling.

Well, after so many failures and so little muscle, this was heady stuff, indeed. My hunk factor rose. And then the "Today" crew began to treat me with the deference hunks think they deserve, and it rose again.

"What did you open with, Remar?" the young soundman said, "I didn't pick it up over my earphones."

All of my life I've wanted to be an expert on openers powerful enough to conquer the most forbidding beauty. Only experts know such lines. But right then, on the beach, with the heady power of hunkdom still on my mind, I could not tell him the terribly powerful words. I only confess them here to protect my conscience and the reputation of the Smith sisters and their mother: "Hi. There's a microphone in my hat and a camera behind that palm tree. Swoon and you're on national TV." The truth works every time.

Our neighbors are big on spot reducing. They have jars of fat-burning cream to melt fat away, two vibrating machines to shake it loose, a rolling barrel to exercise it, an electrical doodad to scare the hell out of it, and three rubber suits to squash it to death and sweat it off. Their bedroom looks like a sex club. Why do they look porkish rather than petite?

Because spot reducing does not work.[1] Hubert cannot just reduce the fat on his stomach or his wife Irma the "cellulite" on her legs, or even her "love handles," which in her case should be referred to as hams. People who sell you creams, clothes, equipment, or doodads as spot reducing miracles are scam artists, all of them. Even legitimate exercises such as sit-ups don't burn fat from specific areas. Sit-ups build your stomach muscles, but the energy from them doesn't come from fat and certainly not from the fat on your stomach. It comes from carbohydrates, the fuel supply of anaerobic exercise.

As with any exercise, if you do sit-ups for at least twenty minutes, you will finally be burning fat, making the exercise aerobic. But you'll be burning fat from all over your body, not just your stomach. Do enough sit-ups to flatten your stomach, and you'll probably die of an overdose of hernias.

But Hubert says their minister, who sells those large buckets of "Descending Dove Secret Fat-Reducing Cream," knows for a fact that fat is burned first from where it was put on easiest. Is he right? Isn't that spot reducing?

He probably is right. Hubert will most likely lose weight first from where he gained it first. But that is not spot reducing.

Our neighbors are just as big on every new fad diet that comes out as they are on spot reducing. They really eat up the ones that promise they can eat what they like or take a magic supplement and still lose weight. Are any of these worthwhile?

Diets that promise you don't have to eat less, diets that make you radically restrict your food intake or restrict the types of food you can eat, and *every single* diet not associated with a sound exercise program *will not work* in the long run. *The only thing that works in the long run is a lifetime change in eating habits combined with exercise.* Diets books aren't needed for that, either; sound books on nutrition are. Please have Hubert and Irma read that again.

But they do lose weight for a while, even though they gain it back. And they have fun reading all those funny diet books. What's wrong with a little off-and-on weight loss?

Any diet, including the worthless ones, can bring temporary weight loss, but temporary weight loss is *worse for you than being overweight.* "If you stay on a very restricted diet, the metabolic rate goes down, and you burn less and less [calories], you are more likely to store fat rather than burn it because you're burning it at a lower level," says Dr. C. Wayne Callaway, director of George Washington University's Center for Clinical Nutrition.[2]

That's bad, but not the worse news. Continually gaining and losing weight can cause your body to "lay down arterial plaque at an accelerated rate," according to Dr. Gabe B. Mirkin at Georgetown University.[3] Have Norma read that statement again, too. Plaque causes atherosclerosis, probably everyone's main enemy in the fight for a good life.

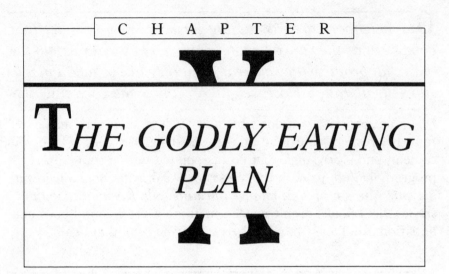

CHAPTER

X

THE GODLY EATING PLAN

Week 17

Grand Bahama Island

I have never been a good dieter. I love food, had long-standing eating habits which made health buffs choke, needed to eat to handle my nerves and anxieties, couldn't stand the tediousness of counting calories, loved fried foods especially, tired quickly of weird diets, and (most important) couldn't stand the thought of giving up forever all of the things that taste good.

To me, "health," whatever that is, and however important it is, was not worth a lifetime of deprivation simply to add an indefinite amount of time to my life for more deprivation.

I, therefore, did not look forward to the dietary aspects of my year, especially after talking with some of my friends who are very serious about their eating habits. One new friend, in her thirties, healthy, robust, and cocky in her beliefs, raised her eyebrows rather condescendingly at me when she saw me drink a cup of coffee. *"My God*, Remar, you *drink* that stuff?" I was going to ask her what she wanted me to do with it, but she answered my question in a way before I could ask it, taking my coffee cup from my hands, walking out the porch door, and dumping my good brew on the grass. She then wanted me to go to her house for a reading of Tarot cards.

"Tarot cards can help us," she said. Uh-huh. When she left, I had another cup of coffee.

Paul, in his forties, was more concerned about the foods I liked to eat. He did not approve of any commercially prepared food what-sover ("Absolutely *filled* with artificial preservatives and unpro-nounceable things that will kill you"). Paul was a vegetarian, too, and thought I should avoid anything that's been alive, including fish ("Fish are absolutely *filled* with lead. As deadly as a bullet").

I played Russian Roulette with a grouper fillet that night anyway, but got real depressed at what these people and others were con-firming to me: to be really slim and healthy, it seemed you had to like pain and probably be a little kooky in other ways, too.

I was curious about all this stuff, but, quite frankly, never thought for a minute that any weirdo or highly restrictive eating plan would work for me, even if it meant my new body wouldn't work.

So I simply started modifying my eating habits as I increased my exercise. (I said this earlier, but repeat it here because it has worked so well for me.) Here on the island, before I began to modify things, my normal food intake for a week would include fried conch (an enormous mollusk, something like lobster meat) at least twice, steak at least once, barbecue always on Tuesday nights at The Tide's Inn at UNEXSO, lobster with nearly a cup of freshly melted butter (butter is cheap here), more fried conch fritters than there are sands on our beach, a thick slice of ham bordered in delicious fat, baked chicken with the skin on it, lots of native peas and rice flavored with fatback, four slices of hot chocolate cake with vanilla ice cream on it, and rum to make it all go down good, as we say here.

I love all those foods (and rum). And there was no way I would give them all up for good, or even for a year. My modifications were therefore planned to shock me as little as possible. I only prepared fried conch twice a month rather than twice a week, and I changed the way I prepared it. Rather than coating it in beaten eggs, I coated it in a mixture of three egg whites and one egg yolk. That cut down my cholesterol from the eggs 66 percent and the difference in taste was nonexistent. I fried the conch in very, very hot vegetable oil rather than animal fat, the native favorite, and before I ate each piece, I pulled off about half the fried batter. The taste was the same, but the calories were much fewer.

I kept eating steak each week, but bought leaner cuts of meat, trimmed them more carefully, and cut my portion in half. Because I eat so many more vegetables, that half portion seems to satisfy me. On Tuesdays at the barbecue, I pull barbecued skin off the chicken and dip the skinless (and virtually fatless) meat in the sauce.

Lobster is on my menu twice each week.[1] Now I melt soft margarine for my dip (better than hard margarine and certainly better than butter), and dip the tip of the meat rather than drown it. The taste is the same. I no longer bury my bread in butter, either. A small bit of soft margarine still enchances the flavor.

I still eat ham sandwiches, too, but I buy ham with the least amount of fat possible, put on about half a thin slice rather than a whole thick one, trim off all the excess fat, use mustard and a touch of diet mayonnaise rather than a thick coating of fat-rich mayonnaise, and munch. Taste buds are funny things. They recognize the taste of the ham, and seem to be happy.

Conch fritters can't really be modified, so I just eat fewer of them. Ditto for my hot chocolate cake and ice cream. Now I have a half piece and one scoop of ice cream on the weekends, and a quarter piece of cake perhaps one other day. The taste is the same, and since I'm always full on things with better value before touching my dessert, my chocolate and ice cream emergency bells haven't set off any alarms. And my rum? I really haven't missed booze much at all.

All of this modificational thinking began to be rather pleasant. Rather than picking up a chocolate cookie without thinking, for instance, I would look at that cookie as an extra one-mile jog of calories that needed to be burned. Walking past the cookie was easier. Rather than drinking a Coke, I drank diet drinks. That 150 calories saved one and a half more miles of jogging. Rather than a sweet roll in the morning, I had a quarter sweet roll with my wheat toast or oatmeal. Four miles saved. Hell, pretty soon I was saving myself a marathon each week.

Modifying, rather than dropping, is becoming a habit now, probably the most important thing to happen to me this year, including the changes in my exercise habits. I think it can become a way of life.

Are *you really saying we don't have to give up all the foods we love to be healthy?*

If your diet is loaded with fried foods, fats, red meats, eggs, and whole milk products, you must modify your eating habits but you do not have to give up anything. Giving up things, as I've said, is virtually impossible because simply living longer just isn't worth being miserable, particularly since most of us have trouble accepting the idea that we will be vulnerable to this damage.

But *modifying* your habits will not make you miserable. In the beginning, it may. Most of us eat more than we want anyway, and breaking that habit can hurt. But try it like this: develop a plan with the kids. Buzbo and Binki, if you haven't noticed, are beginning to look an awful like you two, blimpish. Most kids' bodies mimic their parents' bodies. But Buzbo and Binki are still young enough to learn good lifetime habits now. Can you think of a better thing to teach them?

Developing a plan.   Learn to evaluate your eating habits now. Then write out the modifications to improve them. For instance, eat fried foods one time rather than five times, and always on the same day. Make your red meats the side dish and vegetables the main course. Start skinning your chickens and other fowl. With seasonings, skinned birds actually taste good, maybe even better, since the seasonings flavor the meat, not the skin. Keep skim milk in the fridge. If you hate the taste of skim, try 2 percent; it tastes almost like whole. Then work your way down to skim. Keep fruit around for snacks. Try alternating your daily eggs for breakfast with such things as hot cereals, and when you eat eggs, don't eat all the yolks. Scrambled eggs with the whites of six eggs and the yolks of three tastes nearly the same. (Or four with two, two with one.)

For your plan to work, everyone's got to participate, but try it, stick with it for a month, and soon the new plan will become the habit.

But *will this make me live longer?*

It probably will, but, more important, it will make you feel better. The right eating plan, combined with a modest exercise program, will also help prevent some things more terrible than death. Strokes, loss of limbs due to blood clots, and maybe worse, losing your mind, can all be traced to less-than-healthy eating habits and lifestyle patterns.[2]

The neighbors' preacher, the one who sold them the "Descending Dove Secret Fat-Reducing Cream," says his "Vita-Blasta-Sin" Vitamin Pack will make up for her eating habits. And they've got a year's supply under the sink. Won't that do?

Most people, probably including those two, don't need vitamin supplements. Even if you eat fast foods a lot, that's probably still true. We spend hundreds of millions on vitamins each year anyway because most of us don't have the slightest idea how to judge our vitamin needs. Vitamins are not used as food. They do not supply energy. They aren't depleted by stress. As of yet the only diseases they can cure are deficiency diseases (such as scurvy from lack of vitamin C or rickets from lack of vitamin D), and our country's major nutrition problem is overeating, not malnutrition.[3]

But all of us, including kids, are bombarded with messages implying that vitamin supplements should be part of daily living. In one interesting study of schoolchildren, all of the kids knew about the importance of vitamins, but none of them could name what foods provided them. However, they *all* named several commercial vitamin preparations without any problem.[4]

So how do you know if you need supplements or not?

Generally speaking, if you eat a variety of food types—for instance, eat a salad and fruit juice with your hamburger at Fast Eddie's Burger Barn or choose whole wheat bread for your sandwich and add a salad or vegetable and skim milk—you don't need vitamin supplements.[5] If Norma gets pregnant again (exciting thought, huh), she might need a supplement. Other specific populations may need them, too; for instance, older women and some older men may need calcium, women may need extra iron, and fad dieters consuming fewer than 1,200 calories per day probably need a once-a-day supplement.[6]

But for most of us, remember: it's hard to be vitamin-deficient and it's impossible to clear up your really bad eating habits with any pill. Magic doesn't work.

What about megadoses of vitamins to just chase away colds and diseases and the like?

Most vitamins already contain more than 100 percent of the Recommended Daily Allowances. Some, in their prescribed dosage, contain over 1000% percent. Because the fat-soluble vitamins are stored for long periods of time, you don't need to overload like this. These vitamins (A, D, E, and K) can build up in your body and literally kill you.[7] Excessive water-soluble vitamins simply run through the system, making expensive urine. In spite of various claims for various vitamins by various enthusiasts, there is little to support the claim that megadoses of vitamins ward off illness or hasten its cure.[8]

Well, I've got all those vitamins, anyway, so I'm going to take them. Will it hurt me?

Taken at the proper dosage, no. And the "Vitamins Are Good for You" Foundation, holding their annual meeting in Tahiti, asks me to thank you for taking them.

If the family actually starts exercising and all that jazz, don't we need red meat just to get our protein?

What your body needs is "complete" protein, one that contains all the necessary amino acids. (Amino acids are what proteins and a lot of your body are composed of.) Complete proteins are found in fish, chicken, dairy products, eggs, and red meats. Fish and chicken provide you the protein without as much fat. Low-fat dairy products and eggs are also good sources of protein, but remember that egg yolks are high in cholesterol. To compare, a four-ounce T-bone steak (about half to a third of the size most folks eat) has 30 grams fat and 80 mg cholesterol, one cup of whole milk has 9 grams fat, 34 mg cholesterol; one cup skim milk, a trace of fat, 5 mg cholesterol; one egg, 6 grams fat, 250 mg cholesterol.[9]

Y*ou say this, the people who want to sell you "health" products say the opposite. How does anyone know what to believe?*

You don't need to be a health expert to judge most claims in the health field. These tips, adapted from American Medical Association guidelines, can help you sort out claims about diets, products, machines, and doodads.

• *Is "proof" offered in the form of testimonials or newspaper reports?* Testimonials are not based on statistical evidence, the only accurate evidence, and mean absolutely nothing. Testimonials sound great, but don't ever buy a product based on them. Do you really think a movie star can make a better judgment than you? Think some individual, probably the seller's mother, is scientific proof? Testimonals are often used when real proof is nonexistent. Quoting newspaper reports as proof is just as meaningless. Stories are easy to place. (Since when did you believe everything you read in the papers, anyway?)

• *Do the sellers attack recognized medical authorities? Simply renounce scientifically accepted theories as wrong without saying why? Do they claim the establishment is "holding back" their wonderful discovery or product? Claim their discovery or product is a "secret" from the past or from some lost civilization?* Attacking medical authorities is the oldest ploy. People who use it are trying to establish their own credibility by destroying that of others. These are usually the same people who claim "persecution" from the establishment and simply denounce scientifically accepted information as wrong. Claiming that the establishment is trying to "prevent" a true breakthrough product or treatment is not only old, it's cynical as hell in the way it preys on our normal paranoia of big business and government. Breakthroughs, when they really happen, are welcomed by the scientific and business community because they bring fame and great wealth to many people.

"Secrets of lost civilizations" and other "secret" claims are nearly funny enough to accept, anyway, but don't. These things may do harm.

• *Do they promise "quick" cures or results, fast and easy results?* Clichés are sometimes so nice, and here the cliché "If it sounds too good to be true . . . " fits. If it does, it isn't.

• **Do they use scare tactics to encourage you to buy?** Don't buy anything or accept anything because of emotion. Rational evaluation always works best.

• **Are degrees of the pitchmen from funny-sounding places?** We all feel more comfortable with nice initials around the people we listen to, but don't automatically assume degrees are meaningful. Too often such degress come from unaccredited and/or mail-order schools. In other cases, the degree may be in a field totally unrelated to health or nutrition, say, nuclear physics. So check. Also, if someone claims a "doctorate," for instance, then doesn't name the institution but uses high-sounding terms such as "internationally recognized university," take this as a given: you are dealing with a person who is trying to mislead you.

• **Are they trying to sell you something?** Free enterprise is a wonderful thing, but it's based in part on the right of people to make claims for their products or services. The job of the seller is to convince you of need, whether you have a need or not. Authors like me are just as guilty here as anyone, incidentally. Your job is to evaluate before you spend money.

Can I trust my doctor to answer nutritional questions?

The whole concept of preventive medicine is new. Since proper eating is a preventive medicine itself, many doctors who've been in practice more than ten years don't have nutritional training because their medical school either didn't teach nutrition or only taught it minimally.[10] Find out like this: ask your doctor, casually, if he's been to many clinics or study groups on nutritional science. If he looks surprised at the question and says no, get your nutritional advice somewhere else, for instance from your local government health services division. Lots of good free pamphlets are available.

Some doctors' offices these days have nutritionists on staff. A phone call will help you here. All libraries have hundreds of books on the subject, but look for a book authored by a sound source. Libraries don't (and shouldn't) make judgments on the merits of a book's advice. Major hospitals always have nutritional staffs, and many of these people consult privately. The American Dietetic Association also has a professional subgroup called SCAN, whose members specialize in exercise and sport nutritional needs. The association's toll-free number (800-621-6469) can help you find the right registered dietician for your particular needs.

What's the difference between a nutritionist and a registered dietician?

Anyone can set up shop (or write a book) and call himself a nutritionist. Quacks do it all the time. But a registered dietician has formal training, has passed a national examination, and (obviously) is registered. Ignore "nutritionists." Find a registered dietician.

Our chiropractor cures our ills and keeps us eating those "natural" pills and foods he sells in his office. Do we still have to worry about nutrition and normal doctors?

There are many well-meaning and hard-working chiropractors out there, but you should use them when recommended by your regular medical doctor, and you shouldn't buy "natural" products from them any more than you would buy them from a health food store. Your money is better spent elsewhere.

Many chiropractors also spend a lot of their time learning how to keep you visiting them rather than learning about recent advances in health care. And the majority of them are not trained or equipped to diagnose disease. They are essentially trained to treat the symptom. If you really want to understand the chiropractor's philosophy according to respected members of the scientific and medical community, check out the book *The Health Robbers* and read the section of chiropractors.[11]

What are proteins? Why do we need them?

Proteins are substances composed entirely of amino acids. The body requires twenty different amino acids to survive. Eleven of them are produced by our bodies. Nine of them, called the "essential" amino acids, can't be produced, and have to be consumed. These nine are found in all animal products.

We need about 1 gram of protein for each 2.2 pounds of our

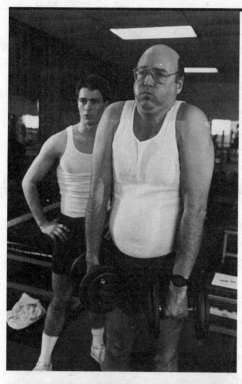

Russ observes my technique with shrugs. He was a little depressed afterwards.

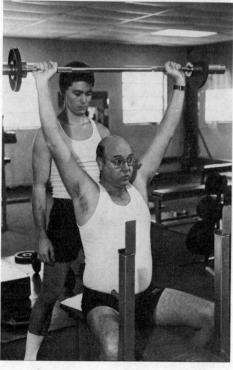

Notice the size of the weight. This is my first day in the gym, January 16. Our gym at the Grand Bahama YMCA is managed by Bill and Marilynn Carle. Both of them are hunks. Russ, my trainer, is already a hunk. I am still a chunk.

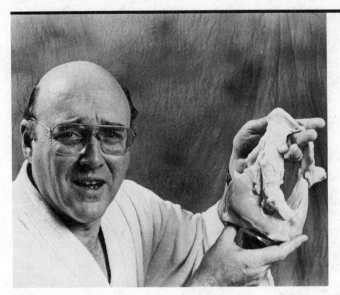

The fat from one piece of chicken. Look at this picture carefully and then read about cholesterol in Chapter 8.

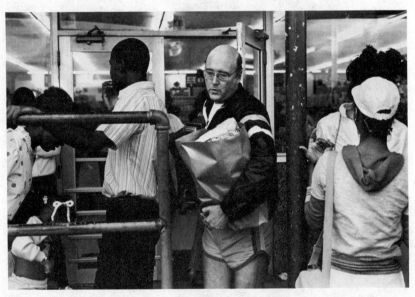

We normally bike to the store, about six miles. A gallon of skim milk is $4.25 here, a small can of tomatoes is $1.09 on sale, so it's easy to eat lightly.

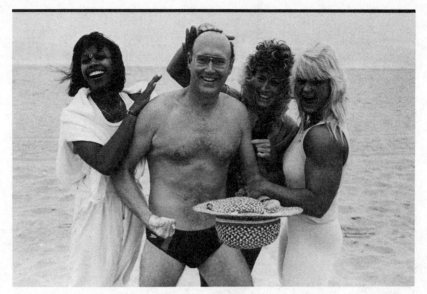

One of the first shots of the new body. Since I'm not a hunk yet, it's possible the camera had a lot to do with the interest of these maidens. I choose to deny that thought, though.

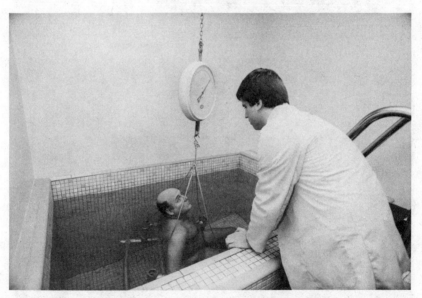

Weighing my fat at the Cooper Clinic in Dallas. Since fat floats, underwater weighing is the best way to determine percentage of body fat. I'm at the clinic for my three-month progress testing in April.

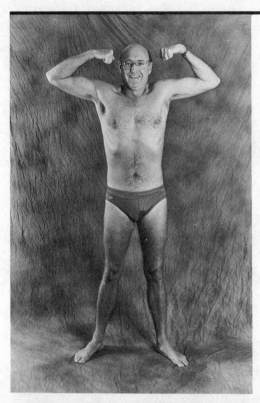

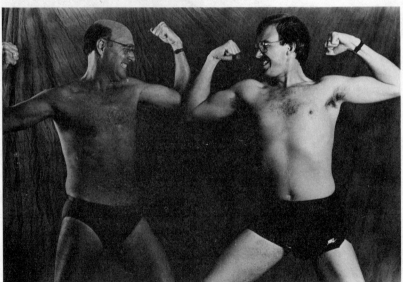

I am making progress. The guy with me is Will McIntyre, my other photographer. Will is married to Deni and thinks he's hunky.

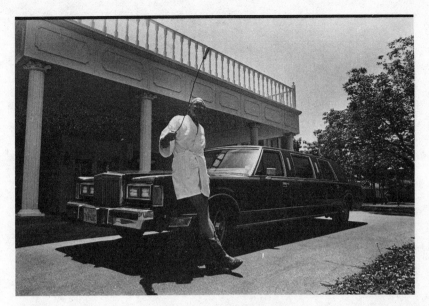

I always dress like this in Texas. The car belongs to the Cooper Clinic.

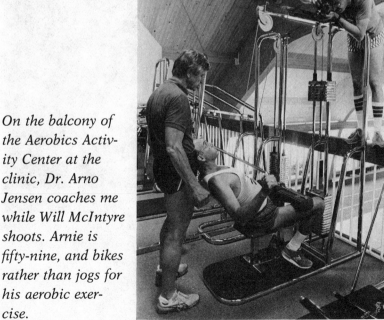

On the balcony of the Aerobics Activity Center at the clinic, Dr. Arno Jensen coaches me while Will McIntyre shoots. Arnie is fifty-nine, and bikes rather than jogs for his aerobic exercise.

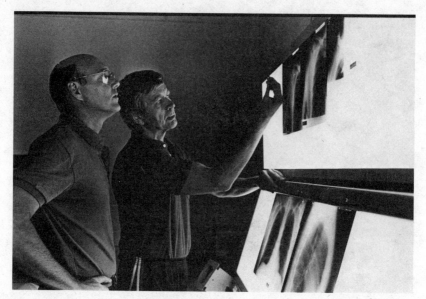

Arnie shows me pictures of my right shoulder. It remained injured for most of the year.

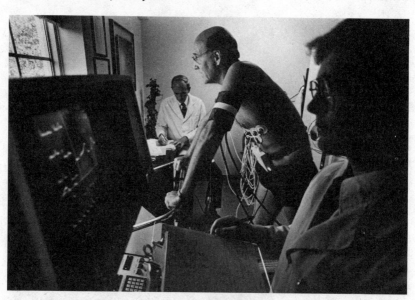

That's Ken Cooper in the background. Ken is my aerobics coach and chief tester. He coined the word "aerobics." My three-month stress treadmill test showed a 50 percent improvement, and moved me from a "fair" to "excellent" category of aerobic fitness.

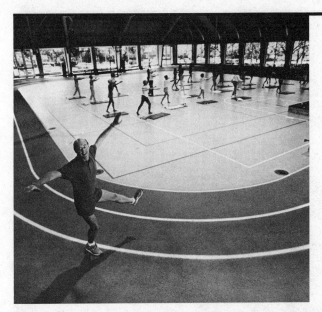

The main gym at the Activity Center. It's here that I watched the young couple playing basketball with their children.

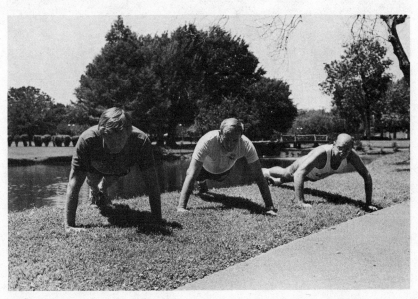

Who has the best push-up form, Arnie, Ken, or me? Push-ups, incidentally, are still one of the best strength exercises you can do.

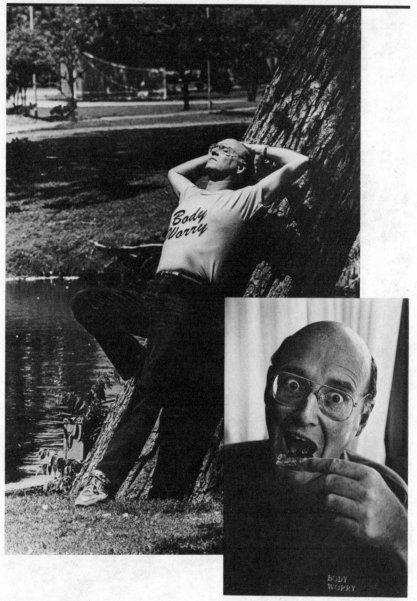

I was hoping a young maiden would stop and admire me. Instead, ducks tried to chase me from their pond. The Cooper Clinic.

Wheat toast with diet jelly tastes awfully good after barium, let me tell you.

weight, the Recommended Daily Allowance. RDAs are determined by a group of nutritionists and other scientists, and are published by the government. They're updated about every five years, and are recommendations, not requirements. Some people might need more, some less. Safety margins are built into RDAs and, generally speaking, they are more than adequate for the general population.[12] Athletes, for instance, aren't considered part of the general population. The normal American diet, you will be happy to know, includes nearly twice the RDA of protein.[13]

If you are a 180-pound office worker, a day's RDA of protein could look like this: one glass of skim milk, two slices of toast, two slices of pizza, three chicken legs, and a lettuce and tomato salad.

How do vegetarians get their protein? Is a total vegetarian lifestyle safe?

The nine essential amino acids are found in plants, but all nine aren't found in one vegetable. That's why vegetarians have to be very careful eaters, being sure to include vegetables which complement each other to provide all nine amino acids. But careful vegetarians receive all the protein they need though they need to eat a lot. For instance, a day's supply of food (1,900–2,000 calories) for a 180-pound strict veggie (no eggs or milk products) would be:

1	cup oatmeal
6	slices of whole grain bread
4	wheat crackers
3	Tbs peanut butter
5–6	cups of vegetables composed of such dishes and combinations as pinto beans with tomatoes and onions over rice, lentil soup, potatoes, carrots, tofu, and rice
½	grapefruit
1	banana
1	peach
4	Tbs raisins
2–3	tsp margarine

What are carbohydrates?

Compounds made up of carbon and water. They come in three chemical forms: monosaccharides, disaccharides, and polysaccharides. In their most basic form, carbohydrates are sugars. Simple carbohydrates (the mono and di's) include the carbohydrates in sweeteners: corn syrup, and honey, and table sugars, for instance, the things we flavor with.

Glucose, the simplest sugar in our bloodstream, is a monosaccharide. All carbohydrates are eventually broken down into it. Glucose is the primary usable form of sugar for our bodies. That's why hospitals administer it intravenously.

Disaccharides, the other "simple" carbohydrate, occur naturally in most foods such as honey, cane sugars, and maple syrup. They are composed of two monosaccharides, logically enough. Table sugar is a disaccharide.

The third form of carbohydrate is called a polysaccharide or "complex" carbohydrate. Complex carbohydrates are formed from long chains of the simple version, and are found in things like fruits and vegetables, grains and cereals.

Why are carbohydrates important?

Carbohydrates in their simplest form, glucose, are the only fuel the brain and nervous system can use. If carbohydrates aren't available, proteins must be broken down to provide glucose. Protein is a precious commodity in the body. It is the most important ingredient of cells, and is seldom used as a fuel. When it is, your body must literally cannibalize itself to feed the brain.[14]

Our mothers boiled everything. Does cooking really make a difference in the nutrient content of food?

Definitely. The nutrient value of vegetables, for instance, can vary dramatically with their method of preparation. Raw is best; steamed or microwaved (easy ways to fix things) is second best, and boiled is a distant third.

What is the nutritional value of frozen or canned vegetables compared to freshly cooked ones?

Vitamin and mineral content in virtually all frozen or canned foods is good, very close to freshly cooked ones. Frozen is equal to fresh, but if you use a canned product, you must use the water it was canned in to get all the vitamins. Unfortunately, this water probably carries sodium with it.

How important is fiber in all this?

Fiber is an indigestible carbohydrate. It's not manufacured by our bodies. It offers us no nutritional value, but adds bulk and water to the solids in our intestinal track, helping to move those things along quicker. Some researchers believe that the quicker waste products move through our systems, the less chance we have to be injured by them. Because we eat cancer-causing things at times, they reason, fiber probably cuts down on our chances of getting cancer by moving those left-over cancercausing things out of our bodies.[15] You already know some of that reasoning from the televison commercials for high-fiber cereals.

There are also indications that some types of fiber may lower cholesterol in the blood—oatmeal, beans, and apples, for instance.[16] *How* isn't known yet, but many researchers think it may be because the cholesterol binds with the fiber rather than the intestinal wall, where it enters the bloodstream.

As of this writing, there is no absolute scientific proof that high-fiber diets lower our risks of either some types of cancer or our cholesterols, but there is definitely enough epidemiological support to make it worth your while to eat enough.[17]

Is there any RDA for fiber? Do I need extra through cereals and the like?

There are no RDAs for fiber, but the Cooper Clinic recommends a minimum of 20 to 35 grams of fiber per day. Thirty-five grams would be roughly equivalent to eating two apples, two servings of vegetables (such as celery, cabbage, or carrots), two slices of multigrain bread, and two other starches such as potatoes or rice. Eating extra fiber in a high-fiber cereal probably won't hurt you and it may help you to obtain dietary fiber more easily.

Does *everyone's body react to salt in a negative way?*

Probably some of the U.S. population is salt-sensitive.[18] The remainder don't appear to be. But, by age sixty-five, 75 percent of us (salt-sensitive or not) end up with high blood pressure.[19] Researchers don't know if that very high percentage is due to the cumulative effects of salt or not, but assume that may be the case. It's probably worth your while, therefore, to be moderate with your salt intake even if you're not sensitive.

How *do I know if I'm salt-sensitive?*

The only definitive way is a test which requires several days in a hospital and constant attention. It will probably cost you over $1500. Doctors have a simpler solution, especially since we all may be salt-sensitive as we get older: they recommend that all people moderate their salt intake and that persons with high blood pressure or a history of it in their family cut down dramatically on their use of salt.[20]

What *type of foods contain salt?*

Sodium (the water retaining element in salt) appears naturally in foods such as eggs, meats, milk, and vegetables. Sodium content is lower when it's found naturally like this. A cup of milk has only 120 milligrams, an egg around 61 milligrams. Three ounces of any meat cooked without salt, 60 to 75 milligrams.

Sodium, unfortunately, is much, much higher in prepared foods. A can of tuna has about 800 milligrams, a McDonald's Big Mac around 1,000 milligrams. Sodium content isn't easy to know at times, and certainly isn't easy to find on labels of packaged foods at times, either, because manufacturers use its more specific names like sodium bicarbonate, monosodium glutamate (MSG, so popular in Oriental cooking), and disodium phosphate. If you are watching for salt in prepared foods, look for any word, however long, with the word "sodium" attached to it.

Is there an RDA for sodium?

The RDA is between 1,100 and 3,300 milligrams per day. Most salt-restricted diets call for under 2,000 milligrams per day, so even salt-restricted diets allow you salt, incidentally. But remember, a teaspoon of salt has 2,300 milligrams.

I am afraid to ask, but what is the general consensus on the effects of caffeine? And what is it, anyway?

It is a drug that acts as a stimulant to the body. In some people it can be an irritant to the digestive system, and some studies seem to indicate that it may be linked to birth defects and cancer of the pancreas. Some studies also show an increased incidence of non-cancerous breast disease in women.[21] All those indications are for very high dosages of caffeine, over 600 milligrams per day. One cup of regular coffee contains from 100 to 200 milligrams of caffeine, a cup of decaffeinated coffee, about 3 milligrams. Sodas have from none to 65 grams. Since as little as 300 milligrams per day has been linked to elevated total cholesterol, Dr. Cooper recommends no more than 200 per day.

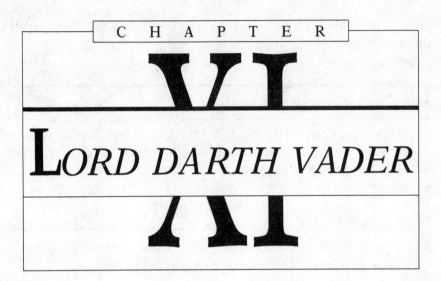

CHAPTER

VI

LORD DARTH VADER

Week 20

<u>*London, Marshalsea Road*</u>

When I was very young and innocent, Superman and his comic books provided me many moments of fanciful safety from real and imagined bullies. At night, after a hard day of feeling picked on or of simply feeling very insecure, I could crawl in those flimsy pages and find more pleasant realities. I could fly in there.

Much later I became a lighthearted fan of Lord Darth Vader, my type of monster because he wasn't really that bad. Even when Vader did away with someone, you couldn't help but like him just a little bit. At least he didn't use bad language or torture people physically. Children understood this. They never felt terror when they saw him, but their skin probably tingled when he swept into a room, the very essence of storybook evil.

My own skin tingled from such memories and thoughts this morning when I first met David Prowse, the man who both played Darth Vader in the three *Star Wars* movies and weight-trained four-time Superman Christopher Reeve. David is my new hunk coach. I flew to London yesterday, after a couple of months of planning, and will spend the next ten days here learning the routines that

112

supposedly make mortals into god types. I think he knows those secrets, too.

David Prowse is the type of person, larger than life in the flesh, we all yearn for when a dark and forbidding alley looms in front of us. He is as manly and rugged as you would expect for one who mingles with mythical characters. His voice, a deep rumble even when he speaks conversationally, fits his frame. He is six-foot-seven, 266 pounds, all muscle. His chest measures 52 inches, the height of many ten-year-olds. He can dead lift nearly 700 pounds. His jaw juts mightily and his brow furrows deeply over thick, expressive, Groucho Marx eyebrows. David does not shake hands, he envelops them, smothers them gingerly so as not to crush them. When I first felt that sensation, I remembered a scene from another mythic classic, when Kong gently sheltered the damsel in his palm.

At fifty, David is very well known in the U.K. in his own right: former British Heavyweight Lifting Champion, an author (*Fitness Is Fun*), an actor in some memorable productions (the bodyguard in *A Clockwork Orange* and the executioner in the BBC's production of *The Balcony*), and an actor in some less weighty productions, too (Frankenstein in *The Revenge of Frankenstein* and Baron Grunwald de Grunt in *Up the Chastity Belt*, a popular spoof movie).

However, David is most recognized in Great Britain as the Green Cross Code Man, a government-sponsored Superman-type character in green tights who appears constantly on British television and in person at hundreds of British grammar schools teaching roadside safety to school children. He travels to these speaking engagements at times in a yellow '69 Camaro with VADERMOBILE emblazoned on the side and a droid just like R2D2 riding shotgun. The droid is green and talks about road safety.

Prowse is a happy man in that car and in the role of Green Cross Code Man, a hero to hundreds of thousands of British schoolchildren and their parents. The children love him because he is as large and strong as children imagine heroes should be, but still very gentle (they run to him without the least hesitation) and not the least bit condescending. Parents thank God for him because, in a country where most children walk to school along roads without sidewalks or traffic lights, his presence as the Green Cross Code Man has helped lower roadside accidents involving children by nearly 50 percent.

We first met in the office of his London gym on Marshalsea Road, not far from the London Bridge. The gym occupies the first three floors of a terrace house. The narrow building looks modest from the outside, and the gym itself is low-key—lots of pine paneling like my gym in the islands, exposed pipes, and different types of free-weight equipment, which looks as if it was picked up here and there (it was).

The basement houses the "heavy" room, all knotty pine and blue carpet, where serious lifters and competitors work out. This room is really the picture gallery. David with *Star Wars* characters, weight lifting characters, and British sports figures; David talking in New York with a group of ladies who watched him film three episodes of "The Edge of Night." Standing behind him in that picture is a then unknown actor named Tom Selleck. There are ninety dumbbells in the heavy room, including a set of eighty-year-old lead-filled dumbbells, and dozens of other free weights and machines.

Upstairs is the "light" room. Sixty by thirty, the walls here are pine, too. Three windows make the room bright and six square columns support the ceiling. Eight mirrors are positioned around the walls. David says this room is for beginners and those who want to work light.

The gym office is equally old shoe. Two Vader statues, one dime-store bought, the other a porcelain mask, sit on a small filing cabinet behind a large Naugahyde chair. Both items are obscured by a toaster oven and electric tea kettle. Piles of folders and books cover a small sofa, several shelves, another filing cabinet, and most of the floor. The wall to the left of the chair is nearly wallpapered with a black-and-white picture of David in medieval costume, javelin in hand, astride a horse. Baron Grunwald de Grunt. On the wall to the left is a charcoal nude of David poised to throw a javelin. A discrete smudge renders the picture "PG."

All of this very low-key exotica—just being with this guy—was fascinating. But as David walked me through the building and finally settled with me in the office, I had only one thing on my mind.

"David, what can you do to my body?"

David was sitting in the large Naugahyde chair in front of the Vader statues. He eyed me very slowly.

"Would you mind taking off your clothes down to your skivvies?"

It is very hard for a person to undress in front of a nearly mythical person, but I did, self-consciously, crossing my arms in front of my chest. He took a tape measure and gauged my wrists and chest and biceps and calf muscles, and though I had been lifting weights for nearly four months, I blushed at the thought of my muscle size. I needed to get my mind off this.

"David, did you measure Superman, I mean Christopher Reeve, like this? Nearly naked?"

"Oh sure."

"How big was he?"

"Very stringy." Good.

"And what about you? Were you ever a weakling?"

"Oh sure. My goal used to be to have fourteen-inch biceps. Mine were twelve." Good. My biceps were at least bigger than David's used to be. It didn't matter that David at that size was sixteen and recovering from four years in a hospital. In moments of great insecurity, everything is relative.

He put down the tape measure, told me to dress, and sat down. I asked the question again.

"Well, what can you do to my body?"

I told you his voice is deep, but it sounded even deeper and nearly spiritual this time. "Remar, I will personally guarantee that by the end of the year you will have a physique you'll have never dreamed of."

I blushed. And then I quickly rumbled through my gym bag and pulled out my tape recorder, shoving it toward him in a quick, jerky motion, as if speed would catch the echo of the words and make them reality.

"Would you mind saying that again?"

David Prowse wrapped his hands, the hands that held *the* light saber and helped sculpt the slender body of Christopher Reeve, around the recorder. He pulled it to him and repeated the promise.

When I replayed the tape afterward in my hotel room, the sound was a little muffled. Those big hands were a bit over the mike, accidentally, I'm sure, but that's okay. Everybody knows heroes don't lie.

Two days later, I lay on the floor of the gym's "light" room, legs painfully suspended in the air, in pursuit of the promised end. David was trying to take my mind off the pain by overloading it with juicy gossip about the *Star Wars* movies.

"What d'ya mean, 'Darth Vader wore white suspenders'?"

From my position on the floor, between grunts, I could see out the three tall windows on the western wall and focused my eyes on the SCAFFOLDING BY SGB signs hung in several places. The whole building is covered in scaffolding. "But no one uses it," David says.

"Been there for three of my sixteen years here." His feet dropped lightly to the blue carpet. Mine dropped like a bag of sand. He still hadn't told me about the suspenders. David answers things when he wants to.

"Delightful!"

We rested a minute before starting the third of five sets of stomach exercises. Five sets each of twenty leg lifts, twenty sit-ups, and one hundred scissors, all done without resting and all done s-l-o-w-l-y. A total of seven hundred repetitions—if I lived through them. David wanted me to do this every morning. As a warm-up to our regular stomach work. Oh Lord.

I stalled for time between sets by asking again about the suspenders. "Did you really wear braces?"

David's eyebrows went up, far up. I've never seen eyebrows that could talk like his. "I did. Had to hold my blooming pants up. The blooming things kept trying to fall down."

Darth Vader shuffling around with his pants around his knees. I liked the image.

"But why white?"

"They didn't show. And they were store-bought. Most things were custom, though."

"Like what?"

"Well," he said as he lifted his legs for the third stomach set, "there were fifteen pieces to the outfit. The briefs were regular. And the T-shirt was my regular extra-extra-large. It soaked up the sweat. I wore a jacket and waistcoat, custom. A jacket with no front, a front with no arms, and a breastplate, all custom-made. And the face and helmet, of course. Custom-made. I wore a codpiece, too. A boxer's codpiece." I did not ask him if the codpiece was custom-made.

"What about the mask?"

"Two pieces. The face was fitted on with straps which tied behind my head. I had a special circular piece at the top on which the helmet fitted." During all this time, David's legs had been suspended above the floor at about a forty-five-degree angle, as if they were frozen there. He looked at my legs, resting on the floor.

"Remar, shall we start? Only four hundred and twenty to go." We began set three. "The most vexing problem," he continued, "was the eyes. The camera could see my eyes in the mask, and they didn't want that. So they put dark lenses over the eyes. So I started viewing things through that triangular mouthpiece, down to the floor. And then they decided they could see through that, so they covered the inside with black gauze. I was essentially blind."

A blind Darth Vader with his pants around his knees. I liked that image even better, and desperately fixed on it as my scissor count approached twenty of one hundred in the third set. Oh Lord.

"David, did you ever want to be Darth Vader's voice, too?"

I told you about David's eyebrows. As I spoke, they recast his face to a more somber look. "I thought I *was*. In the first movie, I learned all the lines, said all the lines. I didn't know they had dubbed over my voice until a friend in California who saw the movie sent me a cable. I mean, I knew nothing about it *at all*." He stopped talking just long enough to watch my leg lifts for a second. "*Slow down, Remar*." David's emphasis on these few words left no doubt in my mind that his voice, when a little irritated, would have been just right for Darth Vader, though perhaps a little British. I promptly told him so. He nodded and continued.

"Then, do you remember in the second movie when Vader and Luke Skywalker were on the gantry and he chopped Skywalker's hand off? My dialogue had me saying, 'Come join me and we will rule the Empire together,' but when I saw the film, Vader said, 'Luke, I am your father.' I knew *nothing* about this at all; it was a huge surprise."

David Prowse is not bitter about his involvement with *Star Wars*, though he was kept in the dark about things like his voice. He is the first person to tell you the movies changed his life and made him one of the most well-known anonymous people on earth, the perfect American Express "Do You Know Me?" commercial.

Now, you may think anyone could have played the part of Darth Vader, maybe a stuntman (even though David had his own stunt-man). But, in reality, *David* is the only person on the earth who did play Darth Vader, and he did it magnificently. He deserves his adulation for those things as much as an astronaut who walks on the moon deserves awe simply for walking on the moon—because the act is so exclusive. I personally think my body designer deserved at least an Academy Award for swagger. And I'm not biased at all. There.

Well, I thought such thoughts as we finished the third set of stomach work and started the fourth set. Only 240 reps to go. Oh Lord. The thought of simply counting to 240 hurt. By now my stomach and legs felt as if they had been sliced by a light saber, though I knew those things never really existed. Darth Vader and

Luke Skywalker fought with *sticks like curtain rods*, a shocking revelation.

David, however, made even that revelation seem unimportant.
"Remar, how much exercise have you been doing?" he asked on
about count number sixty.

"Well, I bike ten miles a day, run about five, walk for miles along
the beach acknowledging the glances of beautiful women, swim a
mile or two, bike to the Underwater Explorers Society, and scuba
dive a couple of times." (I exaggerated just a little on everything,
but that seemed okay at the moment).

"Oh," he said. "And how much do you eat?"

"Only the best, healthiest foods in very sensible quantities. And
I don't snack much and stay away from large quantities and, of
course, too much steak and the like."

"Oh," he said again. "I think that's the problem."

"Huh?"

"You exercise too much. And you don't eat enough. You need to
be eating at least five times a day, lots and lots of carbohydrates
and protein. That's the only way you're going to put on muscles."

I blinked. "But won't I get fat? I mean, David, it scares me to
death to think about eating a lot and exercising less. I'm nearly
handsome now, you know." I said it half in jest and half defensively.
For months I had eaten like a monk and driven myself like a beaver
and the thought of facing flab again filled me with angst.

"Remar, you can't do that much aerobic activity and gain muscle
mass at the same time. Cut out your jogging and leave in your
biking. And do my weight lifting program. And you can eat all you
want without getting fat, if you eat the right foods, of course. You've
got to eat if you want muscles."

My grandmother had a wonderful way of describing heaven: "You
can eat everything you want, *and it will be good for you*." I thought
about that as I happily finished my fifth set of David Prowse stomach exercises. I wasn't in heaven yet, but I was getting closer. A
bigger thrill than any old *Star Wars* movie. Oh Lord.

I *don't have a coach like Prowse, and don't really want to go through all this exercise just for looks. Will exercise do anything for me that's really important? Particularly at my age?*

As we pass early adulthood, many physiological changes begin to take place in our bodies. Earlier I told you about Arno Jensen's success at literally stopping the visible signs of aging with weight lifting. But there are many things which can be altered with exercise. Here are fourteen physiological changes that have definitely been proven to benefit:[1]

Muscle size	Decreases with age, but can be increased or held steady.
Muscle strength	Decreases with age, but can be increased.
Lean body mass	Decreases with age, but can be increased.
Body fat	Increases with age, but can be decreased.
Your heart's pumping ability	Decreases with age, but can be increased.
Your heart's stroke volume	Decreases with age, but can be increased.
The elasticity of your blood vessels	Decreases with age, but can be increased.
Blood pressure	Increases with age, but can be decreased.
Oxygen consumption	Decreases with age, but can be increased.
Lung functions	Decrease with age, but can be increased.
Reflexes	Decrease with age, but can be increased.
Bone density	Decreases with age, but can be increased.
Blood fats	Increase with age, but can be decreased.
Resting energy consumption	Decreases with age, but can be increased.

Our bodies, without disease and the unnecessary complications we place on it, could probably keep us going until we are 115 to 130 years old. Though we can't control many diseases, we can control just about everything else that ages and eventually kills us. "Aging" may have as much to do with sedentary living as it does with our chronological age.[2]

What *is the best exercising diet?*

The same diet anyone should eat: high in carbohydrates, low in fat. An ideal breakdown for most people would be 55–60 percent carbohydrates, 15 percent protein, and 25–30 percent fat.

Will *extra protein help me build extra muscle?*

People who make protein supplements certainly say so, but their proof is always less than impressive. Some physiologists and nutritionists are beginning to think extra protein can speed along muscle growth, when it's combined with the right weight lifting program.[3] But Chris Scott notes, "These researchers, myself included, also believe that protein should come from an increase in your protein food, not pills or powers or liquid protein drinks. So called 'free-form' amino acids don't appear to be absorbed through the intestinal wall [where all protein-amino acids are absorbed] as readily as animal protein. Protein supplements are also extremely expensive, and may put a strain on your liver and kidneys."

Well, *does intense physical activity increase my nutritional requirements?*

When you increase your energy expenditure 40 percent, you generally need to increase your fuel intake 40 percent, if you want to maintain your weight and energy reserves. Professional athletes, for instance, obviously need more fuel than you and Norma at the moment. Manufacturers of supplements have twisted this basic principle a little, however. They like to tell you increased activity makes extra amounts of proteins and other supplements, all handily manufacturered by them, necessary. That is generally not the case. Simply increasing the amounts of food you eat (if you're eating a balanced diet) provides you with the nutrients you need.[4]

Because so many people are pushing supplements, think through the following facts and you'll see why there are probably better ways to spend your money: the RDA of protein for the average nonathlete was established at .57 gram of protein for each 2.2 pounds of body weight. To give us all a big safety margin, that figure was increased to about a gram, nearly twice the amount an average person needs. And the average person already eats twice that, nearly four times the real minimum amount. Because athletes eat so much more, their protein intake is huge.

But *what if you're dieting and exercising or weight lifting really hard? Don't you need supplements then?*

Virtually all good diets always meet your RDAs. Eat a balanced meal when you are trying to lose weight and you won't need supplements. See the how-to dietary section for help.

Our *kids eat those "chewable" vitamins like candy. Isn't that good? Isn't it better to be sure they're getting enough vitamins?*

Vitamin companies like to make you worry about the vitamin intake of your kids. They equate good parenting with a vitamin a day. But good parenting in the nutritional arena shouldn't come from a bottle, it should come from balanced meals. We'll show you how to do that later.

What *about iron-poor blood? Don't women have to worry about it more?*

Some people do have iron-poor blood, an easy thing to know with a normal blood analysis. Highly trained athletes who compete in triathlons and iron man competitions can develop anemia (the loss of red blood cells), but this anemia appears to be short-lived. Iron is important to us all, and particularly important to women. But we need to get that iron from eating right, not from supplements. Because iron toxicity is a real danger, don't take supplements without having a blood analysis evaluated by your physician.[5]

How *important is sleep to our physical health?*

It is important for the function of your central nervous system, but the lack of sleep, oddly enough, doesn't seem to cause significant damage to your organs or cause them to function less efficiently.[6]

Norma *says exercise will be good for our nesting rites. Is she right?*

Some people think high-intensity exercises like weight lifting temporarily raise the testosterone levels in men; others think less-than-maximal exercise temporarily lowers them.[7] No one knows if either of these things is true or important, but everyone knows exercise gives you more strength and energy, and many happy nests have been built on those two qualities.

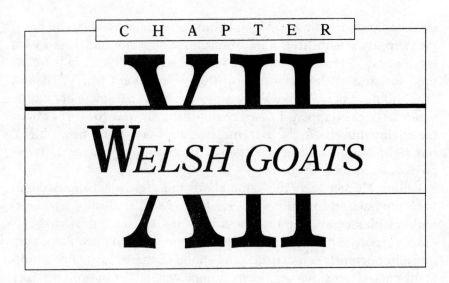

CHAPTER VII

WELSH GOATS

Week 22

<u>*London*</u>

During the past weeks I have worked out in more odd, beautiful, and ancient places in Great Britain than I knew existed—with my trainer, my friend Mary Abbott Waite, my mother, and my gym in tow. I have also come to respect Welsh goats.

The gym, a double set of blue solid-rubber Russian weights loaned to me by David Prowse, fitted neatly in the very back of our silver-blue seven passenger Volkswagen maxi-van. Luggage fitted on top of the weights. At first. As we traveled, our luggage seemed to multiply and eventually filled our siesta seat, the long bench seat just in front of our weights. We learned to nap on top of luggage.

Russell Burd, my trainer and the assistant navigator for our trip, usually sat in the captain's chair in front of the siesta seat. Mother, our trip historian, sat to his right in another captain's chair, piles of books at her feet and a leather-bound log book in her lap, pen at the ready. A red ice chest filled with fresh cherries, plums, sandwiches, and juices served as her footstool.

Mary Abbott, trip navigator, rode shotgun. M.A. is the perfect person to have along if you, like us, much prefer obscure paths to well-traveled roads. She used ordnance maps and walking maps rather than tourist maps. Mary Abbott is also the person who helps me keep my sensibilities about muscles. She is not impressed with large ones. "Remar, if you ever look like Mr. Universe, I'll throw up," she said at the beginning of this year. "Don't worry," I said, "they all have hair." I like Mary Abbott a lot, and think of her words when setbacks happen. I don't really think she has to worry about me having muscles in the extreme. I would *like* to have the problem, but right now would be satisfied with as many muscles as those guys have in their eyebrows.

I think Mother feels the same about muscles in extremus. Mom is seventy-six and proud of it. Her hair is still naturally jet-black, and her glasses are the thickness required to compensate for cataract surgery. She has a steel hip, leukemia, a heart problem, and, more importantly, an attitude that none of these things are significant enough to slow her down. I once coaxed Mom onto a frisky pony when I was about ten, talked her into a hike miles longer than she wanted when I was about twelve, and thought it normal when she and my father let me roam around Europe at age sixteen.

None of this seemed special then. Even when my father bought my twelve-year-old brother and me (at eleven) an old truck to drive around our property, that didn't seem unusual. Now, when I am the age my parents were then, these things and my parents seem pretty unique. A fact I never got to tell my father and have had trouble showing my mother. But true hunks eventually deal with things like that. This trip was, therefore, both a thank-you and a chance for our longest visit in some time, and I did not want my twice-daily workout requirements to interfere with more interesting things like talking and history and beauty and shopping. Early mornings and late nights became my muscle time.

In Salisbury, Russ and I worked out at 5:45 A.M. in the Winston Churchill Room of the Red Lion Inn, a hostelry since the thirteenth century. Winston, in oils, larger-than-life, glances rather demurely across that large, vaulted room at an equally large portrait of the late proprietor of sixty years, a Mrs. Thomas. Mrs. Thomas seems to glance back equally demurely. Some people might construe a liaison from these two glances, but I know better. According to a plaque in the Thomas Suite, Mrs. Thomas "neither smoked nor drank" during her sixty-year tenure as an innkeeper. Winston wouldn't have put up with that.

At Ruthin Castle in northeast Wales, we worked out before an enormous fire in a room built in 1210. The logs were nearly as long as I am tall, and still looked small.

In Windemere, the heart of England's mountainous, unearthly Lake Country, we worked out in a mountainside hotel's billiards room before a full-length lake-view window and an occasional couple who wandered in simply to watch us grunt. "Hear, Hear," one older lady volunteered as she tipped her sherry to us and plopped down into a red overstuffed leather sofa by the window. A retired teacher, she liked to take long walks to restore her energy, she said. The next morning at first light, in the driving rain, Russ and I jogged around Lake Windemere for twenty minutes, mists rolling around us, then retreated to a gazebo above the lake for our stomach work. We shared the space with several drier and more intelligent tame mallard ducks.

On another morning as the sun rose, we lifted weights on the actual battlements of Airth Castle near Stirling, Scotland. The portion we lifted on was over 650 years old, built by the second son of Robert the Bruce. The proprietors here have recently turned the castle stables (only 280 years old) into an elaborate health club, an oddity in Great Britain.

As you can tell, we stayed away from large hotels and cities and spent most of our evenings in imposing old castles, manor homes, or converted mills—like the Arrow Mill near Stratford-upon-Avon, which dates back to at least 1086 when it was valued at six shillings and eight pence. It is now run by the Woodham family, who between puffs and sips actually lifted a few weights with us.

In Ely, close to Cambridge, we worked out *over* the Cam River on a nearly deserted public footbridge. Four students from Cambridge, walking the bridge to reach a favorite picnic spot, stopped to chat with us as we lifted, and as they talked, sculls from their college raced by under the bridge. "Muscles! That's what you bloody need!" the picnickers, champagne in hand, yelled to their puffing colleagues.

It was all delightful, except for the Welsh goats. Mary Abbott, incidentally, says they were sheep, but sheep aren't this mean. We met the first pack in a dew-covered field near Llanwenarth House, a grand, four-guest-room, sixteenth-century manor house in Abergavenny, Wales. The goats here fraternize with Welsh ponies. As we quietly and unobtrusively attempted to enter their field, the goats gave one bleat, which promptly unleashed the ponies in our direction. We chose another field.

Several days later, we had a more serious incident. We were staying at Ardsheal House in Kentallen of Appin, Scotland. Once home of the laird of the Stewarts of Appin, this place sits on a tall cliff overlooking Ben Nevis (the tallest mountain in Great Britain), the hills of Movern, and Loch Linnhe. Russ and I were at the bottom of that cliff, minding our own business, taking in that magnificent view, doing leg lifts on our portable carpets at sunrise, when a single baby goat ambled over to watch us. Though we were in Scotland, I knew a Welsh goat when I saw it, but did not show my nervousness as it eyed us between chews of grass. Goats are like horses in that regard—clairvoyant.

The goat bleated and instantly a protector was at its side, head down, hooves testing the turf. This was a very large beast and its bleat was not a friendly one. As we rose and retreated in slow motion, it moved with us. As we began to trot, it trotted, the thick wool on its body bouncing like springs. When we broke out into a run, it bleated ominously, twice, and ran after us, the brush of wool against our backsides. Russ, young and fast, quickly outdistanced the danger and climbed up the cliff. I leaped up the cliff rocks, gasping for air, just a breath ahead of it.

Later, I dutifully reported our narrow escape to Mary Abbott and Mom. Russ's recollection was somewhat different; as a matter of fact, he even said the animal wasn't really chasing us and wasn't really a goat. "That mother sheep was sort of trotting along with us." I, however, know better. Russ may be my trainer and Mary Abbott may be my friend, but Mom agreed it sounded like a goat to her, and I listen to my mother a lot more these days.

Since Norma and I don't travel with our own gym any more these days, what can we do to help stay fit on the road?

First, think a little more about your eating. Most of us don't think we have much control over our meals when we're not at home, a nice way to eat things like fried grease balls without guilt. But thinking about what you eat and drink away from home is especially important. Many commercial establishments, including the fancy ones, drown food in fats, butters, salts, and God knows what. Here are some tips that will improve your chances of eating a healthier meal.

• If you must have a fried-food fix, pull most of the crust or batter from the food before eating it, and eat smaller quantities. Just a taste of crust will add flavor to the food.

• Eat broiled, baked, and roasted things and season with pepper rather than salt. If you have a blood pressure problem, ask that your food be prepared without salt, and take along your own bottle of salt substitute or one of the other good no-salt seasonings. Years ago, a man who brought out his own bottle at a table would be laughed at by other diners, but now, the feat has a certain *cachet* attached to it.

• If you're in a restaurant that cooks to order, tell your waiter you would like your dishes prepared without butters and sauces. Request soft margarine as the flavorer. Soft margarine is better for you than either butter or hard margarine.

• If you're ordering eggs, ask that half the yolks be removed. Most restaurants are used to requests like this these days. If you normally eat your eggs fried, try poached.

• Eat whole wheat breads and buns, and use soft margarines here, too, rather than butter.

• When you order soups, choose clear ones rather than cream-based ones. Cream soups generally contain more fat.

• Eat more salads and fresh vegetables, and eat them, as I said earlier, as more of a main course than a side dish. If possible, ask that your vegetables be lightly steamed rather than boiled to death. Lightly steamed vegetables tend to fill you up more, since they're crunchy and contain more nutrients than boiled or oversteamed ones.

• When dessert time comes, wait a few minutes before ordering. Give yourself a chance to feel full, since that sensation is a delayed one. When you order, eat fresh fruit or smaller portions of other desserts. Three bites of chocolate cake, if you're already full, are just as satisfying as a whole piece, and might save you 200 to 300 calories and a lot of fat, too.

A*nd how do we exercise on the road? Especially if we don't have time to find a gym?*

Even if you are not a regular exerciser, there are things you can do on the road to keep you fitter. First, ask your hotel if they have a printed jogging map. Even motels are beginning to provide these. A walk will ease those travel jitters, quell your appetite, take away travel cramps, and give you a chance to laugh at all the funny joggers.

Second, try some of these simple exercises. These work as well at the office or at home, too, and will build your strength and endurance, and tone you up if done regularly.

• Squeezing a tennis ball will build your forearm muscle and grip strength, and work out frustrations, too. Keep an old ball with you when you travel.

• Push-ups against a wall will work your chest and tricep muscles. Place your feet as far from the wall as possible for more shoulder work, closer to the wall for chest and triceps. Do a set of 10–20 repetitions four times.

• Leg lifts in a straight chair will build abdominal and hip flexor strength. Sit up straight, grip the chair, extend your legs straight in front of you, and bring your knees to your chest. Straighten them. Do a set of 10–20 repetitions four times.

• For flexibility and toning, place a towel behind your back; use it as if you were drying. Keep the towel as taut as possible, using your own body to create resistance.

If you travel alone on the road, boredom and loneliness can affect you as much as anything. Don't sit in your room or, worse, at a bar. Ask the front desk for the location of the closest gym, and go for a steam bath or sauna even if you don't want to work out. Go bowling. Even go to a play or a show. Keep moving, be active, and think before you eat.

Y*our mother sounds like an active person for any age. But Norma's mother hasn't moved from her special Norman Rockwell rocking chair, except to get her copy of* Soap Opera News, *in ten years. Isn't it too late for her to start exercising now?*

The most dramatic changes in strength and energy and aerobic fitness take place in sedentary older people. According to Dr. Herbert deVries, a noted authority on exercise and aging, a sedentary person's "maximal aerobic power can be improved; the ability of the lungs to function as a bellows improves; the ability of the blood to transport oxygen improves."

But how much can an older person improve? Enough to make life better?

Dr. deVries says that sedentary people over seventy who exercise properly may have a *25–30 percent increase in their aerobic power* within eight to ten weeks!

But how much exercise?

Again, I quote the authority. "Evidence is growing rapidly that we can achieve close to optimal aerobic performance just with walking." The key here, Dr. deVries says, is a program and progress tailored to the capacity of the individual. Before they begin an exercise program, it is especially important that older people undergo testing to determine precisely what they can and cannot do safely. Dr. deVries, incidentally, is a very fit man. His main exercise is surfing ("when the surf's up," he says—just like Troy Donahue) or walking "up and down a hill with my dog Amigo for a couple of hours. Or I run three miles." Dr. deVries is seventy.

Getting really old should not mean a life of inactivity. For most people, it should be the time to get in their best shape. "You may have the body of a seventy-year-old," deVries says, "but you may be able to function like a person twenty or thirty years younger." His book *Fitness After Fifty* is an excellent guide for people over fifty.[1]

What about kids? Do we really need to worry about their activity level?

Out society breeds inactivity, and inactivity is a terribly dangerous habit, especially for kids. And children pick up inactivity cues at a very early age. An awareness of active living is probably the greatest gift you can give your children next to love, so be active with them from the moment they're born. We'll give you some specific programs in the exercise section.

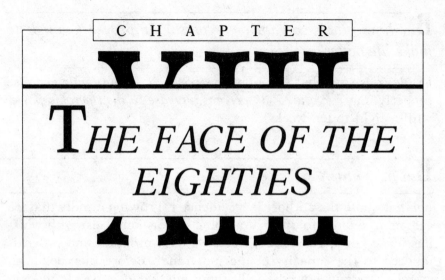

CHAPTER

XIII

THE FACE OF THE EIGHTIES

Week 26
<u>Grand Bahama Island</u>
I returned from England with a back problem, a reinjured shoulder, and a telephone message from the "Donahue" show.

My shoulder continues to react poorly to the amount and intensity of stress our workouts inflict on it. When I first tore my right rotator cuff muscle (one of the three muscles which hold the ball and socket of the shoulder joint in place), that tear healed and scar tissue, zipper-shaped, formed. Scar tissue is abrasive, and as I continued to work out, especially movements which required me to raise my arms over my head, scar tissue rubbed against bone, causing more swelling which eventually affected my shoulder tendons.

If you play baseball or racket sports much, you may be familiar with the pain. It runs along the top of the shoulder when you raise your arm. You cure it by stopping the movements which make it hurt, and the more severe the pain, the longer the rest. If you continue to injure it, you can lose movement in your arm and eventually need surgery.

I'm giving you all these details because injuries are beginning to jeopardize my year. The shoulder injury has nearly stopped my upper-body work for the time being. We have not been able to find a way to work around it, to work muscles from different angles of attack. My back injury is much more painful and has stopped all our gym work. I hurt it on my last day in England, during my last workout with David Prowse. David is such an enthusiastic person about my quest for muscles (and I want so desperately to perform for people who see muscles on me) that I insisted on trying a far heavier dead lift than I have ever attempted, 150 pounds.

A dead lift, as you may remember, is really a leg movement when it's done right. You squat down, grasp the bar, keep your arms and back absolutely straight, and stand up. Because your arms are simply holding the bar, the pressure is on your legs. Do it right, and your legs and your back get stronger eventually. Do it wrong— either try to use your arms to lift the weight, or try to shift the weight away from a hurting shoulder, for instance—and you get hurt. I did both things, bending my arms slightly in the excitement of the moment, then quickly trying to shift the pressure away from my bad shoulder. The pain from the torn muscles in my back was instant and vicious.

Though my back gives me the most discomfort, it will heal faster than my shoulder, within three to four weeks, if I leave it alone. We don't know what will happen with my right shoulder yet. If I have to, I'll just build up my left arm and become a one-sided hunk.

I got to check out the current accuracy of my hunk factor recently on "Donahue." Donahue's staff is all women, it seems, and all bright. They wanted to do a show on the Face of the Eighties, "and we think you would be *perfect* for the show," Marlaine Selip said cheerily when she called.

The Face of the Eighties. Well, that sounded pretty good to me. The phrase wasn't quite as strong as "hunk," but if Phil Donahue himself said it, I could put it on my business cards, like a title.

"Who else are you going to have on?" I asked, masking my excitement.

"The editor of *Gentlemen's Quarterly*. We even want him to dress you in a tuxedo from Saks, if that's okay . . ."

The Face of the Eighties strolling out in a custom tuxedo to the applause of a largely female studio audience and an enormous television audience, all thinking, "If Phil says he's good-looking, he is." As Marlaine spoke and as I imagined my reception, I was talking on the phone right next to my word processor, leaning slightly over the keys. Probably the only reason I didn't drool.

Marlaine then mentioned that the show would borrow me an

expensive human hairpiece to wear just for the end of the show, if I didn't mind trying it on for the audience. The Face of the Eighties asking his fans to vote for his best face, so to speak. Rather than simply saying yes, I let my mind wander out loud. "Yeah, maybe I could ask for thumbs-up for bald and thumbs-down for hair, you know what I mean?" I always wanted to be a director.

Well, after all of this, I arrived several nights later in New York with great hope and confidence. The next morning Lilian Smith from the "Donahue" show picked me up in a car for my toupee fitting. Lilian is pretty, bright, and perceptive. ("You look pretty hunky to me," she said when I asked her my standard opening question, "How 'm I looking today?")

We then headed to Saks Fifth Avenue, and it was there my dream began to fall apart a little. Some of the most handsome, manly men I had ever seen (my age and half my age), literally off the covers of magazines, were already trying on tuxedos in the changing room set aside for "Donahue." I casually asked Lilian who these people were.

"Oh, that's Rich Popejoy, the winner of *Gentlemen's Quarterly*'s The Face of the Eighties contest, and that's Kevin Luke, runner-up, and over there is David Belafonte, Harry's son. They're on the show with you." Lilian mentioned some other names, but I didn't hear her. For a moment I tried to convince myself these guys wouldn't detract from my own hour of glory. Maybe they were going to be my honor guard or something. I (casually, of course) asked Lilian their function.

"Oh, they open the show. And close it. And Rich Popejoy, The Face of the Eighties, is on the panel with you along with the plastic surgeon and the man who had his face lifted and the lady who gives facials and the two men we picked from yesterday's audience to redo, and Bob Beauchamp from *Gentlemen's Quarterly*, of course."

A person could get trampled to death in that group. I forced a smile and made small talk while my tuxedo was fitted. I then introduced myself to Beauchamp, an important and busy man in men's fashion who still had time to walk me through the men's department at Saks for fifteen minutes until he found the right tie and shirt for my blazer. I even laughed a little as I said good-bye to my competition and the rest of the "Donahue" crew. My smile wasn't very cocky, though. I walked back to the hotel feeling subdued and slightly plump.

The next morning at the studio my spirits picked back up a lot.

If you have any ham in you, and I do, a live television appearance in front of hundreds of laughing and clapping people is a thrill. I, of course, tried to look cool. But when the audience seemed to appreciate my physical progress (Donahue showed them "before" and "after" pictures) and then laughed at my request for a brain transplant with the Face of the Eighties, and then clapped even harder when a person in the audience said they admired my determination, I grinned an awful lot.

And at the very end of the show, after the other guys had made their final entrance, marching one at a time up and down the very short runway, Phil Donahue brought me back out. Most of the audience hadn't noticed my momentary absence from the stage, but they all noticed the mop on my head when I returned. I marched up and down the runway just like the pros (I had watched them from offstage, quickly practicing their gait) and, for good measure, even struck a weightlifter's pose in my new hair and tux. I didn't feel the least bit plump. When I asked the audience for their opinion on my borrowed mop and the verdict was for bald, I felt quite muscular.

And do you know who impressed me the most in all of this? After the television cameras were off, when most personalities seem to disappear, Phil Donahue asked his audience to stay seated until he could make it back to their exit. He shook hands with all 250 of them, chatted with them. Hunkiness isn't in the dictionary yet, but that quality should be part of the definition.

R*emar, you're not the only one with back pain and the rest of us don't have a public triumph to help us forget that pain. Will exercise help?*

Lots of people have back pain. Most studies say 80 percent of us suffer from it at some point in our lives. About 80 percent of those who do suffer probably do so unnecessarily, too, for their pain is related to lack of proper exercise, poor posture, obesity, or injury caused by improper movement.[1]

Most back pain is caused by muscle inadequacies. "As we become inactive, our abdominal muscles become weaker, and our hamstrings, the muscles in the back of the thighs, become tighter," says Christopher Scott, the exercise physiologist on my Body Worry

Committee. "A tight hamstring tilts the hips and causes stress on the lower back, the most common area of back pain."

If your back pain is caused by inactivity, "The Y's Way to a Healthy Back" program at many YMCAs probably can help you. The program teaches flexibility and abdominal strengthening, and you don't need to be an athlete to participate.[2]

Two exercises to help you right now, if you're too busy to visit the Y, are:

Stomach crunches. Lie on the floor on your back with your knees bent at a right angle, legs resting on a chair. Cross your hands on your chest. Do not put them behind your head, you can hurt your neck. Try to sit up at a count of one-one-thousand, two-one-thousand, etc., as you do them, but only raise off the floor six inches or so. Do three sets of ten each day.

Hamstring stretches. Many exercises stretch your hamstrings, but this one is easy and safe: lie face-up on the floor with your back flat and your knees bent. Place both hands on the back of one thigh, close to the knee, and slowly pull your leg toward your chest until you feel a slight strain on the back of your thigh. Hold it for five to ten seconds. Do this three times on each leg, daily, gradually extending the leg as you become more flexible. When you can do the exercise with your leg nearly fully extended, loop a towel behind your leg on the calf and use the towel to pull your extended leg to you. These exercises can prevent back pain as well as decrease it. As with any pain, if it won't go away, see a doctor.

N*orma likes the idea of you with hair. How did you go bald?*

Like most men: in the vast majority of cases, baldness is caused by genetics. It's called "male pattern baldness" because it can't occur except in the presence of the male hormones. Just as hormones trigger puberty, they trigger baldness, if that is your particular genetic makeup.

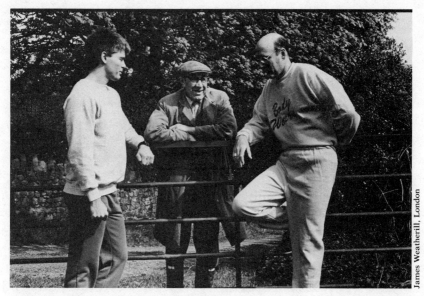

From Dallas to Govilon, near Abergavenny, Wales. Russ and I had been running, or, rather, being chased by a few of those famous Welsh goats, when Mr. Alfred Davis of Govilon stopped by to watch. Running here, even with goats after you, is exhilarating.

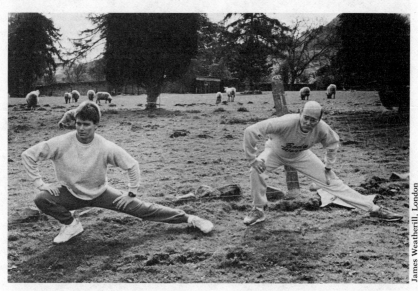

These are some of the famous goats themselves. We are staying at Llanwenarth House in Govilon, a sixteenth-century Welsh manor house, home of Bruce and Amanda Weatherill. If you like lovely manor homes but few guests, you will love this place. But watch out for the goats.

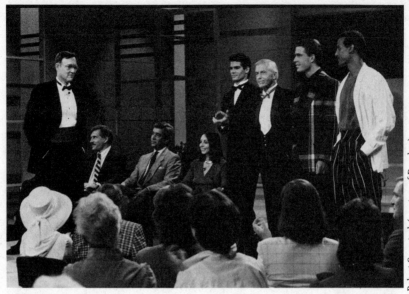

Robert Sengstack (courtesy of Donahue)

Walking the runway on the "Donahue" show. Rich Popejoy, the Face of the Eighties, is the guy with the black hair, the one clapping. Some people think we look like twins.

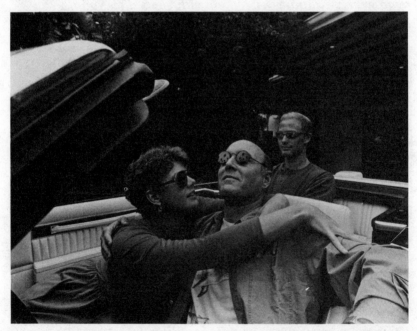

Beverly Hills did not affect me at all, but this mysterious Hollywood starlet could not keep her hands off me at the Beverly Hills Hotel. Chris is in the back seat to protect me from myself.

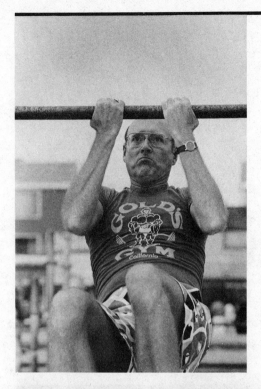

*Muscle Beach, California.
One hundred-and-one,
one hundred-and-
two. . . . I always do lots
of chin-ups before strut-
ting along with the other
hunks.*

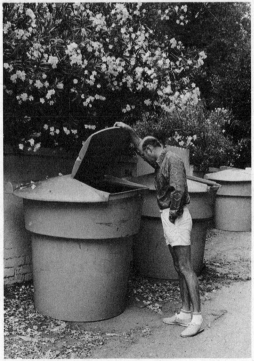

*This is a Beverly Hills
garbage can. They can
be rented for summer
homes.*

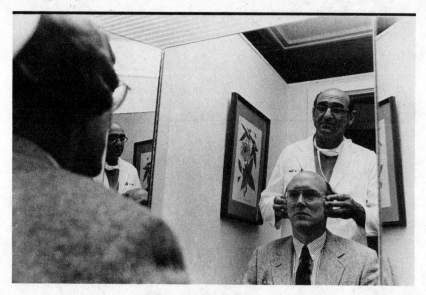

Dr. Frank M. Kamer, Beverly Hills surgeon to the stars, gives me an idea of what my new face would look like if I had a lift. An honest man, he didn't encourage any surgery at this time. I like his hairline.

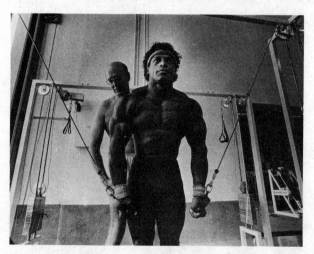

At Gold's Gym in Venice. Tony Pearson takes a lesson from me. Tony is a former Mr. Universe.

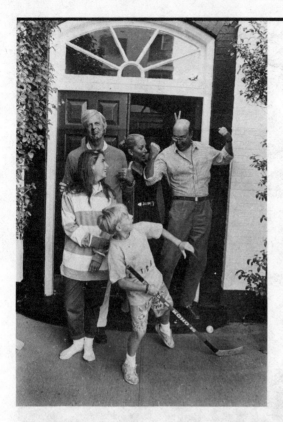

The Plimptons: George, Freddy, Medora, and Taylor. Everyone's impressed with my muscles but George. I think he's jealous. George encouraged this book, and took a particular interest in the size of my stomach.

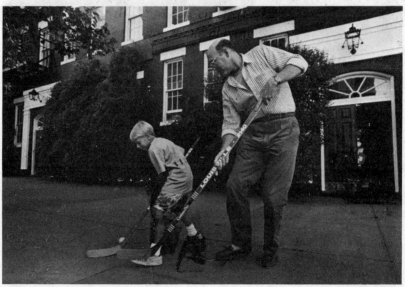

Taylor is a special friend of mine. In the islands, I take him diving. In New York, he coaches me on my hockey skills.

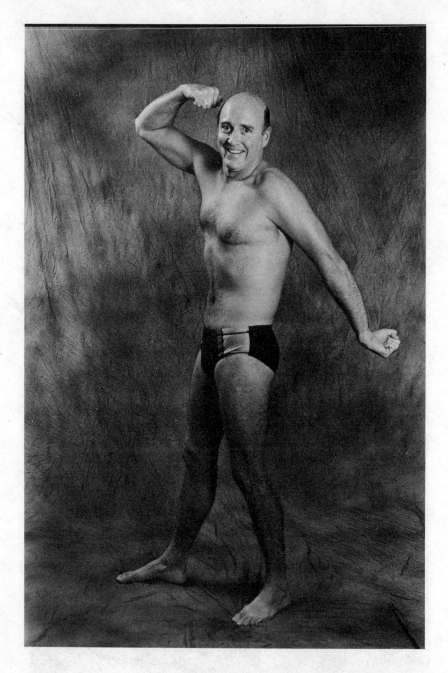

September in New York. I am still not a hunk, but small muscles lurk. I really don't have posing down yet, as the position of my left wrist indicates.

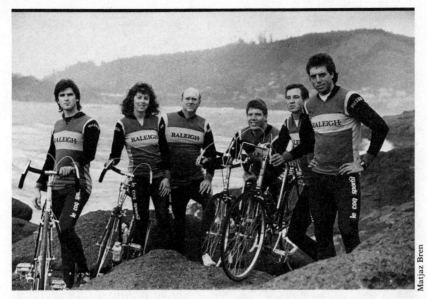

It's really hard to look happy when you've been biking over ter-
rain like this. Near the Devil's Punchbowl in Oregon, with Bret
Anderson, Anne Knabe, Martin Engel, Steve Buettner, and Dan
Buettner. I biked about forty miles of their 18,000-mile trip.

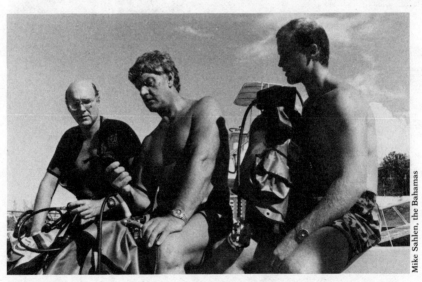

September, back on the island. I've gained weight as I've tried to
put on muscle. David Prowse, the man who played Darth Vader
and weight-trained Christopher Reeve, checks his air before a
dive. David is one of my hunk coaches, and has come to the island to check my progress since May. Christopher Scott, my exercise physiologist, watches.

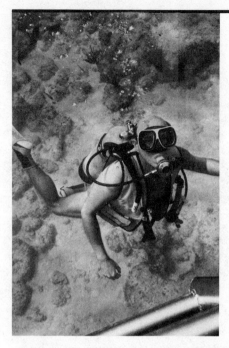

Scuba diving on the shallow reef. I tried to dive at least once each week.

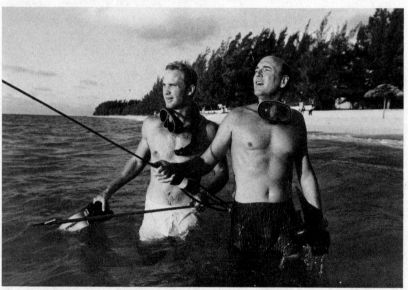

Many days at sunrise, Chris and I would head out to spear lunch. We're both pretty good shots now. And how do you like the way my body is coming along? Late October, and a lot of my extra weight is off again.

Is there any definite way to prevent it from happening?

Absolutely, without question. Castration before hair loss begins prevents baldness nearly every time. It's not recommended by the AMA, however, as a cure.

What actually produces hair?

Each hair is produced by a follicle. There are about 100,000 on the average head. An individual hair grows for about three to five years, about an inch every two or three months. After all that growing, the hair actually rests for another three months, then falls out. If your follicle is healthy, a new hair begins growing in the same place immediately.

So what happens in male pattern baldness?

Most of us would say the follicle "dies." Actually, it's still there but your particular genetic code turns it off. The man who discovers "the switch" to reactivate these retired follicles will make billions.

Does hair ever fall out from "lack of circulation"? That's what the man said who sold Norma the full-head massager.

Baldness isn't caused by lack of circulation, or lack of "follicle food," or vitamins. Healthy hair follicles transplanted into a bald spot grow very well, for example, until their programmed time to die. If you transplant hair from the back fringe which never dies to your balding hairline, for instance, those follicles will produce till you die.

Do you mean individual hairs seem to have a predetermined life span?

Yes. If you transplant a hair follicle from an area that is already balding to an even balder spot, you'll probably lose that transplanted hair, too. Hair seems to have a mind of its own when it comes to life span.

How much hair loss is normal?

The normal person will lose thirty to sixty hairs a day. At any one time, about 90 percent of your hairs are growing, and 10 percent are resting and thinking about falling out.

Can't sickness and the like cause baldness, too?

High fever, childbirth, major illness, some surgical procedures, and severe emotional distress seem to affect hair production and loss. Very low diets (under 800 calories) can affect it, too. A very, very few men suffer baldness caused by treatable medical problems; only a knowledgeable physician, usually a dermatologist, can make these diagnoses.

What about all those things to rub on the scalp and encourage growth? Aren't they real?

There is absolutely no scientific evidence to support the value of vitamin rub-ons, biotin, inositol, and virtually all other "miracle" applications. (More about the possible exception, minoxidil, in a moment.) Applying a male hormone to the scalp may help a dying follicle to recycle one last time, but it will then die.[2] A few other preparations may get those follicles which produce little one-sixteenth-inch fuzz to grow to one-fourth-inch fuzz, but this makes you look like a peach, not a man.

Doesn't washing hair too much encourage faster fallout?

No. You don't lose hair if you overwash, but you do lose friends if you underwash.

Is it worth using very expensive shampoos?

It's worth it to the manufacturers only. Washing it with virtually anything this side of acid will not speed your rate of hair loss. Some conditioners and hair sprays or even a perm can help you achieve a fuller look with what you've got, if you want to spend as much time as Norma in front of the mirror.

Are there really a lot of quacks in the hair business, or am I just being overly suspicious?

It's hard to be overly cautious with your money in the hair field. Like other quack areas, the quack remedies for baldness prey on false hope. They try to build their claims on "scientific fact," or at least scientific-sounding fact. For example, some quacks claim they have products "formulated by specialists" or, at times, doctors. Others offer testimonials (as worthless in this area as they are in weight loss) and "money-back" guarantees. There are two problems with "money-back" guarantees from quacks: the words alone make many trusting people assume the sellers must be honest, which most of them aren't, and the guarantees themselves are worthless. Most simply don't refund money. Trusting people, therefore, buy because they take advertisers at their word. They are taken because the word of quack advertisers is worthless. In the hair area, incidentally, many of the people taken aren't simpletons. Every man with a bald spot will try a funny product at least once, and most of those guys are too embarrassed to seek their money back when the spot grows rather than shrinks.

Quack remedies seem to fall into four categories. You might want to see which one you like the best:

Remedies taken orally.   Absolutely none of these over-the-counter things work at all, but they may have side effects which can jeopardize your health.

Remedies applied to the scalp.   All of these seem to be based on feeding your hair follicles. Hair follicles don't eat. Such topical products don't work.

Appliances. Things to help massage your scalp, or "wake up" your follicles. A scalp massage feels great without a special follicle enhancer, so save your money.

Clinics. All manner of places offer themselves as specialists in the treatment of hair loss. Some claim they are "doctor supervised," but most have little to do with science. Virtually all clinics recommend an extended series of expensive treatments or visits which not only won't put hair on your head but will also scalp your wallet.[3]

What about hairpieces? Are there any that really look natural?

Nothing is sadder than a man who makes a fool of himself with a hairpiece without knowing it, and so many of us do that. But there are hairpieces that make you look like the man you so richly think you deserve to be. They are expensive, however, and, since they can't rejuvenate themselves, take constant maintenance and must eventually be replaced.

What's the difference between a natural one and a funny one?

No off-the-rack pieces really look natural. The shape of an individual's head and hairline is so personal that wigs (full-head covers, essentially) and hairpieces (partial covers) need to have that hairline individually designed. The hair itself makes a difference, too. Real hair is virtually the only thing that really looks natural.

Where do I find a good designer?

You need an artist, not a mass-produced hair center. Use your Yellow Pages for the first selection. Visit each center, and then ask for clear pictures of their products installed. Look at the hairline. If all the pictures have hair dropping over the hairline, the pictures are probably covering something unrealistic.

I have a hairpiece in my closet, from my appearance on the

"Donahue" show. I planned to bring it out for special occasions, but haven't used it yet. Yes, it looks real and, yes, I feel great with it on for a while, but eventually tire of looking like something other than the genuine thing. Hairpieces are probably the best-looking, certainly the safest, and maybe the least troublesome artificial hair procedure out there. The best are virtually undetectable. But all of them still are somewhat like an actor wearing a mask, and I'm not personally comfortable with that yet. I show my vanity in my search for muscles.

What about hair weaving?

From the pictures in the paper, this looks good. The "before" and "after" pictures are a seemingly honest visual testimonal, and draw folks to hair weaving centers in droves. The reality isn't always quite that nice, however.

From the pictures and accompanying words, hair weavers seem to imply they weave artificial hair in with your remaining hair. A concept which sounds morally nicer to those of us who worry about pretending about hair. I am one of those people. And phony hairs among the real does sound a little more straightforward than totally dishonest hair.

Hair weavers don't do that at all, of course. Hair weaving is simply a method of attaching a semipermanent hairpiece to your head. In most cases, the "clinician" or "trichologist" (fancy words with absolutely no medical/scientific/training basis) makes a plait of the client's remaining hair, usually with a reinforcing string woven in. A hairpiece is then permanently secured to the plait.

There are several problems with the hair weave approach. Because the bases of these hairpieces are loosely woven, hairlines are poorer than with traditional hairpieces. Much more importantly, it's hard to clean the scalp under the hairpiece. Skin infections are fairly common. Even if you don't contract an infection, hairpieces take attention. Since the plait of natural hair which serves as your anchor grows, you have to return to your hair weaving center for adjustments regularly.[4]

Hair weaving clinics list the pluses as being able to wear their pieces at all times—in bed, shower, pool—and without fear when a damsel runs her hands through it. Nearly all the TV commericals for these things use the "damsel's hands in my hair" ploy to hook us, a smart but cruel thing, since the greatest fear of any toupee wearer is having the wig discovered at the moment of erotic potential. Even this image isn't really accurate. Since woven pieces are anchored around the sides but not at the hairline, they don't fly off, they simply rise up like the vinyl roofs of old cars moving down the highway.

Or worse. We all got a big laugh not long ago watching a scuba class in the UNEXSO pool. One poor, unsuspecting soul had no idea his perma-weave headpiece was serving as a catch basin for his exhaled breaths. At each exhalation, ole perma-weave would rise and fall like a fast-talking clam shell. So much for this man's swimming guarantee.

How about hair implants?

"Hair implants" is another term which misleads us. It is generally used by sellers who plan to anchor your hairpiece with actual sutures in the scalp.

In a hair implant, a number of suture loops (made of nylon-type material) are fixed permanently in the scalp. The hairpiece is then attached to these suture loops. The drawbacks here are the same as with weaving, but with the very big additional drawback of foreign bodies sticking through your scalp. Infections are always an eventual danger. All those openings in the scalp receive daily stress from the tugging of the hairpiece, and are perfect little doors for bacteria.[5] Add to that the difficulty of keeping the scalp under the hairpiece clean, and you begin to wonder if users of this procedure are stupid rather than vain like the rest of us.

Some practitioners attach locks of hair to an individual suture, supposedly a more natural-looking approach that's easier to keep clean. But this procedure still requires placing foreign matter through the scalp, and the scalp treats all foreign matter as an irritant. There are usually more infections here, too.

But don't these procedures require a doctor? Doesn't that mean the procedures are safe?

A doctor is required to put in the sutures. The "clinic" staff does the rest. You normally see your regular doctor when and if the infection problems begin.[6] If this procedure interests you, check with an AMA office close to you and the Better Business Bureau about the reputation of the clinic.

What about the procedures that use skin to hold a mop on?

The technique is called "tunnel grafting." Two skin loops are constructed on the front and back of your head and serve as anchors. This replaces things like plastic sutures to hold the mop, but the skin loops themselves are as vulnerable to injury as the artificial sutures themselves. Tunnel grafting also provides only two anchors for the hairpiece, which can make it shift a good bit more.

What about actual artificial hair implants?

These things are being done in Rio. Thousands of actual artificial hairs are implanted in your scalp, over 10,000 for a full head of hair. That's 10,000 potential infection spots.

But that's not the worst of it. These hairs fall out on a regular basis, and have to be surgically replaced. Since each hair costs a dollar, keeping hair like this can cost you $15,000 a year. Plus airfare and hotels and lots of doctors bills. But that's not the worst of it. Most of these hairs don't seem to like the heat too much. In the wrong conditions, they melt. Oh God.

The medical horror stories about artificial implants would make Stephen King blanch. Go to Rio for the girls, instead.

How about hair transplants? Those things really do work, don't they?

This seems to work extremely well for many patients, but picking the right surgeon is very important. Just as a number of balding men aren't good candidates for transplants, a number of doctors who practice the procedure aren't good candidates for your trust.

In the most common type of hair transplant, a small plug containing four or five follicles is punched out of the donor area (usually down low on the back of the head) and placed in a punched out place in the site to be filled in. It takes about 200–300 plugs to fill in a normal receding hairline, a two- or three-step procedure over time.[7]

Does this work if you are really bald?

If you're really bald, with only a horseshoe fringe of hair, say, you probably are not a good candidate because you have few of the right trees available to cover a lot of desert. Donor hairs must come from a relatively permanent place, usually the nape of the neck.

How do I find a good doctor? Norma's preacher says he knows one who also communes with the spirits.

Since doctors are just people, there are doctors who practice scams and/or sloppy medicine. Since poor results will always be highly visible, think before you plant. If possible, talk to people you know who've had transplants. If possible, look carefully at hairlines of these folks and make a judgment on how natural their new hair really looks. Trust your judgment on the esthetic issue; don't trust the newly planted person's judgment. We all tend to see through those rose-colored glasses when our own looks are involved.

If you can't find some transplant patients themselves to talk to, call up your regular doctor and a good local dermatologist for recommendations. Find at least two potentials, if possible. If you'd like, ask your barber for some ideas. Barbers are the priests of hair lore, so you may listen to what they've learned from any confessionals, but don't automatically take their word as correct. Some less-than-scrupulous hair doctors pay barbers for referrals.

Actually interview the doctors, if possible. Look at pictures of their work. Try to talk to some of their patients in the waiting room, or over the phone. Successful patients are nearly evangelical in their loyalty to a good doctor; victims of failed plantings are equally as vehement in their disappointment.

What is "scalp reduction"?

A doctor, using a balloon-type device inserted under the skin, stretches the scalp. He then cuts out as much of the bald spot as possible and sews the new edges together to provide as much hair cover as possible. Not everyone is a candidate for this, including me. Stretch my scalp enough to cover my bald spot and my ears would be on top of my head.

What about minoxidil?

Many are touting it, and since minoxidil is expected to receive the approval of the FDA, a blessing the Upjohn Company, its producers, are very optimistic about, millions will probably buy it. Something, at last, from other than quacks. Upjohn has applied for the name Regaine Topical Solution.

Upjohn sponsored studies at twenty-seven centers around the country. The research there was certainly objective and scientific, the good news; but the results so far haven't been that promising, the bad news. Safety is also a question you might want to think about.

Minoxidil did grow hair, usually in men just beginning to go bald (mostly men in their early twenties). Seventy-six percent of the men using the product showed hair growth. But only 40 percent of those felt their new hair growth was moderate, and only 10 percent felt it was dense. Placebos, incidentally, in some instances, were just as effective as the drug.[8]

Dr. Arthur P. Bertolino at New York University Medical Center, using a formula parallel to Regaine, found only 10 percent of the patients have a "cosmetically significant improvement." He also found the solution works best if a bald patch is no larger than four inches across and at the back rather than the front of the head.[9]

How safe is it?

Minoxidil is a very powerful blood pressure medicine, which has various side effects, including impotence, in some users taking it to treat high blood pressure. Even though the solution applied for hair growth is only 1–2 percent as strong as the blood pressure medicine itself, the solution must be applied as long as the user wants hair growth. The long-term effects of the solution can't be known yet.

Why can't I just get some minoxidil from my doctor and apply it myself? Won't that be cheaper than waiting for the real stuff?

Regaine will probably cost about a thousand dollars for a year's prescription.[10] It really isn't that expensive to make (and has been around in blood pressure form for quite some time), but Upjohn is no fool when it comes to the price balding people will pay.

Doing it yourself isn't the way to go, however. Because oral medications like minoxidil are suspended in other solutions, and since self-medication isn't easy to control strengthwise, mixing up home remedies could do you harm.

What are you going to do, Remar?

No one would like to have a real head of hair more than I would. During the year, I've looked for it a lot, but real hair just doesn't exist for most of us (yet) unless we were born with it.

If you are determined to have something close, anyway, find the simplest, easiest-to-maintain substitute. If you decide to have a transplant, virtually the only reasonably successful and safe procedure other than mops, don't expect perfection. Regardless of what you do, don't be discouraged. Lots of new surveys show that bald is becoming sexier in the eyes of women (foxy and smart women, I like to think) every day.

Norma says my teeth are yellow and cracked and crooked. And I'm afraid the gap in the front nearly reminds me of the width of her hips. Other than that, they look fine. But, what can I do with them?

A lot of interesting things are happening in people's mouths these days, and most of them are pretty good.

Bonding.   It isn't related to modern sex, but it is one of the most popular and relatively inexpensive procedures for fixing chips, discolorations, cracks, and even gaps between teeth. In the procedure plastic resins are applied directly to the surface of teeth already treated with a mild acid solution. The coatings are hardened with chemicals or ultraviolent light, and then polished.

Bonding normally costs only a third to a half as much as having teeth crowned, but there are a few disadvantages. The procedure is usually only good for five to seven years. And the bonded surfaces themselves are vulnerable to hard wear and staining. Smoking, coffee, tea, nail-biting, ice-chewing, raw carrots, and corn on the cob can all be hard on the process, for instance.

Capping/Crowning. These procedures involve grinding down teeth and then seating a crown or cap on the stub. For years, these have been the best methods for fixing broken or badly damaged teeth, and are still the most durable. The cost, of course, is higher.

Implants. These are certainly the hot thing in dentistry, but the long-term durability and effectiveness of the procedure are not known yet, regardless of what your dentist says. In implants, a titanium screw is implanted in the jawbone and allowed to heal. Then a gold-and-porcelain tooth is attached to this support.

Implants are usually done only when other procedures such as root canals are not feasible.[11] Before you rush in here, ask your dentist for the names of patients who have been sporting implants for a year or so.

Adults Wearing Braces. Orthodontics involves the movement of teeth which are fixed in bone, and it's become a popular and nearly trendy thing with many adults. The process has a few drawbacks, though, so think about them before opting for a metallic or plastic smile: adult jaws are full-grown and their bones denser than children's. Adults' bones don't respond as fast as children's bones, therefore, in terms of healing or recontouring. Because of that, adults have to have more overcrowded teeth removed and more supplemental jaw surgery than most children.[12] Both procedures cost and both can lead to the chance of infection.

Adults also have a higher incidence of gum disease even before orthodontic appliances are added to the mouth. The appliances make it harder to keep teeth free from plaque and gums healthy.

My eyes don't match. What can I do to make them look better?

Sciences advances, but not that far. Here's a rundown on the things that may help.

Eyeglasses. The greatest advance is those glasses that don't show that you are wearing bifocals and trifocals. I got my first pair four years ago and only my opthalmologist knows.

Hard Contact Lenses. These things are durable, long-lasting, easy to clean and care for, and can correct all types of vision including astigmatism. They take your eyes quite some time to adjust to, however, and have to be taken out nightly. Some people never adjust.

Soft Contacts. Your eyes usually adjust easily to them, so they can be worn quickly with little discomfort. Although they don't fit all eye problems, the newest lenses reportedly work with very near-sighted people or people with astigmatism, problems older soft contacts couldn't help. However, soft contacts must be carefully cleaned in special cleaning equipment and are fragile. Improper cleaning can result in eye infections. Soft lenses can rip or tear, and have to be replaced more frequently than hard contacts, perhaps every year.

Extended-Wear Lenses. When the FDA gave its blessing to extended-wear lenses, both the manufacturers and the customers alike began to drool. Thirty days without fooling with your vision sounded like a miracle to virtually all of us who need help to see.

The real world of extended-wear lenses hasn't been that perfect. These lenses are very, very thin, as little as .002 inch in the center, and are extremely susceptible to tearing. Most people go through several pair a year, an expensive habit.

Most doctors don't even recommend that the lenses be worn for thirty days (two weeks seems to be the limit), but wearing them even for two weeks can lead to the deposit of eye protein, clouding the lenses and causing eye irritation and at times infection.

Extended lenses also seem to be more difficult to fit for the best vision. Before choosing an eye center for these, try to talk to several people who've been dealing with the center for a year or two.

Why don't I just forget glasses and have my eyes operated on? Aren't those radial keratotomies the best thing?

Since radial keratotomy is essentially cosmetic surgery on the most precious thing you've got next to life, your eyes, please read this carefully before letting a scalpel touch them.

This surgery to correct nearsightedness (myopia) involves making eight to sixteen slashes in a pinwheel on the cornea. It remains very controversial surgery, with its proponents arguing that it is perfectly safe while many opthamologists (doctors with advanced training in eye disease and surgery) maintain a wait-and-see attitude. These opthalmologists argue that it is the long-term results that matter, not the short-term results—particularly on something as valuable as your eyes.[13]

Isn't it safe if the government lets them do it?

Surprise. The government has no regulatory authority over the testing and approval of any new surgical procedures, unlike its authority over the approval of new drugs and medical devices. Deciding whether a new surgical procedure is effective and safe enough to use is left to the surgeons who perform the operation and the various peer review processes under which they operate (hospital boards, professional societies, etc.)

Radial keratotomy, however, was so controversial that, in a rare move, the government funded a five-year study on the safety of this procedure. Called PERK (Prospective Evaluation of Radial Keratotomy), the study was conducted at nine medical centers around the country, most university-related.

A number of independent doctors already performing this surgery didn't like at all the intrusion on their business of the PERK study and the accompanying keratotomy moratorium recommended by the American Academy of Opthalmology. They claimed doctors at universities and institutions were curtailing their rights to practice medicine. They sued. As in many lawsuits, the persons conducting the study decided it was cheaper to settle than fight, agreed to pay a quarter of a million dollars in damages to the plaintiffs, and also agreed to release a statement suggesting that radial keratotomy was an acceptible treatment, based on the results of the first year of the study.[14] That statement was released to the press and, of course, the public took it as a blanket endorsement.

The results released after four years of the PERK study, however, are not very encouraging. In fact, they'll probably come as a surprise to many prospective patients who are familiar with the glowing reports in the popular press and the newspaper advertising claims of some radial keratotomy clinics. The Harvard Medical School *Health Letter* summarized the four-year results as follows: "Between one and four years after the operation, only 6 percent of the treated eyes retained the correction achieved by the operation. About 20 percent had shifted back toward nearsightedness, and over 70 percent had tended to become more farsighted. The drift away from normal vision was regarded as significant [enough to require correction with lenses] in about one-third of the patients."[15] Even though the surgical techniques have changed since these operations were done and the studies of these techniques are not finished yet, the Harvard folks feel that the message is that "good results after one year won't necessarily last a lifetime."[16] They recommend caution until the long-term results of these new techniques are in.

Remember that physicians performing this surgery can claim the procedure is safe, and they may be splendid surgeons, but if you are among those whose improved vision doesn't last or those who have problems, no lawsuit can correct your vision.

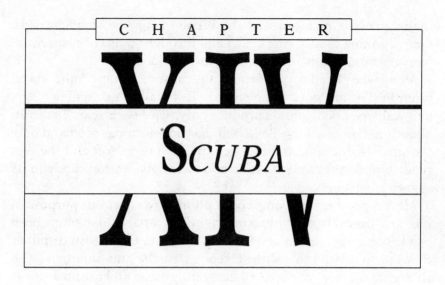

CHAPTER XIV

SCUBA

Week 29
Grand Bahama Island

On our island, the heat begins to leave about thirty minutes before sunset, taking with it the color of most things, depositing it in the clouds, it seems, which turn from threatening and dark to the colors favored by hip designers. I'm sure this happens many places, but it seems special here. This time of day is my favorite for pleasure biking.

My bike is a Royal Enfield ten-speed, bright red, with a Sears speedometer which read 897 miles this morning. That's five and one half months' riding. My pedals have toe clips with leather straps. Clips, I was told, make your legs work on the upswing, increasing your pedaling efficiency by about 30 percent. They make you look very serious, too. But toe clips grip very tightly, and at stop signs, when I needed to drop my foot to the ground to keep from falling over, my toes would stick, and I would fall, in slow motion, to the ground. My clips are now for show.

I usually ride for about forty-five minutes. Grand Bahama's infrastructure—broad, four-lane avenues and hundreds of miles of other roads and canals—was designed to support half a million people. Only 40,000 live here permanently, so the biking along most major roads is pleasant and the biking along the smaller roads, many running close to the beach and through stands of casuarinas, banyans, and palms, is dreamlike at this hour.

Along what I call my "A" route, the most handsome route, cocoa plum bushes are now being staked out by all of us regular bikers and walkers. Cocoa plums produce only twice each year. The fruit, about the size of a Ping-Pong ball, has an enormous seed and only the smallest bit of flesh, but when the flesh turns soft and the skin reddish-pink, the taste is exotic and sweet, like cotton candy in its sugary elusiveness.

All this good taste dooms cocoa plums to a short but purposeful life, and quarrels over plucking rights at a particular plum bush can become vegetarian versions of California Gold Rush disputes. Some people avoid this with stakeouts, usually grandmothers, who sit during the day near favored harvesting areas to chase away birds and people.

My method of collecting is called hit-and-run. I pick just a few plums from each bush, dropping them down my shirt, then move on before any alleged proprietor can catch me. If my strategy works, I look pregnant before the ride is over.

Much later in the season, when the easy pickings are over, we all go much farther on the unpaved real backroads of Grand Bahama, really the prettiest parts of the island, and bring out large bags of plums. Going toward the East End, the best plum areas are along the deserted beach road to Old Freetown. Bushes here are jungle-thick, the plums seem meatier, and the flesh tastes unusually sweet, especially if you're lying on your back under a palm on a isolated beach. Bikes will only get you to the beginning of this road, incidentally, for it quickly turns to very fine and deep sand. At that point, we hide our wheels in the brush and start walking or, if the tide is low and the moon right, speed along the wave-packed beach.

Whether I'm pleasure biking at twilight or on a serious plum expedition, I usually end my days at the Tide's Inn, our island's scuba-diving hangout. I start my days there lots of time, too. The Tide's is upstairs at UNEXSO and is the type of place that likes people in bathing suits and T-shirts, even at night. Chairs here are blue canvas directors' chairs, the decor fishy (including two stuffed sharks, the standard gallows humor prop at every dive spot I've seen in the world), and the food very informal. One large wall is virtually covered with the names of The Underwater Explorers Society's members. At night, videos related to diving play constantly on a wide-screen television.

At least once each week, I bike to UNEXSO about an hour before sunset, grill a couple of hamburgers with friends or eat a couple of spicy Bahamian beef patties, and then grab my diving gear for a night scuba dive.

To many people, scuba seems like an awfully exotic and dangerous sport, like I think of skydiving. In truth, it's a peaceful, easy sport, very good for nonathletes like me. It also has great brag potential with nondivers. ("Sharks? Oh sure, I see a lot of them." The diver then yawns.)

But even good shark stories don't have as much brag potential as night dives. Look at ocean water at night and it looks *solid black*. God knows what lives down there, big, grouchy, and hungry, just waiting for a juicy human. Most experienced night divers, including me, encourage those thoughts in the uninitiated, supposedly for good-natured amusement. I really think we're venting our own embarrassment at the memory of the fear we felt the first time and might still feel. After hundreds of night dives, I still wonder about the things down there just before jumping in that cool blackness. Sharks do feed at night, you know.

But in my hundreds of nights dives (note the casual brag), I've only found beauty down there. Leave your diving light off as we do most of the time, and night diving is like swimming into the early evening sky, when you can still see but stars are out. Many of the smallest undersea creatures create their own light. Simply move your hand through the water and that movement creates bioluminescence, like the sparks of sparklers coming from your hands. Look in the distance and see a small chain of lanterns floating by, salps. Turn on your light and look for sleeping fish. Some of them, like parrot fish, sleep so soundly you can actually pick them up and swim around with them under your arm.

Lobsters and crabs carouse at night. Bahamian lobsters don't have claws, but they do have long tentacles. They roam the ocean floor and coral heads freely, occasionally side by side, brushing against each other gently, using their tentacles like blind men's canes, moving with the jerkiness of a happy old couple trying to make it home after their first night on the town in years.

After about forty-five minutes of gliding around with carousing lobsters and the like, most of us, excited, return to the balcony at the Tide's. We talk loudly if any nondivers are around, soaking up their looks of admiration at our bravery, and we invariably fall prey to the lore magnification syndrome, a syndrome fisherman in particular know very well. With each repetition of a good story, things grow. If a person was lucky enough to see something unusual by himself, the thing *really* grows. I personally grew a nurse shark, about as dangerous as bad breath, from two feet to seven feet in three conversations, probably a record.

A good deal of drinking goes on during this time, especially if the dive has been blessed with at least one dramatic moment: riding a large turtle, or spotting a school of large eagle rays, for instance. I'll even have one beer myself, now. But around eleven, I wander back through the Tide's, past the backgammon games, then past the table where Fritz and Dave and Jack, my friends who live on sailboats in the harbor, are solving world problems, then out the back gate. I bike home in less than five minutes.

I usually have a juice at the house and stretch out on the softest sofa on my porch. My house isn't fancy here, but it's spread out and islandy. The porch, about twenty-seven by twelve, is really a part of the living room, since I seldom pull the glass wall shut which separates them. Large, leafy plants fill both rooms. Ceiling fans turn most of the time. From my position on the softest sofa, I can watch curly-tail lizards, the terror of tourists, scurry around my deck, just outside the porch and under a large banyan tree.

My island lifestyle, while it doesn't yet include a hammock on the beach and tropical maidens at my beck and call, would fulfill most people's island fantasy. But life here is very down-to-earth, too. Things stay in perspective. A nice definition of what "normal" should be. I've thought about that a lot in the last few days, for I soon leave for the land of the "abnormal"—Hollywood.

Are biking and diving both aerobic exercises?

Diving really isn't exercise at all. Moving under the water in a weight-free environment doesn't provide enough resistance to do you good aerobically. But it's a great activity, aside from the fact most divers wear bikinis. Biking, on the other hand, is one of the very best aerobic exercises. It's nonimpact (unless you wear toe clips and fall, like some bald people I know), can be performed as well in your home with a stationary bike, and is fun since it brings back lots of childhood memories.

You eat all that natural island food, that's why you're healthier, isn't it? Norma and I should go out and buy those "free-range" eggs and organically raised vegetables, shouldn't we?

The people who usually benefit from the "natural" phenomenon are the people who sell the products. The health food industry takes in billions each year, and with all that money comes the power to advertise and create even more false awareness of the supposed benefits of health foods.

First, there is no legal definition for most of the terms used by this industry. The sellers can therefore use virtually any terms at will. Second, "natural" businesses use down-home labels and nature scenes to imply their products are simply better because of this down-home quality. But foods raised on animal fertilizers don't have any more nutrients than ones raised on chemical fertilizers. And "natural" vitamins have exactly the same chemical composition as laboratory-produced vitamins.[1] The one real difference between "natural" products and regular products is the price: health foods cost approximately 50 percent more.

What about food preservatives? Are they all bad?

Preservatives are added to our foods for many reasons, including improvement of food quality (to fortify and enrich), maintaining freshness (which can preserve the nutritional value), and simply adding consumer appeal (such as color, flavor, or sweeteners). Preservatives at times may cause problems because they are biologically active. They go through extensive testing before being used commercially, but the pressures from manufacturers and potential users is so great that some preservatives are probably approved before they should be.[2]

Does reading labels help here?

The nutritional information on packaging can be an enormous help to you, if you get in the habit of reading labels. The habit can scare the hell out of you, though, if you really learn what some of the ingredients do. Unfortunately, manufacturers also make it hard at times even to know what the real ingredients are. For instance, they can add ingredients which are compounds themselves, but they are not required to list the ingredients in the compound. Say your quick-fix macaroni and cheese box dinner lists cheese as one of the ingredients. It need not say what went into the cheese.

At least you don't have to worry about additives and preservatives with things like fruit, right?

Oranges, bananas, even nuts have been altered with gasses, colorings, and other "enhancers." If you really don't want anything unnatural, take the coverings off. If you want to eat the coverings, wash and scrub the fruit well.

Norma says it's okay to eat lots of sugar, since the sugar manufacturers are advertising how "natural" it is. And I saw that beef is really "natural," too. Are you telling me we can't accept those nice folks' claims?

Sugar does contain "only" sixteen calories in a very level teaspoon, and it is "natural" in some sense, too, I guess. What the ads don't tell you, of course, is the fact there's no nutritional value in sugar, and that one soda contains nine teaspoons of this nutritionally useless, natural thing. The sugar isn't bad, as we noted earlier (I love it), but the calories won't help you.

The beef people are taking the same approach. Since cattle roam free and happy (from the way it looks on TV), their natural state alone must make it better for you. All beef contains saturated fat, such a close friend of coronary heart disease. When you eat beef, eat the leanest cuts possible.

Milk cows are being promoted for their naturalness, too. The "realness" of their milk is supposed to make it better for us. Unfortunately, whole milk has 4 percent fat. Stick with 2 percent or, even better, skim milk, which has all the nutritional value and virtually none of the fat.

Even honey bees are being abused. Honey does taste great as a sweetener, but its sugar has virtually the same chemical makeup as regular sugar, and it contains more calories per measure since honey takes up less space than sugar granules.

O*ur local health food store, Mega-life (Howie Makabuck, prop.) sold us some special herbal rejuvenating juice, which we can drink or put on our hair. Is all this herbal stuff okay?*

Herbal remedies are not regulated by any government agency, so no standards exist. They contain natural chemicals that can very definitely affect the body. The *Journal of the American Medical Association* warns doctors the products may be the culprit in signs of food poisoning. Herbal products are sold many times by "pyramid" or "multilevel" type companies; the sales meeting and person-to-person selling style of such companies allows many questionable claims to be made orally by salespeople while shielding the company from responsibility. The head office can claim, "Oh, we didn't authorize them to say that," though in staff or distributor sales meetings they may have done just that. Although the products are required by law to carry a label indicating that they do not replace the services of a doctor, such face-to-face selling techniques keep these outrageous claims flowing.[3]

And unfortunately, the products sell as if they did you some good. They don't, and may do you real harm.

W*ell, why doesn't the government prosecute the sellers?*

Government agencies don't have the time or money to prosecute many false claims. As William Jarvis, president of the National Council Against Health Fraud, has observed, "You've got a line of quacks 3,000 deep and taking them one at a time, some of them are going to die of old age before [the FDA] gets to their cases."[4] Further, in this particular area it is often hard to document the false claim since, as we've noted, so many claims are made orally, usually at sales meetings where potential sellers are whipped into emotional frenzies that would make Elmer Gantry smile. Truth is very seldom a part of these meetings, and the message spread there is passed on by the individual sellers to innocent (and usually older and less-educated) victims. Listen to what one reporter heard said at such a meeting, and decide for yourself how much fact and how much hyperbole is present:

> What this product does is *awesome*. This will normalize blood pressure, reduce the plasma and cholesterol level in the blood, reduce the buildup of plaque inside the arteries, stabilize blood pressure. If it's high, brings it down; if it's low, brings it up. *Incredible*. Nothing else like it in the world.[5]

Scumbags like the people who say such things make fortunes, and obviously couldn't care less who they hurt. Stay away from herbal remedies, and stay far away from the people who try to sell them to you with a smile. They are not your friends.

Now before you sling a cup of Red Zinger at me, let me say that many herb teas are indeed tasty. But beware of teas which are supposed to have "medicinal" properties and are said to treat several conditions. If overused, even such common herbs as chamomile, ginseng, or sassafras (often used in teas) are toxic.[6] You need to know what you're really drinking in an herb tea, and an herbal enthusiast is not the person to get your information from.

What are some other favorite quacktics out there?

Here are a few fun techniques and gimmicks in the world of food and/or supplement quackdom:
• Assertions that food from supermarkets is unhealthy.
• Instant, computerized nutritional evaluations where supplements are sold. Sounds like a nice idea, but remember the purpose of the evaluation is to promote the supplements.
• Claims of effortless dieting through starch blockers or fat melters. Though some of these products have been banned, similar new ones are always popping up.

If *a product quotes an article, isn't that a sign of an upright seller?*

A number of magazines will publish anything if the author buys an ad. In quackdom, articles are written constantly for public consumption, and then quoted as if they were scientific papers. A generally good rule for judging the integrity of a magazine is this: if all of the articles in a particular issue are positive about products, services, and treatments advertised in that magazine, you are probably dealing with a sleazebag publication. If the magazines also rail against conventional products, treatments, and services—and rail against established authorities—you can bet your flea powder you are dealing with people who put your dollar above your health.

We *read in* Mega-life *magazine about a really neat way to really check your nutritional needs by psychic testing and hair analysis. You mean the article might not be scientific?*

Psychic testing and hair analysis aren't the only bizarre "tests" out there. "Pulse" tests for nutritional needs are popular. Certain blood tests, which claim to spot food allergies and which go under names like "cytotoxic testing," "leukocyte antigen sensitivity testing," and "food sensitivity testing," are even more popular and in clinical trials have been found just as worthless.[7]

I *bet you don't like bee pollen, either.*

Bees are nice, and honey is nice, but promoting bee pollen as the world's "most perfect food," as some sellers do, is about like promoting wasps as friendly.

But there are worse things out there. For instance:

Spirulina.   Sold in pills or powder, spirulina is a blue-green algae that grows in brackish ponds and lakes. In its pure form, it's a source of protein with many minerals and vitamins. But quacks claim more power for it. They claim that phenylalanine, an amino acid found in it, can switch off hunger pangs in the brain. Un-huh. Some nutritionists feel that large amounts of spirulina can be dangerous, and that the excess uric acid in the product may cause kidney stones or gout.[8]

Glucomannan.   That wonderful "secret" of the Orient. This stuff comes from the konjac root, and is supposed to speed the food through your digestive tract. Ergo, eat more without gaining weight. Buy it and, ergo, you are taken again. Since the konjac root has been eaten for many years in Japan, glucomannan is marketed as a food, incidentally, though the FDA has tried to change that.[9]

HCG.   This product comes from the urine of pregnant women, and is approved by the FDA for treatment of "certain problems of the male reproductive systems and in stimulating ovulation in women who have difficulty conceiving." That's not why some diet clinics use it, though. They claim that injections of this hormone will help you lose weight. Both the FDA and the AMA say the product is useless for that purpose.[10]

Q*uack products and quack remedies must cost plenty in money and suffering. Why can't we put an end to it?*

Though we Americans are an educated people, quackery and health fraud do thrive. The practices presented in this chapter are only a few of the hundreds of scams, schemes, and false hopes sold every day. Some device sold as the "latest breakthrough" is often just a new twist on a practice which may be hundreds of years old. Quackery has always been with us and probably always will be, as long as disease and suffering exist. When our current scientific knowledge cannot help or treatment seems too slow, our instinct is to do something. As I was working on this, serendipity led me to a passage from Tolstoy's *War and Peace*, which states reasons for quackery's continued existence that are as valid today and tomorrow as when they were written in 1869. One of the young heroines has fallen ill and her concerned family brings in practitioner after practitioner and doses her with various useless nostrums in an effort to help. Tolstoy writes of these practitioners:

> Their usefulness did not consist in making the patient swallow substances for the most part harmful (the harm being scarcely perceptible as they were administered in small doses), but they were useful,

necessary, indispensable, because they satisfied a moral need of the patient and those who loved her, which is why there will always be pseudohealers, wise women, homeopaths, and allopaths. They satisfied that eternal human need for hope of relief, for sympathy, for taking action, which is felt in times of suffering. They satisfied the eternal human need that is seen in its most elementary form in children—the need to have the hurt place rubbed. A child hurts himself and at once runs to the arms of his mother or nurse to have the hurt place kissed or rubbed. He cannot believe that the strongest and wisest of his people have no remedy for his pain. And the hope of relief and the mother's expression of sympathy while she rubs the bump comforts him.[11]

Today we often cannot believe that our scientists and physicians, the "strongest and wisest of our people," have no answers. So we listen eagerly to anyone who promises hope—the charlatans, the quacks, the pseudohealers.

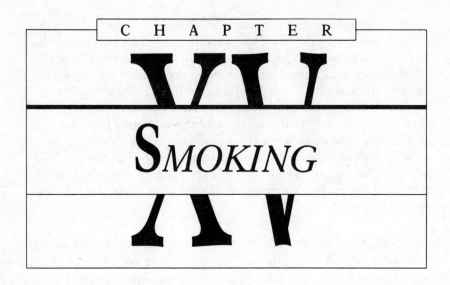

CHAPTER
XV

SMOKING

Grand Bahama Island

I was rummaging through the library at UNEXSO and found a copy of John Fowles's *The Magus*, a great book which brought back an unusual memory.

Except for a rabbit tobacco cigarette or two when I was learning about adult things at twelve (rabbit tobacco grows wild in many parts of Georgia, and we would pick, dry, and roll our own), I had never smoked a cigarette until reading *The Magus* in August 1971. Thirty and balding, I was visiting friends in Bermuda—islands held a special attraction for me even then—and on the day I smoked my first real cigarette, I was sitting in a fighting chair of a forty-two-foot sport fisherman, my feet propped up, a pipe in my mouth.

I had not smoked the pipe long. A friend had given me two in New York several months earlier because she felt they made me look "distinguished," and since I just loved that thought, I had learned to hang one constantly from my lips with the most practiced casualness. The damned thing would never stay lit, though.

Anchored near a wreck several miles from shore, I had been able to keep my pipe lit as I read *The Magus*, however, and found myself puffing more than ever as the novel drew me in. A mystical, by-

160

zantine tale, *The Magus* also took place on an island, and as the plot became even more complex, my pipe tobacco ran out. Right by my feet, on the rail, was a pack of Kool menthol. I remember the pack had only two or three cigarettes in it (even a slight breeze would have blown it seaward), and I remember thinking what a stupid place the rail was to place something so light. So I picked it up, looked at the word "Kool" for a minute, and pulled out one cigarette. Until that moment, I had not smoked cigarettes because I did not want to do what all my friends seemed to be doing and also wasn't quite sure how to keep the cigarette from looking "funny" in my mouth. Some people looked very laid-back when they smoked. My image, I feared, would probably be more like Mr. Peepers sucking a straw. Until that moment I had also hated the smell of cigarette smoke. It reminded me of claustrophobic meeting rooms and miserable colds.

I put the Kool in my mouth anyway, lit it tentatively, turned my eyes back to the book, and inhaled, deeply. And saw stars. That Kool was the most powerful, and oddly wonderful, drug I'd ever taken. I tried to read, but could not for an instant. And then I began to read and puff. The few cigarettes in the pack were gone within the hour. I rummaged through the galley and found a full pack.

That night, when we returned to shore, I bought my own. Benson and Hedges menthol. And through that pack and the next, I pretty much smoked for the instant high the cigarettes gave me, savoring each puff for another charge.

At first, the rush was the only reason I smoked. A nice, legal drug trip. Then the immediate pleasure seemed to diminish, and something for a while as nice replaced it: cigarettes gave me something to do when I was nervous or restless or insecure or frustrated, and at that time in my life, I was many of those things a lot. I did not think of my new friends as addictive, however, and enjoyed them fully.

I didn't think of them as too unhealthy, either; though, at times, logic made me wonder. During the early seventies, there was a lot of press about pollution in the air and its deleterious effect on health. Oil or coal power plants in particular were damned in the polution debate. It did cross my mind a few times that directly inhaling smoke from a cigarette had to be something like sticking your head in a power plant smokestack, but the thought went away. I smoked rather happily for five years.

And then I started paying attention to the press about smoking and health. The articles made me think, but I needed the habit then, and I sided more with the tobacco industry spokesmen than alarmists. I mean, could responsible businesses like tobacco companies really sell things they knew would kill? Because my smoking habit was such a short-term thing (What was five years? All the press talked about "long-term" dangers), I didn't worry too much but did start telling myself that one day I would quit. Especially on the mornings my throat tasted like the muck from a horse stall. I switched to lower-tar-and-nicotine brands.

By 1978, during regular physicals, doctors started telling me rather casually that I should quit smoking. None of them seemed to make it life-or-death, but all seemed to say if smoking was bad, it would get you with cancer. No one mentioned heart disease at that time.

But as I read more on smoking, as my cough developed, as cigarettes became a necessity even when my mouth and throat burned, my real problem with cigarettes started to bother me. In 1979, visiting my friend Jerry Preston, a nonsmoker, I for the first time got out of bed at 3 A.M. and drove around a strange town until I could find someone to sell me a fix. The next day, I deliberately ran out of cigarettes again to prove my willpower, but the cigarettes won again. I drove to a corner market, didn't open the cigarettes as I drove back (self-control), then sat on Jerry's wonderfully open and green Florida porch (the only place in the house he allowed smoking) and slowly drew in the first deep breath. It tasted so damn good, but was followed by the bitter aftertaste the mind can deposit when it loses an important battle. The damn things were stronger than my will. Self-esteem went down a little, then.

The quitting attempts started. I went to a hypnotist. She was expensive. "That's part of the therapy," she said, a really great line, as she took my money and tucked it in her cleavage. I made it about an hour and kicked myself for being such a weak-ass. I bought some of those graduated filters. Aside from the fact some people thought the filters made me look like a bald FDR, they did nothing to help me. My self-esteem notched down.

And then, while I was again visiting Jerry in Florida three years later, my mother called and asked me to fly home, a problem with my father's health. Mom isn't nervous or dependent, and the tone in her voice scared me. Dad had developed a blind spot, and simply did not want to move or talk.

We knew Dad had emphysema. His doctors had forced him to give up cigarettes for pipes twenty years before. We knew it had slowed his activities down, too. But we didn't really think he was too sick. I walked out of the house with my mother and father the next morning, pausing for a moment because he wanted to look at the yard, and drove to the hospital. By three that day we knew he was dying of a lung cancer that had spread and formed an inoperable tumor in his brain. He died in two weeks. I smoked a lot the day of his funeral.

My habit became more self-destructive then. I smoked more when I was worried the most. I smoked more when I sat down at the typewriter, and a lot of my time is spent at typewriters. The thing really won, and even on the mornings when my cough sounded an awful lot like my father's, I lit up. For me, the most destructive thing about cigarettes (I thought) was their ability to quietly take away your self-respect.

I tried dozens of times to quit. In mid-1983, a low-stress time, I actually made it three months without smoking, but never once quit thinking about cigarettes. The first puff was more sensual than an orgasm. In December 1984, my continual throat problems sent me back to a doctor for about the twentieth time in four years. This fellow had given up trying to convince me to quit smoking. But on his office wall was a recent article about the dramatic health changes even in very old people who quit smoking. I liked that. I had pretty much decided that thirteen years of smoking—how did that many years go by?—had already done its damage. But if the article was right, even people who had smoked *fifty* years could change physiologically by stopping.

Without much thought I asked the doctor for a nicotine gum prescription, and without any resolve I chewed the first piece as I drove home. Out of curiosity. The gum tasted absolutely terrible, and it burned nearly as much as smoke down a raw throat. But for the first time in years I did not smoke for two hours. I didn't want to. That scared the hell out of me, so I instantly lit up a cigarette and thought about really trying to quit one more time.

My plan was very cautious. Rather than swearing off, I'd simply go hour by hour and see what it felt like. Each time the urge came for a cigarette (and they came very frequently. I was smoking over three packs a day), I chewed and the urge went away. The first full day I chewed twenty pieces. For the rest of December I chewed nearly that many every day. But I went through the Christmas holidays without smoking once. Several members of my family smoke a lot, but I even made it through the holidays without preaching at them. I wasn't at all sure my smoking habit was ended. There is no hunger like the hunger for nicotine, and I didn't believe gum could really take that away.

And then a favorite aunt was taken to the hospital with pneumonia. Edna, seventy-one, had quit smoking five years before. Her pneumonia wasn't that bad. It only prevented her from using around 30 percent of her lungs, a loss anyone can stand with healthy lungs. But my aunt had already lost 40 percent of her useful capacity because of emphysema. And she could not live very well on the remaining 30 percent.

Edna, her eyes bulging from the strain, was gasping for air when I first saw her in the hospital. Her daughter was trying to hold her hands down, trying to prevent flailing hands from jerking out tubes. My aunt was suffocating. Down the hall, three other people were dying the same way, tubes down their throats, respirators replacing lungs, all of them smokers at one time in their lives. And during the time it took for my aunt to die, two of those people died also.

I used my gum a lot that week, too. But I also decided not to smoke again. And though I kept gum in my pocket for nearly a year, using it for about six months until my physical and emotional dependency habits left me, I haven't smoked yet.

Now, finally, two significant things have happened. *I don't miss cigarettes anymore*, even in down moments or moments of stress. The emotional addiction has left. And, more important, I feel pretty damn good for finally taking control of my life when it comes to at least one vice. Quitting smoking was really the beginning of my remake. Anyone who can do that can do anything.

N*orma quit smoking with the help of something she calls her tantric yoga research partner. She says quitting makes food taste better. Is that why she gained forty pounds?*

Smoking over long periods does dull your taste buds, and quitting does seem to bring some of them back to life. Don't forget, I started my blimp imitation after quitting. But many psychologists think emotional cravings rather than physical ones are the reason people gain weight when they quit. Whatever the cause, smart smokers have always used that as an excuse not to quit. I certainly did.

Smoking certainly couldn't be as bad for you as being overweight, right?

Wrong. Smoking is *always worse for you than being overweight, if you have a choice of the two.*[1] And you don't have to gain weight, either, if you substitute other things for that part of your life. Starting an exercise program at the time you quit, for instance, can usually control your weight problem.

Who smokes, anyway? Haven't most people quit?

According to the American Cancer Society, 33 percent of all American males over twenty are cigarette smokers; 28 percent of women smoke.[2]

What is cigarette smoke, anyway?

It is a mixture of the air around you and the various gasses, liquids, and solid particles produced or given off when tobacco burns. The solid matter is collectively called "tar." Cigarette manufacturers love to put the word "tar" in quotes, because they like to imply no such things exist, (and therefore can't hurt you) and, in part, they are right. "Tar" isn't the stuff you pave with. It's composed of thousands of compounds, including hydrocarbons, organic acids, alcohols, nicotines, and, to a lesser degree, radioactive lead and polonium. Virtually all of these things are toxic,[3] and this is where the cigarette manufacturers' cute use of quotes around the word "tar" is misleading. "Tar," as we've defined it, is a lot worse for you than the tar your foot may pick up on the beach.

The gasses in smoke include carbon monoxide, carbon dioxide, and significant amounts of cyanides, acrolein, nitrogen oxides, and ammonia.[4]

How specifically does smoke damage the lungs, if it does?

Think of your lungs as a big tree. The major airway, the trachea, is the trunk. It branches into smaller and smaller branches and twigs, the bronchi and bronchioles, and finally into leaves, small air sacs called alveoli. Much as the leaves of a tree present a surface area for carbon dioxides in the air to be absorbed, the alveoli, loaded with oxygen, present their surface area to oxygen-starved blood. As blood cells absorb the new oxygen, they cast off an equal amount of carbon dioxide, which is carried out through the branches of our lungs and expelled.

Alveoli are hard-working, rather single-minded, and very, very fragile. So fragile our bodies produce special cell linings just to protect them. One type of these special cells secretes a mucus to prevent alveoli injury or irritation. Another type cell grows fine hairlike structures called cilia. The cilia are like an efficient fly-paper-coated conveyor belt. They trap anything that lands on them, irritants and germs and the like, and move them along until they reach your mouth. When you cough sometimes, you're finishing their work.

Unfortunately, cilia cannot handle the toxins in smoke *at all*. Inhale some for just thirty seconds and your cilia become paralyzed for at least fifteen minutes. They cannot trap and repel other irritants, germs, and particularly the particles in the smoke itself. Continue to expose them to smoke, and they die. They literally fall off and are replaced with cells which cannot protect your alveoli from foreign matter.[5]

While your lung tissue is losing these defenses, it builds another defense by producing special fighter cells (alveolar macrophage) which battle the tars and also attract white blood cells to fight off the smoke attack. But the enzymes and chemicals produced by these cells to help fight off the smoke attack are not very selective in their battles. They accidentally traumatize lung tissue, weakening the alveoli and robbing the small airways of the elasticity vital to proper expansion and contraction. Ultimately, the alveoli collapse and die. As with any traumatic injury like this, your body forms scar tissue to cover the injured area. This thick tissue begins to block the tiny passages in your lung. Those portions are now dead. Your body labors to operate with less surface area for feeding your blood.[6]

At that point, you have emphysema. And it was at that point that my aunt Edna lost her chance to live. She died of one of the chronic obstructive pulmonary diseases, COPD, as the doctors refer to them: uncomplicated bronchitis, chronic bronchitis, and emphysema. Studies indicate that 80 to 90 percent of all COPD is caused by smoking.[7] COPD is also known as COLD, chronic obstructive lung disease.

I *don't like scare tactics, and I don't like alarmists, either. So what diseases does smoking definitely cause or contribute to?*

What I present here is cold fact: cigarette smoking is the most important preventable cause of disease and death in the United States.[8]

Smoking is the major cause of lung cancer. It is a major cause of coronary heart disease; diseases of the arteries (there are many); bronchitis; emphysema; cancers of the larynx, oral cavity, esophagus, pancreas, and bladder. Smoking, combined with things like alcohol, certain oral contraceptives, and other inhaled elements like asbestos, also dramatically increases the risk of certain other diseases.

Women smokers who use oral contraceptives increase their risk of heart attack approximately ten times over women who do neither. They also increase the risk of certain kinds of cerebral hemorrhage.

Smoking during pregnancy represents a major, controllable threat to the health of unborn children. Smoking during pregnancy slows the growth of the fetus, doubles the chance of low birth rate, and leads to more spontaneous abortions and fetal and infant deaths.[9]

H *as anyone actually tracked how many people die each year from illness and disease directly related to smoking?*

Yes. According to the U.S. Office on Smoking and Health, three hundred and fifty thousand Americans die *prematurely* each year from diseases directly related to smoking.[10] These deaths account for one in six of all deaths in the United States each year.[11] Smokers are ten times as likely as nonsmokers to die of lung cancer.[12] *At the same time,* smoking increases the risk of cancer of the larynx by five times, cancer of the mouth by three times, cancer of the esophagus by four times, and doubles your risk of cancer of the bladder and cancer of the pancreas. Your chances of getting emphysema as a smoker are thirteen times higher, and your chances of getting heart disease are doubled.[13]

The U.S. Surgeon General, in a report based on comprehensive study of all research in the field, says more than three-fourths of deaths from diseases of the heart and blood vessels are positively associated with cigarette smoking. These deaths represent almost half of all deaths from *all* causes.[14]

And, if all this isn't enough to make you squeamish, let me continue: smokers experience a coronary heart disease death rate 70 percent greater than nonsmokers. Heavy smokers—over two packs a day—have a 200 percent greater chance of dying. For men under fifty-four, smokers experience a coronary heart disease death rate three times that of nonsmokers of the same age.[15]

How *does smoking bring about damages other than lung damage?*

Those "tars" seem to be the major cancer-causing elements. Nicotine, an oily alkaloid in tobacco, actually affects the cardiovascular system. It literally raises your systolic blood pressure and cardiac output, increases the levels of free fatty acids (which leads to diseases of the arteries), and probably increases the stickiness of "platelets," the things that stick to your artery walls, eventually blocking them.[16]

The carbon monoxide gas in your smoke (about 4 percent) does something more interesting. Your blood has an almost suicidal love of this poisonous gas. If your body needs 200 units of oxygen, the blood will accept 1 unit of oxygen and 199 units of carbon monoxide, it it's available. Your heart, among other things, does not react well to that type of treatment.

But *isn't there a point of no return when it comes to quitting? If someone's always smoked, isn't it cruel to make him or her try to stop when the damage must already be done?*

Even if you have been a two or three pack-a-day smoker for fifty years, your body will respond dramatically to a smoke-free existence. Specifically:
• Your risk of dying from heart disease drops the day you quit smoking and in the majority of cases eventually becomes no greater than people who have never smoked.

• If your lungs haven't already been damaged, you are unlikely to have more lung-related diseases than nonsmokers. If your lungs have been damaged substantially, the damage will not increase.
• Blood circulation in the brain will probably increase.
• Even people over seventy have dramatic increases in the amount of blood and oxygen reaching the brain, which reduces their chances of stroke. Smokers over seventy who quit also reduce their chances of things like Alzheimer's disease.
• The skin doesn't age as fast.
• Ulcers heal faster.[17]

Does smoking lower-tar-and-nicotine cigarettes help at all?

Probably not. Studies indicate that smokers keep the supply of nicotine in their blood reasonably constant.[18] When they switch to lower-tar-and-nicotine cigarettes, they subconsciously take bigger puffs more often. Some people actually take in *more* tar and nicotine, because they take bigger and more puffs, and smoke extra cigarettes, to boot. Thank your cigarette manufacturers for this nice marketing ploy.

What about smoking cigars or pipes instead of cigarettes?

A recent study found that smoking four or more pipe bowls or cigars exposed the smoker to smoke equivalent to smoking ten cigarettes.[19] Research also shows that pipe and cigar smokers are at higher risk than nonsmokers for cancers of the mouth and throat.

Some other things you don't want to know:
• Nicotine is so deadly that one drop in the eye of a rabbit will kill it instantly. Keep your cigarettes away from your rabbits.
• When you smoke, changes instantly take place in heart rate, skin temperature, blood pressure, peripheral blood circulation, brain waves, and hormones affecting the central nervous system.
• Nicotine qualifies as an addictive drug, just like heroin: it affects brain waves, alters moods, and serves "as a biological reward that elicits certain behavior from both laboratory animals and human volunteers."[20]

If all this is true, how can cigarette companies stay in business without the hell being sued out of them?

First, people are starting to sue them. I wish we had a central place to send money to support more suits, too. Second, cigarette companies are defending themselves with the most cynical defense. As they continue to present cigarettes as manly, just great for the outdoorsmen, and oh, so right, they tell the court, "Smokers should know smoking will kill. Don't those fools read the warning labels?" Doesn't that legal strategy make you respect those guys?

How do you know if you already have lung damage?

A test of lung function called spirometry can measure the capacity of your lungs as well as their efficiency and flow rates. By comparing your results to a "population" of the same age, sex, height, and percentile rank on performance, physicians can tell if you have lost part of your lung function and how much. This is the test that told me I had lost some lung function. You can have one as part of most physicals these days. If your doctor can't help you here, call the respiratory therapist at your local hospital.

Will I actually feel better the minute I quit?

No. As a matter of fact, you'll probably feel awful, and if you were a heavy smoker, you'll feel really awful. Withdrawal symptoms associated with smoking can be nearly as traumatic as symptoms from heroin for some people. But the pains do go away.[21]

What works?

Many things really do work, but they're all based upon the following understandings and, most important, upon a person's real desire to quit.

1. Understand specifically what cigarette smoking does to you. Reading these pages may make you light up, for instance, which is okay. But if it doesn't also make you want to really try to break the habit, go visit any hospital's respiratory unit.

2. Be objective with yourself. How much do you really smoke a day? Mark down each cigarette, and the number itself may scare the hell out of you. Write down the number and the reason you're smoking (wake-up smoke, cup of coffee, nervous energy, etc.) and you may better understand your particular physical and psychological dependencies.

Different analysts may use different names, but all of them break down the types of smokers like this:

• Smoking for stimulation: to pick you up, keep you going, wake you up.

• Smoking for physical pastime: you like to doodle, play with pencils, like the ritual of lighting up.

• Smoking for pleasurable relaxation: because you enjoy it.

• Smoking to reduce tension: when you are angry, uncomfortable, or upset about something; when you are blue or depressed.

• Smoking to satisfy craving: having a real, openly addictive, desperate need for a cigarette when without one.

• Smoking from habit: lighting up without even being aware of it; you let the cigarette burn up in the ashtray or light another without realizing you've already got one going. You light up like clockwork.[22]

Knowing what factors influence your smoking may help you select the best methods of breaking the habit. For instance, if you have addictive cravings, quitting cold turkey is apparently more successful than trying to taper off.

What's available to help someone quit?

Whatever the method, all of these are based upon cold turkey or tapering off.

Help Groups.   There are two kinds, nonprofit and for-profit. Most have some success (remember, it's really up to you in the end), but watch out for rip-offs in the for-profit outfits. Some of these guys charge as much for one group session as a good shrink would charge for an individual visit. Some don't like to tell you how they work without signing you up first, and some put a really high-pressure sales job on you. Before choosing a group, call your local office of the American Cancer Society, the Heart Association, or the Lung Association for some recommendations.[23] Check any for-profit outfits with your Better Business Bureau and local medical association, and don't pay a lot of money in advance, though some outfits will tell you that's part of the therapy (just what my hypnotist said). Generally speaking, group support really helps a lot of people.

Hypnosis.   I've personally had a bad experience here, but some people swear by it. There's no accurate scientific data to support either case. Some reports suggest a high initial quitting for a short time before backsliding. If you are the type of person who responds well to biofeedback and other meditation-type techniques, this might work well for you.

Aversion therapy.   There are lots of these, and they all make me a little queasy. Aversion therapies supposedly make the smoker associate unpleasantness or pain or discomfort with smoking. Therapies range from electric shock therapies at clinics to self-aversion tactics such as rapid smoking to the point of nausea or sticking yourself with a pin when you want a cigarette. If you are big on things like this, I know where you can get a great catalog of whips.

Acupuncture.   Acupuncture itself works for many things, and it seems to work for some people here. Acustaple—that's right, staple—is touted by some people, too, but traditional acupuncture fans don't think much of it.

Exercise.   You can't smoke when you're exercising. Cigarettes don't taste as good when you smoke after exercising. And exercising does take people's minds off their habit. A regular, moderate exercise program can help you quit. Jog each time you want a cigarette, for instance, and you'll probably be running marathons soon.

Gadgets.   Filters and other over-the-counter toys don't seem to have an identifiable track record.

Nicotine gum. It does not work for everyone, but it does work for some. In the usual prescription, each piece of gum contains 2 mg of nicotine, about as much as in two regular cigarettes or three to four "light" cigarettes. The directions tell you to chew each piece for at least twenty minutes when you feel the urge for a cigarette.

This product is in gum form so that it can be absorbed through the linings of the mouth. Because it doesn't give the immediate "hit" to the brain smoking provides, the manufacturer claims it does not seem to create addiction since the "hit" is missing.[24]

The gum certainly seemed addictive to me, however, but it was an easier addiction to break.

People seem to have better luck with gum when it is used with a support group and counseling. In two studies, 47 percent and 30 percent of those who had taken the gum as part of a larger plan were still not smoking after one year. (Those numbers are very good, but in the same study, 20 percent of the people given placebos rather than real nicotine gum had also quit for a year.[25] Does that tell you anything?)

In that same study, only 10 percent of those people given nicotine gum independent of a support group quit for a year; 10 percent of those given a placebo quit, too.

Well, *after all this, if I quit smoking, will I have fun kicking people who still are weak?*

The most rabid evangelists seem to be reformed smokers, but please don't be like that. Smoking is probably the hardest and most important battle anyone can fight for their health—ever.

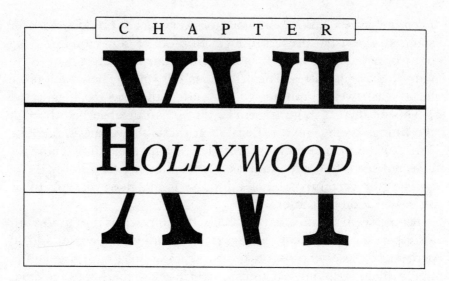

CHAPTER XVI

HOLLYWOOD

Week 36
Grand Bahama Island

I leave the island tomorrow for the month, a tour for a consumer book of mine. In between radio and TV shows (about eighty), I'll work out at a lot of different gyms, try to eat right, exercise some, and fly a lot.

My last trip off-island wasn't fast but it was weird. To Hollywood. Beverly Hills. Right by the Yoga Tantra Center and the Bowser Boutique, which share the same building, and Jaxon's Dogramat, where the dogs are really clean. This place is Garrison Keillor's Lake Wobegon gone wrong, I am afraid.

I flew to California for something I thought only happened to people in movies, to meet the folks who have bought the movie rights to my life. What they're really interested in, of course, is my search for hunkdom, but I prefer to think they actually care about some other important events, too, such as the time I won the state championship for playing solo tuba. I played "Till Eulenspiegel."

Now, I know a movie isn't an important thing, and know I probably won't recognize even myself in the finished product, if, indeed, it makes it to the silver screen or television tube (most things don't).

I also know Robert Redford, my choice for the hunkified me, may not be available for the part. I think he's going to be busy that week. But I was still excited. Though a film doesn't make you good or happy or important or even rich, it does make you immortal in some way, like a good granite monument, and it does impress all the people you grew up with, which is worth something.

Christopher Scott went to Hollywood with me. I finally stole Chris full-time from the Ariel Human Performance Center in Miami. Gideon Ariel, of course, is one of my advisers. Gideon's place, a combination gym, health club, and preventive medicine center, is very fancy and impressive.

The center's star physiologist, Chris is bright, decent, enthusiastic, and very down-to-earth. As we pulled up the long, limousine-lined driveway of the Beverly Hills Hotel, to the Hollywood community as Buckingham Palace is to Royalists, I started getting a little excited at the thought of the movie stars strolling around, the deals being made as producers "took" lunch in the Polo Lounge or "did" meetings in one of the poolside cabanas. Chris didn't sense any of this. He got out of the white convertible I had rented to make the right theatrically understated statement, walked right past Harvey Korman without a double take, and absentmindedly turned to me and said, "Remar, can I get on over to the library at UCLA? I've got to get that article on free fatty acids and plasma."

I nodded yes and walked up to the reception desk, slightly nervous but masking it well. As I said, very powerful things happen at this hotel, and normally only very powerful people stay here, and you don't just walk up and say "Hi" at the registration desk, you say something that quietly indicates you're a part of the show business power structure. I had asked a friend for tips.

"Yes, Sutton. Checking in. Any telephone calls?"

You don't say your first name and always ask for phone messages, in a low-key voice, my friend had said. For a minute, I didn't think it would work. The very distinguished-looking man behind the counter made a quick glance to check out my famous quotient, obviously failed me there, smiled a practiced smile, then signaled to an assistant with one hand as he searched for the "S" telephone messages with the other. He found nineteen messages there with my name on them.

Nineteen messages at the Beverly Hills Hotel, before you check in especially, means something. The distinguished-looking man stepped in front of the assistant he'd summoned and smiled genuinely, placing the messages before me carefully, as if rough handling would show disrespect to the callers.

"Oh *yes*, *Mr.* Sutton! Welcome back!"

I did not remind him this was my first visit, obviously did not tell him how many of those calls were plants. I simply smiled. Low-key, of course. That afternoon I bought some reflecting sunglasses.

The next morning, at about seven, Chris picked me up for an hour's aerobic work in hilly Beverly Hills. When I'm in a new city, especially one with a different terrain or climate, I try to scale back my exercise program. Lots of walking to allow for in-depth sightseeing seemed right for here, so I give you a quick sight-seer's review:

• Some of the houses are pretentious to the point of tackiness, but all of the yards are lush, beautiful, and better-tended than most people's children. I'll bet there are more gardeners in Beverly Hills than there are commercials in a year of made-for-TV movies.

• Virtually all of the gardens have lots of small but serious signs announcing the name and threat level of that particular garden's security service. Where I come from, a nice sign saying SECURITY PATROLLED is considered pretty neat, a definite status sign. Here, they don't fool around. ARMED RESPONSE is the favorite wording, ARMED GUARD ON PREMISES was the most prestigious, and I honestly became a little nervous when I absentmindedly picked a leaf from a tree next to one of those signs. We decided to jog a little after that.

• People here have a lot of garbage, as evidenced by the size of their garbage cans, about five by four feet. One of these rather handsome things, embossed with the name of the city, is provided free to each residence. Some residences have several. I wanted to lift a lid or two, see if these people's garbage actually had odor, as they say, but thought it best not to tempt those signs again.

There must be many moral lessons in all of these things, but, because I hope to visit Beverly Hills again (a reporter's curiosity, you understand) I would appreciate it if you would draw your own conclusions.

After our walk, I did a hundred leg lifts and a hundred stomach crunches in my room, then quickly showered and slowly dressed for my big meeting. I had to look just right. The "Today" show had decided to film it. Will and Deni McIntyre (you see their pictures all the time in *People*) had decided to shoot it. And the first part of the meeting was to take place in the Polo Lounge itself, the sanctum sanctorum of Hollywood dreams. After about six changes of clothes, I decided on a look of studied insouciance, that look so prevalent in men's fashion magazines. My pants were wrinkled. I wore a tie, but pulled loose at the neck. My shirt was striped and my coat an understated silk tweed. No socks, of course. I don't even think the bellmen wear socks at this hotel.

I then practiced some deep breathing to help me relax, and, at about ten after eight, entered the Polo Lounge. Aware that these people were buying the story of a man who said he cared about health as well as hunkiness, I ordered the most wholesome breakfast: one skinned, roasted chicken breast ($7.50) and a quarter piece of melon ($3.50) and a glass of fresh orange juice (a bargain at $2).

During breakfast and the subsequent ceremonial filming in the gardens with TriStar Pictures and Green-Epstein Productions, and a final meeting at ABC Television (filmed by "Today's" NBC crew, a funny twist), I did my best to be myself and at the same time not visibly affected by the strange conversations going on. I understood it when my injuries were talked about as "good" for the story. ("Do you think you might have some more?" one of the guys cheerfully asked.) In an odd way, I even understood it when my heart disease was presented as a positive thing. "We're talking about a guy who could die here," one man said to the ABC bigwig—a show-business-sized dose of exaggeration (I hope). That might improve the story, but I won't like the ending, let me tell you.

I enjoyed most of my Hollywood adventure probably more than I want to admit. There is something disturbingly tasty about so much attention, so much glamour, so many powerful illusions. I do not think, however, any of it will change the underlying me. Though these days I do have an overpowering desire to put on my sunglasses before shaving.

R*emar, you were in the land of hot tubs, exotic massages, and "meditation." What about those things?*

All of the "hot" things—saunas, steam rooms, hot tubs, and whirlpools—can be fun, especially if you're with the right person. Except for whirlpool-type machines used in treating some injuries, they really don't have any proven health benefits other than the relaxing (or stimulating) feeling that may arise from your presence in one.

There are some potential problems with them, though. First, don't use one if you suffer from heart disease, diabetes, or high or low blood pressure. You shouldn't use one if you're under the influence of drugs, including alcohol, anticoagulants, antihistamines, stimulants, vasoconstrictors, vasodilators, tranquilizers, or narcotics. Pregnant women should be extremely careful, but then, they shouldn't be in a hot and sultry place anyway. All of these things apply, unless you have an opportunity to take a famous Hollywood starlet in one of these things to be wicked. And on that note, let me warn you that the next few pages are written from the author's point of view as a man, and as one who has always dreamed of a body good enough for a little potential sin. Ladies and children might therefore want to skip to Chapter 17.

The problem with hot tubs, saunas, whirlpools and the like is the heat that's associated with them, logically enough. When the body heats up, it sends extra blood to the peripheral regions, which requires extra pumping, which places a strain on the heart. The blood is sent to the skin to help dissipate body heat, which doesn't happen, incidentally, when you're sitting in 104 degrees of steaming water with a Hollywood starlet at the Beverly Hills Hotel, for instance.

Getting out of these situations can be tricky, too. If you should feel a need to stand up quickly and exit (for instance, if the Hollywood starlet's boyfriend, the stuntman stand-in for King Kong, should arrive), you could faint. That's because much of your blood has been pumped to the body surface to help cool it. More blood to the surface means less blood to the brain.

On second thought, using these things can be damned dangerous. But if you're going to use them anyway, make sure the water is changed daily (chemical reactions and bacterial growth can happen quickly there), and/or the thermostat in your tub or steam room is operating properly.[1]

What about massages?

These, too, are wonderful when administered by Hollywood starlets, if the door is locked. Massages actually have health benefits, too, including improved circulation, elimination of waste products, stretching of muscles and tendons, and rehabilitation of soft-tissue injuries.[2]

Massages aren't a cure-all, though. Never massage a severe injury, or a site where there is hemorrhage or infection.

What about biofeedback and other weird stuff like that?

Biofeedback is one of several relaxation techniques that actually do help some people. All the techniques help to identify what being relaxed really is and assist gravitation toward that state. Mind-over-matter. And since so many health problems can be brought on by mental problems, like the high blood pressure that comes from the tension that arises when a Hollywood starlet's boyfriend finds out your room number and is beating on your door at 2 A.M., think about giving one or more of these things a try sometime:

Biofeedback. This is the term used to describe a way in which information is being received from the body. Practicing it initially requires equipment to determine heart rate changes, skin temperature, muscular activity, brain wave activity, and skin conductance. Now, believe it or not, we can control some of those processes with our mind.

Biofeedback can be thought of as a three-stage process: information, such as your heartbeat, is measured. That information is converted into something you can understand, such as your heart rate. You are trained to literally think your heartbeat down, something you can actually see happen.

Biofeedback has served many uses: it's worked to relieve some headaches, high blood pressure, asthma, and ulcers.[3] It is not a cure, but it's not a snake-oil-salesman-type thing, either. If you'd like more information, call the Biofeedback Society of America, or a local university psychology department.

Meditation. It isn't only for monks or weirdos, and it's free—rare when it comes to anything having to do with health. Meditation is simply a mental exercise which helps you focus your attention on what you want to acknowledge rather than the things that demand to be acknowledged. It teaches you to use the mind to relax the body. Beware, though, of meditating groups or organizations which resemble religions and charge you gobs of money.

Autogenic Training. This uses the body to relax the mind, the opposite of meditation. It teaches you a type of self-hypnosis that induces a feeling of heaviness and warmth in the body. Now, look deeply into my eyes. That's what I said to you-know-who at the Beverly Hills Hotel.

Progressive Relaxation.   This teaches you to tense up a specific body part and then relax it. What you're trying to do here is get the feel of yourself in both the tense and relaxed state. You can progress from body part to body part, and the tension phase can be especially fun if you've escaped from the Hollywood starlet's boyfriend and rendezvoused again with your meditational object in a hot tub, where the temperature is always rising.

All of these types of self-help mind disciplines are interesting to know about, even if you aren't particularly into mind games. Your local library can provide you some good information on each.

I *travel a lot to places as strange as Hollywood, and I feel more strung-out on those trips. What can I do to lessen the strain?*

Dr. Eric Goldstein, Ph.D., a stress management specialist in Miami who works with me at times, and Chris Scott have some good advice on stress and travel-related stress.

Changing time zones.   Three nights prior to flying, begin to switch your body's timing. If you are flying eastward, go to bed an hour earlier each night, and rise earlier, too. If you are flying westward, go to bed (and get up) later. Try to also move your meals to coincide with the new time zone.

Handling long trips by plane.   Sleep as much as possible on a plane, but when you're awake, make your time productive. Take a book or work with you. Take your own tape recorder and tapes, and create you own "space."

Handling strange environments.   Make them as familiar as possible. Take along a picture or a familiar object. Dr. Goldstein has worked with well-known athletes who take along stuffed animals.

When you're away, also keep your concentration and focus on the present, on things you can do right then.

Here are some good exercises for managing stress:

Diaphragmatic breathing (a fancy word for breathing deeply) can relax you. Breathing usually becomes shallow and rapid during stress. Deep breathing counters this reaction and better oxygenates the blood. Place your hand on your stomach, above the navel. Breathe in slowly and very deeply, holding your breath for one or two seconds. Breath slowly out through your mouth—the slower the better. If you're breathing correctly, your stomach will *rise* when you breath in and fall when you breathe out.

Try the Progressive Relaxation technique I mentioned a minute ago. It works anyplace, in any position, with the exception of what is commonly known as the the starlet reflex syndrome I also mentioned earlier. Tense a muscle group (for instance, your shoulder muscles) for several seconds. Then relax them. Be conscious of the different sensations. Recognizing muscle tension will make it easier for you to tell your body to relax.

"We can't change many stressful situations," Dr. Goldstein says, "but we can change our reactions to those situations in ways that will help us." For instance, at all times walk, don't run, from the Hollywood starlet's boyfriend.

DALLAS TO THE DEVIL'S PUNCHBOWL

Week 38
Dallas, Texas

I am in Dallas, one of the last cities of my month-long book tour. This is an especially busy tour, too. My weekdays usually start at 4:00 or 4:30 A.M., when twenty-four-hour room service brings me decaffeinated coffee, wheat toast, and oatmeal. Invariably, whatever city I'm in, my toast is accompanied by three mini jars of "gourmet" preserves, which aren't on my eating schedule right now and therefore go instantly in my goody bag before they tempt me.

This trip's goody bag already contains twenty-seven mini jars, and lots of other things nice hotels give you, too. The bag probably weighs fifteen pounds, a good weight for morning exercise, but instead I drop to the floor before pouring a coffee and do very disciplined push-ups. Right now I can do fifteen perfect ones before my shoulder begins to hurt. My feet then go on the bed and I do one hundred crunches in four sets. These two exercises, which take less than five minutes, can help keep your body physically toned.

After exercise and breakfast, I work at my portable computer. My most productive writing hours have always been before sunrise, and these hours on tour seem to be especially good ones. But by seven I'm usually showered and dressed. If my day calls for only radio or newspaper interviews, I wear very informal clothes. For TV, I put on the blazer and slacks that comprise my dress wardrobe.

Invariably by seven, a car picks me up for the day's interviews. A writer can always tell how his publisher likes him by the way he gets around for interviews. Four years ago, I had to catch cabs. Two years ago, ladies in very small cars picked me up, sometimes with their kids in the backseat. This year, the ladies are driving Mercedeses and Cadillacs, have fruit waiting in the car for me, and drop their kids off at private schools. I don't know if I'm doing better or the ladies are doing better.

By nightfall, after five to seven shows, my escort drops me back at my hotel. This tour, I am staying in hotels with some type of health facilities. Though at times I don't want to, each day I make myself change and head to that facility. At first, I felt a little uncomfortable walking in elevators and through lobbies dressed so skimpily. But after looking at the bellies and tired faces of many men checking into nice hotels these days, I feel nearly smug. It is not easy to work out when you're tired and strung-out, but invariably those are the most satisfying workouts.

Before this year, my hotel routine while on book tour wasn't quite that satisfying. Tours are lonely things, in a way. People, cities, and shows become a blur; it's hard to sleep with time changes and all that adrenaline pumping through you from having to be "up" constantly; hotels, even nice ones, lose their charm quickly. I spent my free time by the television with a beer in my hand. No more.

Here in Dallas, it's especially easy to be good healthwise. I'm staying and exercising at the Cooper Clinic, where all my testing this year takes place. Everyone walks or jogs between buildings, the only alcohol within sight is rubbing alcohol, and food is so wholesome-looking it probably blushes at the thought of cholesterol.

A couple of thousand families belong to the clinic Activity Center, a handsome place. The gym itself is vaulted wood, glass-walled, and large enough to host several activities at once. A balcony filled with free weights and machines overlooks the gym floor. Fast-paced, pleasant music plays constantly. One wall is lined with the total distances logged by many center members in their particular sport. I don't want to make you feel wimpish, but Louis Patrick Neeb, forty-five, has jogged over 50,635 miles. Marcia Goldenfeld has swum 3,246.66 miles.

Last evening from the balcony I watched people in their seventies doing aerobics with people in their twenties. At the other end of the gym, a couple about twenty-five and their two children, no more than two years old, were playing basketball together. The father held his daughter high and threw the ball with her, then the mother, blond, tanned, and athletically fit, chased it with their son. "Good! Nice catch!" The parents seemed to be having as much fun as the kids, and I could not help but think how lucky those two children were.

This morning, between interviews, I went back to the clinic for my ninth-month physical. My doctor this trip was Arno Jensen. I told you in Chapter 7 some things about Arnie (you will remember him as the fifty-seven-year-old hunk), but I'll tell you more here. Arno personally doesn't like to jog. Since the Cooper Clinic was founded and is run by the man who started the world jogging, that's pretty much like being a Cardinal who doesn't support the Pope.

Arnie, however, definitely believes in fitness (including jogging for some). He trains on his stationary bike hard enough to beat out every single jogger his age ever tested on the stress treadmill at the clinic—enduring thirty-two minutes! Until the last test, that is, when a man beat him by ten seconds.

Arnie told me this trip his lean body mass has increased again. At forty-one, Arnie was 18 percent fat. At fifty-seven, he is now 9.6 percent fat. He eats like that proverbial horse, too. And he really does draw the looks (unrequited—he's happily married) of twenty-year-old beauties when he works out on the balcony overlooking the gym area. I had heard of this from others, but experienced it myself this trip. I like Arnie, but I don't like to stand by him in the gym when the ladies are around.

My own physical state continues slowly to improve in most areas, however. Since my last exam in May, I've added 2.7 pounds of muscle. Though I would like more muscle, Bob Stauffer's words of many months ago are true: good definition makes for a great look. And working with my body is doing more for me emotionally and stamina wise than I had ever imagined. Arnie Jensen made me feel pretty good about my growth, too. Arnie has added only fifteen pounds of muscle in seven years, which maybe makes me hunkier than him in the muscle-gaining area, right?

The fats in my blood continue to decrease, too. My "good" cholesterols are rising and my bad ones falling. At the Cooper Clinic, the ratio of good to bad cholesterols is the most important measure of interior health, and my ratio has dropped from 7.2 to 6. To be really healthy, mine needs to be below 5. My triglycerides, another fat, have also dropped marginally. My count is now 173, getting closer to my recommended maximum of 124.

The one really disappointing test result was my percentage of body fat. In May, when I was still restricting my calories to lose weight, that percentage had dropped from 30 percent to 15 percent, a point under my "ideal" percentage of fat, according to the docs. This time, after eating five special meals a day to help feed my muscle growth, it's up to 21.5 percent. I am not fat, but the new ripples on my stomach are looking a little smothered. I'm therefore going on a diet which weight lifters use to "rip down" for contests.

Just a few moments ago, I received a phone call from some friends near the Devil's Punchbowl along the Oregon coast. They're completing 3,000 miles of an 18,000-mile bike trip, and I, with the thought of excess fat creeping back on my nearly healthy and beautiful body, have decided to spend my weekend biking with them a little bit. How spontaneous have you been lately?

Depoe Bay, Oregon, three days later: Is anyone interested in taking over an Alaskan gold claim? It's a pretty piece of land, I'm sure, a big claim right on Canyon Creek—1,320-by-1,320 potentially gold-rich feet in the midst of Fairbanks Township itself, and dutifully registered on Page 240 of Book 490 at the Fairbanks office of the Alaskan Department of Natural Resources.

The claim is owned by my young friends from Minnesota, Spain, and Yugoslavia. They don't have time to mine it right now, since they're still 15,000 miles away from their final destination, Tierra del Fuego (the "Land of Fire") at the very tip of South America. Their trip is an extraordinary athletic endeavor and has interested me since I heard about it many months ago. No one has ever biked from Alaska to the tip of South America before. If fortune is with them, they will cross 100 miles of roadless jungle at the Darien Gap (bikes on their backs), pedal across the driest desert on earth, the Atacama in Chile (where it hasn't rained since the sixteenth century), and bike the length of every troubled South American country you've seen on television.

On this very misty, fog-shrouded day, however, the eight of us are spending the weekend at a cliffside cabin on the Oregon Coast, and as the others go about individual chores, I can watch sea lions climbing rocks with some effort, then beating their flippers together enthusiastically, occasionally using a flipper to wipe a brow, it seems. A small deep-V-hulled boat keeps circling about a thousand feet beyond the shoreline, six well-wrapped people on its bow, watching for a whale to surface and blow again. The whale likes this particular cove, for he's been in the vicinity most of the morning. The music as I watch and the seven others work is Simon and Garfunkel's "Bridge Over Troubled Water," much more my music, you would think, than my young friends'.

Dan Buettner, twenty-six, of Roseville, Minnesota, chased me down at the Cooper Clinic with this biking invitation. I have known the four Buettner boys and their parents for five years, and have often wondered how Roger and Dolly keep their sanity with such an independent crew. Dan studies and bikes throughout Europe, honing his writing skills, for months on end, on virtually no money, with the casualness of a person walking down a street. His knapsack usually includes several classical books, and his first stop in any city is at a newstand to buy some newspaper with American stocks listed in it.

Tony, twenty-seven, runs a ski-related business in Colorado. Nicky, seventeen, is still at home, but planning his first solo hiking trip of Europe. Nicky just told his parents he feels "confined" by normal life. And Steve—right now downstairs in the garage working on the group's bikes—plans to return to Spain after this little biking diversion to continue his international studies. All of the boys are black-haired, rugged, tall, and handsome. Roger and Dolly are proud of their kids and their independence (they taught them to love being active in the outdoors) and at the same time are scared by it.

Dan thought up and largely organized this particular bicycle trek to first promote friendship among nations and secondarily to set a Guinness record. To those ends, many municipalities and governments here and south of the border are helping the seven along, and the group meets lots of people (and has even saved the life of a seriously injured kid in an automobile accident), and each bicycling mile is logged.

But because I know Dan and have now met the group, I don't for a minute think these five guys and two women are doing this primarily for nobility or records alone. Above everything else, they are doing it for sheer adventure, the *energy* of it, about the best reasons in the world to do anything, I'm coming to believe.

I had intended to spend this weekend working off a few pounds, escaping from the pressure of touring, and listening to the exciting experiences 3,000 miles of biking must have already generated. I thought I might pick up a few tricks real jocks use to keep in shape as they bike halfway around the world, too. But as I watched and became a part of this weekend, I was more fascinated by these people themselves, not just their adventure.

Martin Engel, twenty-seven, and Anne Knabe, twenty-four, are both second-year medical students. Anne, slender and quiet-natured, is the only woman biker, but she was accepted by the others with a natural assumption of equality which would make Gloria Steinem proud. She appears to be the group philosopher.

Martin is tall, broad-shouldered, and equally quiet. From a family of mountaineers, Martin is an encyclopedia of outdoor facts and a beaver when it comes to storing things. The one pot used to cook virtually all the group's meals since their cooking utensils were stolen in Seattle is a five-quart Boy Scout pot Martin received when he was thirteen.

Bret Anderson, twenty-four, is probably sick of hearing it, but is all-American-looking, the type of young man you expect to say "sir," which he did until I told him to knock it off. Bret is studying international business, but I enjoyed his knowledge of the guitar more.

Last night, after a dinner of fresh crab and salmon, and chanterelle mushrooms picked less than a mile from the cabin, Bret sat with his feet propped up and played classical guitar as we ate freshly picked grapes for dessert. He then joined Matjaz Bren, the group photographer, in a chess game. A Yugoslavian, Matjaz, twenty-four, taught English at a school in Morocco before immigrating to the States, and plans to join the foreign service here eventually.

At about nine last night, Rafaela Salido came upstairs from helping Steve Buettner work on the bicycles. Raffi, an attorney from Spain, has dark eyes and hair, freckled cheeks, and one of those smiles which seems to make her look at once shy and very naturally happy. She and Steve are the support crew for the trip. They joined Dan and me in Scrabble. Anne and Martin were lost in books, occasionally coming back to the world to kibbitz our game.

This quiet time seemed to be important to the group. After 3,000 miles of sleeping together in a ten-foot camper and eating breakfast, lunch, and dinner from a community pot, privacy becomes a discipline if you plan to keep your sanity. This weekend in a borrowed cabin was the last planned break before South America.

But then Bret pulled a tango tape from the group's music case and placed it in the recorder and for the next hour the men from Minnesota and Yugoslavia and the Bahamas took turns dancing tangos with the medical student from Minneapolis and the attorney

187

from Spain. I didn't know how to tango, felt awkward with these wonderfully relaxed young people who danced dances from my generation's dreams, but eventually felt like the eighth person on their team. I must tell you it was a totally unexpected and enchanting evening.

We biked together this morning for about 40 miles along the Oregon coast. My biking on Grand Bahama is flat and easy, not at all like the hills here, and I had never biked so far before without a break. At the start of my year, the thought of biking 4 miles to Freeport scared me. But today, even though it nearly killed me at times, I kept up with the group, even taking the lead twice. And when it occasionally crossed my mind that these nice folks might be going easy for my sake, I pushed the thought away faster than my wheels could spin. Appearances, I decided, were as exciting as reality.

I fly out in the morning for a day in Seattle and then an overnight flight to Grand Bahama. My friends continue south for another 15,000 miles. I worry some for their safety, but I envy and admire them, don't you? And I think their resourcefulness will get them through. It's like that gold mine claim that's now for sale. When my friends were told only miners have access to the first 500 miles of rutted road from Prudhoe Bay, Alaska, south, they simply went and filed a mining claim. The claim's good forever—as long as someone works on it two hundred hours a year. And I have calculated that two hundred hours of work on a gold claim will work joff about ten pounds of fat and put on about three pounds of muscle and, you know, that's worth about as much as a good strike.

After eight months, my interests and friends in life are changing somewhat. Active people interest me a lot more, and more important, I think I interest them. I am reminded of much new research which states that being active and involved in life has as much to do with longevity as simply exercising. If that's the case, I'm going to live a very long time, I've decided.

Before we dig for gold, Norma wants us to have physicals. *Should we? And what should they do to us?*

In the opinion of many, the best preventive medicine specialist in the country is Dr. Cooper, so my answers here are based on his recommendations.

If you consider yourself healthy and are under thirty, physicals every two or three years are fine. Between thirty and thirty-five, have one every two years. During these years, have at least one resting electrocardiogram simply as a reference point for the cardiac changes that come later in life.

If you are over forty, have a thorough physical, including a maximum performance stress test, every year or eighteen months. After fifty, definitely have a physical every year.

Should women have different physicals?

They should have the same basic examination, but should also have a baseline mammogram between the ages of thirty-five and forty. Between forty and fifty, have one every one to two years, depending on you family history. After fifty, have one every year.

Pap smears should be started before age twenty and should be done no more than two years apart.

This may be a dumb question, but what's the big deal about physicals, other than the doctor making money?

As Dr. Cooper says, virtually all our major health problems start out small. That's the reason regular physicals can be important. And if you are in some of the high-risk categories we talk about in this book, physicals can definitely be lifesaving.

Okay. So what constitutes a good physical?

Obviously, if you have definite things wrong with you, or if you know you're in some high-risk groups, your physical should deal with those areas. Obviously, you should be honest and nonblushing when you talk to the doctor, too, though most people lie and blush. Don't worry about sounding like a hypochondriac and don't leave out a detail.

Now, with that said, here's a rundown on a good, comprehensive physical.

A complete health and medical history.   How you feel about yourself, your health history, your family history, social history (your interaction with people, not those fancy clubs you and Norma belong to). Histories lead the doctor to potential problems, and make you an individual rather than some type of health statistic.

Standard measurements allow comparisons to statistical groups and are the basis for measuring changes in you. For instance, blood pressure, weight (or, more important, body fat), heart rate, pulse, circumferences (is your stomach larger than your chest?).

Examination of your head, eyes, ears, nose, throat, neck, and lymph nodes. And on down toward the toes.   Part of this isn't bad (like checking your chest) and part of this is godawful. The prostate exam for men, pelvic exam (and pap smear) for women, and a sigmoidoscopic exam (something the size of a telephone pole is inserted in your rear end) are terribly important, the best ways to determine prostate, cervical, and colon cancers. Because those cancers are brutal ones if left untreated, put up with the pain and embarrassment of these tests, and make sure your doctor administers them if you are over forty.

Central nervous system tests, like when the doctor hits you with that little hammer. Your reflex (or lack of it) might be a sign of things like multiple sclerosis, spinal cord damage due to disease, and, believe it or not, syphilis.

Blood and urine tests.   Probably the best windows to the function of many organs.

X rays may not be necessary, depending on your age and physical condition. They are important in judging the condition of your organs, lungs, and skeletal system.

Treadmill stress tests.   They can help detect the presence of heart disease and determine your system's physical limits. You can't fool a treadmill.

A meeting with the doctor.   Detailed written reports and letters are good, but a consultation with the doctor is a must.

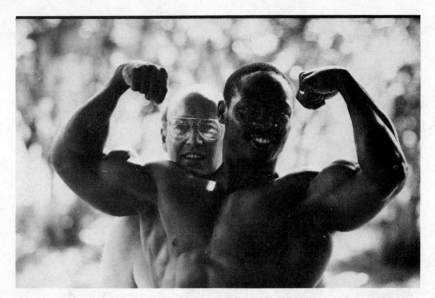

Henry Charlton has been the guest poser at many world body-building events. The most famous Bahamian bodybuilder, Henry works out regularly with us at the YMCA.

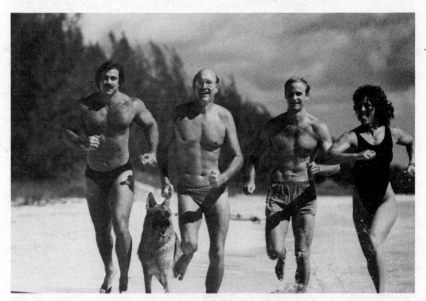

We were supposed to have our tongues out for this shot, but only the dog Sai and Marilynn listened. Bill and Marilynn Carle are the managers of my gym, and both hold bodybuilding titles. Her most recent one is "Miss Southern States 1986."

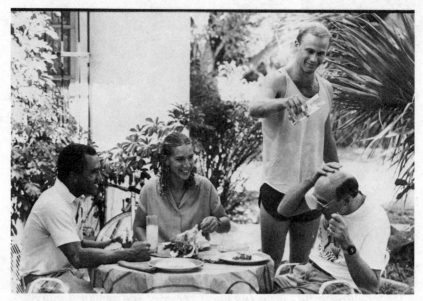

Ollie and Pam Ferguson join us for breakfast. That's a conch shell on the table, and one of my seven bikes in the background. Ollie is a supervisor at UNEXSO, and Pam a member of my exercise class.

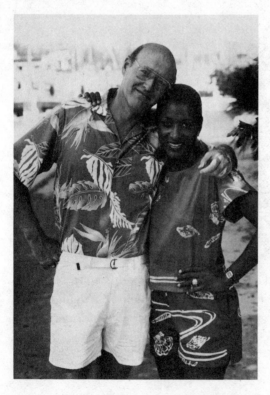

November. Marva Monroe, administrative director of the Grand Bahama Promotion Board, works out and jogs with me. In the brains and looks department, she's the female equivalent of what I want to be.

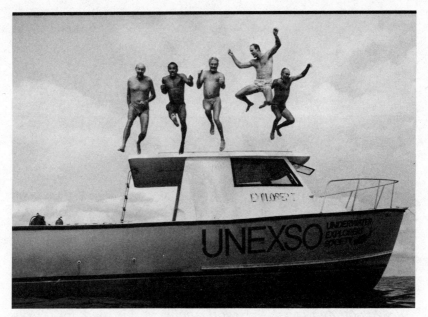

Banzai! I can't tell you how my energy level improved during this year. I jump off boats all the time now. Ollie Ferguson, Mike Sahlen, Chris, and Ben Rose (of Ben's Caves at the Lucayan National Park) join me as we calmly step off the boat.

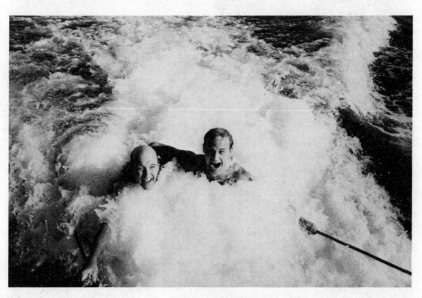

Called "Burfing," this sport requires a strong arm, a fast boat and a tight bathing suit. We don't tell women the last requirement.

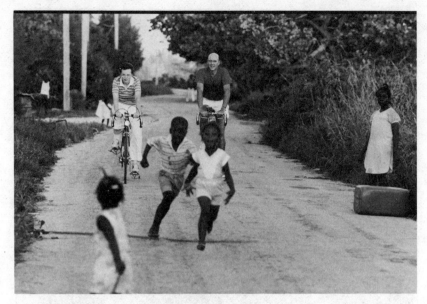

Mary Abbott and I won't reveal the name of this road, for it's on the way to our secret cocoa plum patch.

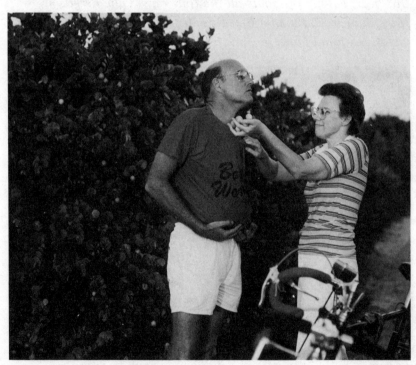

The proper way to transport cocoa plums. They taste best in pancakes on Sunday morning.

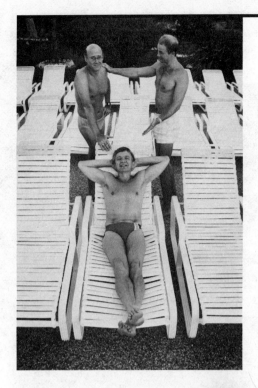

I really do like Arnie Jensen, but I hate it when he steals all the maidens' stares.

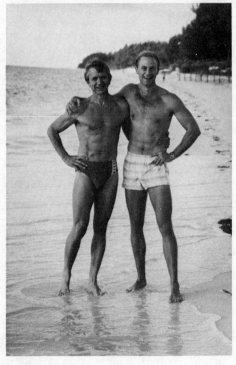

Arnie and Chris. These two could be brothers, though they're thirty-four years apart in age.

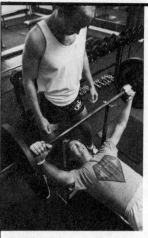

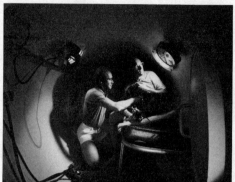

(Left) Notice the size of the weights, and the smile on my face. A November picture.

(Right) Kurt Alcorn and I spent six hours pretty much like this in the recompression chamber. Mortality isn't an abstract idea in a chamber.

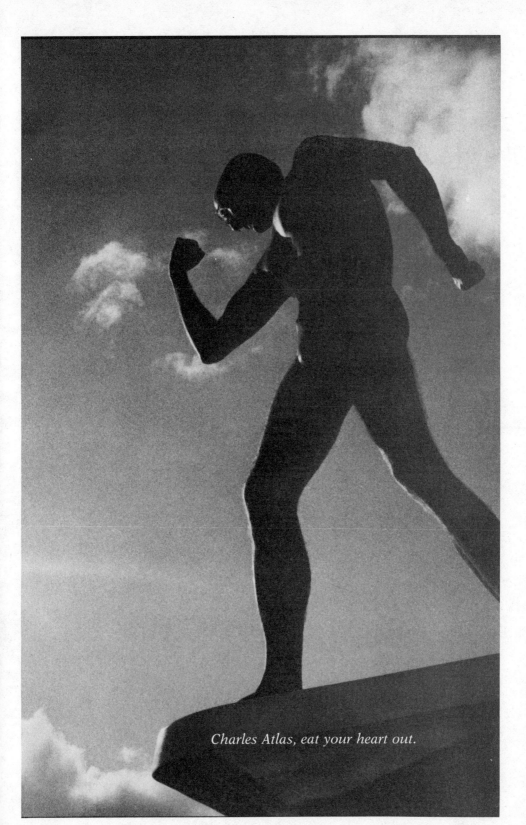

Charles Atlas, eat your heart out.

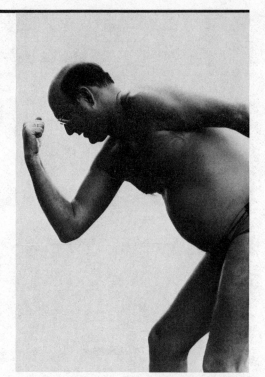

Day 1

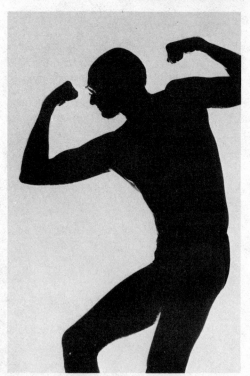

Day 300

Physicals are a hassle. They're expensive. But they are the linch-pin of preventive medicine.

Looking into the future.   Would you like a preview of what the doctor will say to you? If you're gutsy and really honest with your-self, this test may tell you a lot. Run your answers down the right margin, or use a sheet of paper.

1. In the course of your normal activities such as getting in and out of chairs, mowing the lawn, doing chores around the house, do you become winded or fatigued?
2. Do you frequently wake up fatigued?
3. We talked earlier about ways to judge the amount of fat on your body: the pinch test, looking at yourself naked in the mirror without trying to suck it in, remembering your shape in high school if you were lean, and thinking about the sizes of clothes you wear now. Lock yourself away, release the stomach, and give yourself an accurate blubber reading. If you're close to high school size already, you shouldn't be reading this book anyway, so give it to a real person. Or go on to Question 4.
   • Are your stomach and chest about the same size? (Ladies, this means *chest* for you, too.)
   • Is your stomach larger than your chest?
   • Are you much more "filled-out" than you were in high school?
4. Do you eat fried foods, gravies, dishes prepared with a lot of butter, creams, or sauces more than once each week?
5. Generally speaking, are your breakfasts composed of eggs and bacons and/or sausages and hams?
6. Are your lunches usually fast foods or foods fried and/or breaded?
7. Generally speaking, are your favorite dinners composed of red meats, fried foods, foods with sauces?
8. If you eat red meats, do you leave on a portion of the fat?
9. For dessert do you choose cakes, pies, and other baked/sweet items over fresh fruits?
10. Do you smoke?
11. Do you smoke over two packs a day?
12. Do you drink more than two drinks a day?
13. Do you drink every day?
14. Do you think of your work situation as stressful?
15. Do you have high blood pressure? (If you don't know, stop here and find out).
16. Has your doctor ever told you to "watch" your blood pressure?
17. Do you take any prescribed or over-the-counter medication for "nerves"?

18. Do you ever experience tightness in your chest, usually associated with pain?
19. Are you over forty?
20. In your perception, are any of your parents, grandparents, aunts, or uncles seriously overweight?
21. Do any of your parents, grandparents, aunts, or uncles have "adult-onset" diabetes?
22. Have any died from diabetes-related complications?
23. Have any of your parents, grandparents, aunts, or uncles had a heart attack or coronary heart disease?.
24. Have any of your parents, grandparents, aunts, or uncles had a stroke?
25. Have any had cancer?
26. In your personal time, do you seek inactivity rather than activity and interchange with others?
27. Do you seem too busy to exercise, or avoid actual exercise?

The only crystal balls in medicine, the only things that in any way help doctors predict your future well-being, are the patterns of your past and present life—your genetic inclinations, your intakes, your activities and attitudes toward your own body and mind.

If you answered yes to many of these questions, most doctors and health specialists would rate your future prospects for health and general well-being as less than optimal. If you answered yes to virtually all of them—for instance, if the questions show you're overweight, eating wrong, inactive, smoking, drinking too much, and from a family with a history of health problems—virtually all doctors and health specialists would fear for your health and perhaps your life. Your chances of serious premature health problems and an earlier death are astronomical.

I do not mean to be melodramatic about this, but in reality serious disease and death *are* pretty melodramatic, aren't they?

But if you decide to make a change for the better, you can. That decision never seems very dramatic or exciting, which may be the problem. Arnie Jensen says, "It takes ten minutes to convince someone to have his stomach removed, but ten years to convince him to change his lifestyle." It has taken me more than ten years to make that decision, but I have made it. And, I promise you, if I have, you can.

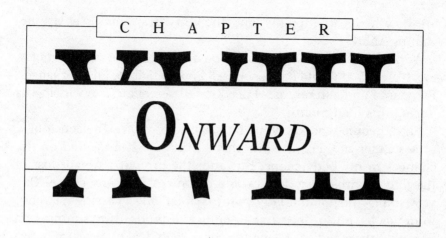

CHAPTER XVIII

ONWARD

Week 42

<u>*Grand Bahama Island*</u>

As I started my remake nine months ago, my intentions (and my dreams) were of a final book chapter which would detail the end result of hunkification. I envisioned the chapter as rather X-rated. Perhaps a racy excerpt or two would appear in *Penthouse*, and the last words on the final page would be a quote from some beauty who had shunned my old, blimpish body but, on a subsequent swoon walk, caught a vision of the new me (so muscular even the biggest hulk would shudder a bit) and fell prey to my animal magnetism. I expected she would say something like, "Remar makes every beautiful girl a fallen woman."

Of course, the months didn't quite go like that. They did bring changes in my body and more notoriety than I had thought possible. I am very proud of the new, leaner, tighter me, too. I worked for every damn change, and, by God, I plan to keep working. And I'm finding that a little notoriety is worth about two inches on your biceps. But I still am somewhat insecure about my looks and, at times, feel as fat as I ever looked. Probably always will. I haven't fallen in love with exercise itself, either, whether for vanity (sit-ups) or health (jogging). I do it, however, because the end results are now believable for me, and the activities themselves are becoming habit.

As the body has changed, my mind has undergone some changes, too. I knew that would happen, but did not anticipate all the changes. For you to understand that, I need to tell you about a few incidents during this final month.

First, people who knew me fat seem to have grown accustomed to a slender me. For a while there, everyone commented on the changes in my body shape. But after the dramatic weight loss of the first months, very few people commented on my shape. One very young and popular lady on the island made a passing reference to my looks, but in the same breath said minds always impressed her more than bodies. Though I took a good deal of pleasure in her thinking, an affirmation of things deeper than flesh, I was a little disappointed she hadn't made some comment like, "Boy, I wish my dad looked like you." Or at least wanted to feel my stomach muscles. You know, tentative fingers on the firmness there, as she looked deeply in my eyes. I mean, I did lose nine inches on my belly. I went from pear-shaped to slender, from forty-two to thirty-three.

I went from nervous to confident in the gym, too. The biggest, hulkiest lifters were saying things like, "Hey, brother, you're whipping that devil, aren't ya!!!?" And my muscles did seem to reshape themselves though they haven't yet grown enough. People use the word "tight" to describe my body now. My back, which used to look like a slab of bacon, is lean, slightly V-shaped, and ripply with small muscles when I flex, which I do a lot if anyone is looking. My chest really developed. Nine months ago, my breasts sagged so much they embarrassed me even when I was alone, but now, by God, I look pretty good there. My stomach is just beginning to have the washboard effect so highly prized, I am told, by young maidens.

My shoulders are coming along, too. Nine months ago, they were nonexistent. Now, as I type, I can see a pleasant curve on both arms. And probably most interesting of all, my new tight state has really affected my face. Several people assume I've had a face-lift. An older man on the island asked me at a party for the name of my plastic surgeon. I did think about a face-lift, and some hair, too. I'm not dead set against either procedure, but I've decided they're not right at this time. I have worked for all my changes this year, and even though some of them may be minimal, they are all mine, a part of my body.

I'm not trying to say foreign hair and surgical procedures are

more vain than my own pursuits, either. As my looks have improved, I have discovered mirrors. For so much of my life, I've
avoided the truth of those things with the determination of a vam-
pire avoiding a wooden stake. But now I kind of like them. I've
found a way to flex my right bicep as I shave, and after a shower
I dry off in front of the full-length mirror rather than a blank wall.
I even decided Paul Harvey's headline, written at the beginning of
my new year, was going to be at least a little prophetic rather than
simply funny because of its impossibility: FAT MAN INVITES US TO
WATCH AS HE TRANSFORMS HIMSELF INTO BRONZE GOD. I worked on my
tan a lot.

And then, on a very beautiful blue-skied Bahamian day two weeks
ago, an incident happened which made me confront the real substance of this year—and my life, too.

Scuba diving has always been my very best tranquilizer. A diver
doesn't need to worry under normal circumstances, and after the
thousands of dives I've made in fifteen years, normal circumstances
make breathing underwater as natural as breathing on the surface.
Therefore, when Chris Scott and I went on a seventy-five-foot dive
a couple of weeks ago, a last-minute decision to pass the time while
my friend and editor Mary Abbott Waite hooked up my new laser
printer, my mind was on fish and coral canyons and caves.

At the end of every dive with the Underwater Explorers Society,
all divers, including the most experienced, normally come back to
what is called the ascent line. It's a large rope with a forty-pound
weight on the end dangling from the stern of the boat. The rope,
which hangs within ten feet of the ocean floor, is used by divers to
carefully control their ascent rate. This ascent from the dive holds
the only potential danger for sensible divers.

As you rise, the pressure on your body is lessened, since less water
is over you. At seventy-five feet, for instance, the average depth I
was diving, your body experiences close to four "atmospheres" of
pressure—this means that the pressure of the water is four times
as heavy as the pressure at sea level of air on your body. The water
above you is as heavy as the distance from the edge of space to the
surface of the water times four. You don't feel this pressure because
liquids and solid matter don't compress.

But gasses are affected by pressure; they compress under heavier
pressure and expand under lighter pressure. My problem began
here. Rather than rising very slowly, hand-over-hand on the ascent
line, I decided at the very last minute to practice what is known

as an emergency free ascent (EFA). In an emergency ascent, a diver forgets the first two basic rules of diving—(l) breathe all the time and (2) rise no faster than your slowest bubble—and rushes to the surface, blowing out continuously on one breath. EFAs in a way serve a real purpose: they let a diver know he can have an out-of-air emergency at great depths, even 120 feet or so, and still make it to the surface in one breath.

But statistically, EFAs are dangerous. Because the very rapid ascent forces gasses such as oxygen and nitrogen to expand very rapidly in the body, the pressure of that sudden expansion can very occasionally force air through the lung tissues themselves into cavities around the lung, the tissue area around the neck, or the tissue around joints. These particular types of problems may cause a lot of pain, but normally don't kill you. If the air enters the bloodstream itself, it may kill you. When an air bubble enters your bloodstream, it travels along the interior walls of your arteries without incident for a millisecond or perhaps even a number of seconds or minutes, until the bubble, traveling in progressively smaller blood vessels, is larger than the vessel.

At that point, the bubble sticks, usually in an artery in the brain, blocking the circulation of further oxygen-laden blood to the precious tissues there, much like a clot. Brain tissue is most intolerant of oxygen starvation. Within four or five minutes, if the blocked area, now a clot, is not cleared, the affected brain tissue dies.

Because of these dangers, no scuba organizations actually teach EFAs any more. Diving students practice swimming horizontally for long distances on one breath rather than vertically.

They taught EFAs when I learned to dive, however. And on this day, I decided it was time to practice it. Quite honestly, before starting to rise, I looked to make sure none of the instructors from the Explorers Society were watching me, for any of them would have lectured me for the foolishnesss of it.

But no one was watching me, and I had broken this rule, gone against these odds so many times before without any consequences. I dropped my regulator to my side, raced to the surface nearly eight stories above me, my head tilted back to allow expanding air to flow freely from my mouth, and broke through the surface with the practiced aplomb of a dolphin rising for air. At some point during the ascent, an air bubble entered my bloodstream.

Because I do dive so much and have very low air consumption, my dive was longer than most of the divers, and the boat was nearly rigged to pull anchor as I climbed aboard. I felt great, and chatted with the ten other divers around me. For about a minute.

And then the pain began. It started in my back, directly under my right scapula, a pain so hot I began to sweat. For several minutes I attributed it to a muscle pull. But as *The Explorer I* entered the Bell Channel near port, the pain began to move. I remember feeling very alone at that moment. Muscle pulls don't move. I also did not want to tell anyone. Very experienced divers are at times foolishly proud, and I did not want to alert people with a false alarm if my pain was a muscle pull, and, even more foolishly, did not want to face the worse alternative: that I was in the midst of a diving accident, especially one caused by my mistake. I went to the bow of the boat, away from people, and began to breathe deeply and slowly.

As the boat pulled up to the dock, my symptoms were beginning to resemble a heart attack. Pain under my rib cage. A lightheadedness. Very spotty vision. I walked from the boat quickly, up a ten-foot gangplank, and stood alone by a bank of scuba tanks, confused, and for the first time really afraid. For, as I stood there, and as the pain made it hard to breathe, an overwhelming feeling of doom settled on me, as heavy and suffocating as any I want to experience before I die. And then I had the oddest thought. It seems so very funny now, but it did not then. I was going to die and would never see my new laser printer at work.

Mike Sahlen walked by me with two empty scuba tanks. Mike is the Explorers Society's underwater photography expert, and on this very unusual day, he walked by at the right moment. "Mike, don't say anything yet, please, but something's really wrong with me," I said.

"What, Remar?" He stopped walking, as if an invisible wall had stopped him. I told him about the pain. He sat me in a nearby chair, then walked away, very calmly but very quickly, I remember. I could not see very well by then, and the pain was moving up my back toward my shoulder and neck, and I suppose my head and brain. It was a grudging pain. It stuck in one place, and then it moved.

I don't think I had sat for more than thirty seconds when Mike returned with Steve Watson, one of UNEXSO's diving supervisors. Even as Mike and Steve walked to me quickly, other diving instructors were beginning to initiate a diving emergency plan. Diving accidents are not time-forgiving accidents. Any problem is considered the most serious problem until the actual accident is diagnosed. People moved quickly, therefore.

Steve talked to me first, asking questions which sounded as casual as the briefing airline stewardesses give before a flight, but as important to me as that stewardess's orientation toward an escape door in a crash. John Englander joined us. John is the president of UNEXSO, a special friend, and as he, too, asked me the most innocent questions, another instructor placed an oxygen mask over my face. Pure oxygen is critical in diving accidents, since it helps to get more oxygen to oxygen-starved areas, such as the brain, and helps to reduce swelling. We walked to John's office, an instructor carrying my oxygen bottle, another walking by me, watching me closely. I did not know it then, but they all were prepared for me to pass out.

John already had Dick Clark, one of the world's authorities on diving accidents, on the phone. As I breathed oxygen, John described my symptoms. I could not hear Dick. But when John looked up at me and the instructors watching me and said, "Okay, we need to take him down," I was so very glad Dick was at home Saturday. And when John said, "Bubs, we need to take you down to 165 feet," I was especially glad he was home. That depth in treating diving accidents is normally only used for embolisms, air in the blood, blockages of the brain, things that can kill you.

In diving accidents, the most important, and at times only lifesaving, treatment, is called a recompression chamber. A chamber recompresses the air around you, taking your body and its gasses back to pressures similar to the depths of the ocean, the great pressure recreated there squashing things like air bubbles traveling in the bloodstream until they disappear. Because diving is such a statistically safe sport, and because chambers and the treatments are so expensive, chambers are scarce.

But there is a chamber at UNEXSO less than twenty feet from the docks. Four of us walked from John's office toward the chamber room. As we walked, others were cutting off the supply of air used to fill the scuba tanks and redirecting it to the chamber. Marian Wilson grabbed a gallon of orange juice from the Tide's Inn restaurant, while two others checked oxygen bottles and attempted to locate Doc Clement, the chamber's official doctor.

Kurt Alcorn, a new instructor in his twenties, red-haired, freckled, and quiet, volunteered to enter the chamber with me. Kurt's job was to watch me, take my pulse, listen to my lungs, take my blood pressure, administer resuscitation if I should pass out from either the embolism or oxygen toxicity.

The chamber looks like an iron lung. Made of steel, its interior is four feet ten inches by eight and a half feet. It has two locks, one bed like an ambulance stretcher, a sound-powered telephone, and two small portholes. There is nothing electric inside it. Nothing flammable. No paper, no loose metals. Because of the great pressures created in chambers, the oxygen in the air is concentrated, and can flame up. No one has ever survived a recompression chamber fire.

Kurt and I spent six hours in that very close space. I was wearing an oxygen mask most of the time and could not talk. But I thought a lot. I had no control over my life whatsoever in that chamber. The four people just inches away, turning levers and controlling oxygen and air flow, ruled my life more completely than any jail tender ruled a prisoner's life.

A foolish, thoughtless decision had put my life in jeopardy. Because of that decision, my life was literally taken out of my control, and though I trusted the people running that chamber, I could not help but wonder what would happen to us if they turned a lever the wrong way. Or if an exhaust valve should rupture. Explosive decompressions turn people into spaghetti. And then I thought about people who've had strokes. An embolism is really like a stroke. What if the chamber hadn't been there? If I had died, that would have been the end of it, I guess. But what if I had been paralyzed? Left with a mind that couldn't will a body to do things? Any debilitating illness is probably like being isolated in that chamber, only worse. The thought reminded me of the red-and-white land crabs prized as a delicacy by most of us on the island. The crabs have powerful claws which give them mobility and protection. But when land crabs are caught, all of their appendages are broken off before the crabs are carried to local markets. The crab bodies sit on market shelves and the only way to know they are alive is to watch the jerky movement of their eyes.

And then, as the pain left me, as the air bubble in my bloodstream was crushed by the great pressure in the chamber, my mind went back to the sense of doom which had overcome me only minutes before as I stood on the dock. That moment defined "regret" for me in a way I cannot define for you. What was happening to me had been in my control and I had botched it. How many times had I made emergency ascents, ignoring the fact they were dangerous? Why did I think the rules didn't apply to me? Because of the chamber I was a very lucky person, was given a second chance to correct a needless risk. From that day on, Remar Sutton would rise to the surface at the lazy pace of a sea slug.

At five-thirty that afternoon, I crawled out of the chamber tired, somewhat sore, and feeling very mortal. Mary Abbott and Chris drove me home, and though it still sounds stupid, I went directly to my office to watch my new laser printer work.

My diving incident—I won't call it an accident, because it wasn't— gave me an opportunity to think about the elements of risk I confront in my own life, particularly concerning my health, and reminded me more forcefully than I wanted to know how many of those elements are under my control. Until this year my concerns about health were as immediate as my concern about an embolism. Rules of cause and effect didn't apply to me. Let me assure you that a confrontation with death reminds you they do.

But we don't think about the rules until we see the problem. Not long ago, as I walked on the beach, a bikinied man who looked sixty, and had a belly that made my former body look svelt and a cigarette hanging from his mouth, yelled, "Hey, aren't you that swoon walker or something?"

I said yes, as he dropped a few ashes on the sand and coughed. "You know, I give your articles to all my friends," he continued. "The out-of-shape ones."

"Oh, really? What do you do to keep in shape?"

I tried not to sound sarcastic, and obviously succeeded, for the man simply continued talking. "Oh, nothing. I used to be a football player, you know."

"Oh? When was that?"

"Twenty years ago. I'm forty-two."

The number fit his waist much more than his age. I walked on, slightly uncomfortable, because the man was me before I began to face reality.

Under his denial, he probably thinks about his health and shape like I used to, too: things were too bad to really correct; damage was already done. Those thoughts are wrong, however. Too late is when you are dead.

My last official swoon walk is without doubt the proof of that, too. I walked to the beach with the "Today" show in tow and Anastasia Toufexis, health and fitness editor of *Time* magazine, pad in hand, waiting for me on the beach. With that level of press around, it's hard to cheat.

I was, therefore, a little more nervous than usual. Under normal circumstances, swoon walks are as much mental fantasy—how we want to perceive ourselves—as they are reality. Even during my first swoon walks, when little children kicked sand in my direction, I could at least pretend. In my later walks, I simply cheated, sending an emissary to the beach before my walk to make sure all beautiful maidens knew that the proper swoon just might get them on national TV or, at the least, in my column.

At first, I thought a little cheating would work for my final walk, too. My friends had gathered up about forty of the youngest, most beautiful girls a man could imagine this side of a morals charge, reminded them of the camera, and whipped them into a frenzy of anticipation. The girls were even given "before" pictures to provide them the proper perspective on my body. For very significant events, I try to think of everything.

And on camera, there's no question every single girl swooned as I strolled down the gauntlet in a new, fire-red mini-bikini. No man could dream of a better reaction, and no director could feel better about his production, and for a minute there I had trouble remembering if life imitates art or art imitates life. Frankly, I didn't care, either.

Anastasia, however, was real concerned with the veracity of my final moment of glory. After the cameras were off, and as the girls began to drift back to their boyfriends, all young enough to be my children, she began to ask them unsettling questions: "What do *really* think of that body?" she asked eight or nine of the girls. "How old do you think Remar is?" she asked others.

And then, to my horror, she asked all the girls to compare my body to their father's body. How would they react if their father had walked down the beach like this?

Anastasia was behind me when she asked the first group of girls these questions, and for an instant my insides quaked. I could not turn around. As Anastasia asked the questions, the girls began to giggle and then laugh.

Right then, I knew how that famous king without any clothes must have felt when truth finally arrived in the form of a young kid's innocent words. But then the girls began to talk: "Wow, I *wish* my dad looked like that," a couple of them said. "And how old is your dad?" Anastasia asked. One girl said thirty-eight, the other forty-two. I, of course, am nearly forty-six.

"And how old do you think Remar is?" Anastasia asked. For an instant, I wanted to pull her off the beach quickly while I was ahead in those conversations, but stopped myself when the first girl said, "Oh, I'd guess around thirty-four or thirty-five." I blinked, then turned to the prettiest girl. Good looks and health run in families, and I didn't think there could be a chance her dad would be a dud. "Tell me the truth," I said, "do you really think I look better than your father?"

As I spoke, there were probably a dozen women standing around me in a circle. Behind the young ones were four or five ladies in their forties, and behind them a few ladies in their sixties. As the beautiful young girl picked my body over her father's, all of the women chimed their agreement, and I swept my eyes to each of them, fixing their faces and their admiring glances in my mind as permanently as it holds my name. That was a life-changing moment.

I didn't want to leave the beach after that. For about an hour, I roamed it casually, comfortably, and, quite honestly, with a good bit of pride. I know, of course, that I'm no real hunk. I never really wanted to be, if you want to know the final truth. I simply want to feel good about myself. And perhaps a little rambunctious at times.

I came back to my house, pulled out a letter with a picture attached to its top left corner, and dialed the number at the bottom of the page. I received this particular letter some time ago, and have hesitated to take it seriously, since it's from one of the most heavenly looking women, about thirty, I've ever seen. I do not know this particular woman yet. And I have never accepted an unknown woman's invitation to "spend a few days" at a very exotic tourist destination. And I am not sure if I am going to do that with this particular woman, either, since her line was busy, and my line, after practicing it a dozen times, doesn't sound quite right yet.

But I will tell you this: after a year of working hard, eating right, and living a fantasy, very few things would surprise me anymore. I hate to think of the trouble I may get into soon.

Muscles and Health,

Remar Sutton

PART II

THE
BODY
WORRY
PROGRAM

START UP

If you have thoroughly read the first part of this book, I already like you and think you are very smart and possibly good-looking. You are courageous, too. Reading about all the things that can go wrong with your body, your health, and your mind when you live a godly life, much less a sinful one, makes Stephen King's worst nightmare seem like a fairy tale.

That is why you are going to like this section of *Body Worry*. Because in exchange for a very small amount of time, it is going to show you how to make comfortable changes in your living habits that will literally transform you inside and out. After you've done a little diagnostic work on your eating and activity patterns, the program won't require more than thirty minutes six days a week, and part of that time you'll be doing everyday things, anyway.

Now, I know "just" thirty minutes a day sounds like just thirty minutes in a dentist's chair, drill turning. You don't have the time for that right now, am I correct? Or the courage to endure the pain? And anyway, you were thinking about donating thirty minutes a day to your neighbor, who's planning to run for President, and you think that's more important.

Stop those thoughts right now. The time is there. And you must find it, for the sake of your own health and well-being, and for the

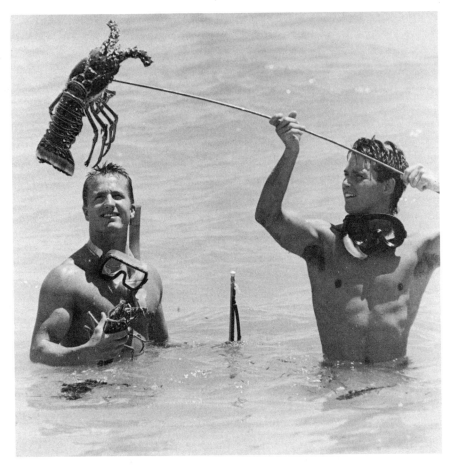

The North Shore of Grand Bahama is inhabited by lots of "crawfish" like these. In one afternoon, Eric and Russ bagged nineteen.

sake of those people you love. The transformation of your health, and even the transformation of your outward appearance will impact on those you love as much as it will on you.

The transformation will happen to every single one of you, too— *if* you will devote that thirty minutes a day and *if* you will be patient. Here "patience" is defined as at least one year from the day you say go. Now, that may seem like a *really* long time right now, but compared to the years it took your body to reach its current state, it is a wink. And though you may not believe it, this isn't going to hurt much anyway. As in any meaningful venture, there will be bumps along the way, but in time what you begin here will become as natural as driving a car.

All *the terrible things you've got to do*

Any of the pieces of the Body Worry program will make you better than you are. But you must do the program as a whole if you plan to hold me to my no-money-back guarantee of a new you. And the package plan isn't that complex, either:

1. Thirty minutes of aerobic activity three times a week. You are already an expert at one of the activities: walking. But you may like our water or biking or jogging programs, too. We show you what to do, and how to mix and match an activity with your particular interests and fitness level. And even if you can't now walk ten feet without resting, you can be *jogging* within a year if you want to. Right now, that may seem like an awful punishment for a job well done, but do not despair. Your body and your mind will tell you it's worth it.

2. Thirty minutes of strength training three times a week. You can do it at home watching television, if you like, and you don't really need equipment. If you wish, do fifteen minutes when you rise and fifteen before you retire. Strength training will take the softness from your flesh, make your bones stronger, shape your stomach, and make everyday tasks easier. Regardless of your age or condition, you'll be able to do these movements, too.

3. Modifications in your eating habits. This book is not about dieting, and it's certainly not about giving up all the things you love. It is about gradually modifying the way you choose foods and the way you eat them, so that you can continue to enjoy eating— even eat deliciously bad foods sometimes—without too much damage to your insides or too much expansion of your outside.

Doing the homework to really understand where you are now takes patience and about four days of record keeping and then evaluation, but after that, the going is easy and the desserts taste as good as ever.

4. Learning the secret Mantra. The only weight loss programs which really seem to make their authors a lot of money (not that I care about that) are the ones written by people with "secrets"— quacks, spiritualists, or what my daddy used to call "funny people."

Well, they laughed all the way to the bank, and, as an experiment, I would like to know what that laughter is like, too. Everything I've said so far in this book, therefore, will fail, and you will get really fat if you don't fix my Mantra in your inner and possibly cosmic consciousness: "Moderate Up and Moderate Down." It can be conveniently abbreviated as "MUD." MUD means looking for opportunities to moderately increase your general activity and intake of healthy foods while also looking for opportunities to moderately decrease the bad things you do.

MUD opportunities are all around us: Take the garbage out yourself rather than having someone else do it; try nibbling on a strawberry rather than a doughnut; do a push-up against a wall when you're restless rather than have a drink; when you have a drink, have one less. MUD thinking is probably more important than all of the well-planned programs in this book. It is the basis of a really healthy mental and physical life. And MUD thinking doesn't really hurt at all. Start thinking that way *right now*, and implant that Mantra firmly in your mind. Now, let's begin to MUDdle our way through the plan.

One thing before we get to work

What condition are you in right now? You must know the answer to that question before going any further. The steps which follow will help you answer it accurately.

In addition, you're going to need a good spiral-ring notebook pretty soon to record this personal evaluation and to start charting your future, so you might want to get one now before reading further.

What about a physical?

- If you answered "yes" to many of the questions on pages 191–192, if you are over forty, if you have any known health problems such as high blood pressure, if you are really a sedentary person (regardless of your age), you should have a physical before going on any further. Page 190 gives you the elements of a really complete one. *Turn to the health questionnaire on page 191 and list all of your negative health factors (those questions answered "yes") in your notebook.*

- If you have the time and the money, you should probably have a physical anyway. Benchmarks are important in any physical fitness program, and you will want to know your body's true but depressing state at the beginning of your program in order to really appreciate its state a year from now.
- Whether you have a physical or not, you should know these things before going on further. *Put the results in your notebook.*

Your maximum exercising heart rate at several levels of difficulty. Your maximal heart rate—the number you should *never* go above— is roughly 220 minus your age. *Compute that number and put it in your notebook.* Generally speaking, you should never, ever push yourself even close to that level. Therefore, compute your maximum exercising heart rate at 60, 70, and 85 percent of that rate and *put those numbers in your notebook.* Your goal is to eventually exercise for thirty minutes of constant work at 60+ percent (but not more than 85 percent) of your maximal heart rate.

Your blood pressure. A machine at a drugstore is better than nothing. If it indicates high blood pressure at all, go to the magazine rack, pick up something interesting (but nothing that will set your blood coursing), and read for ten minutes. Take it again. If it's still high, you *must* go see a doctor. Do not undertake any exercise program without doing so.

Your cholesterol count. You should know these numbers as well as you should know your blood pressure. Have at least a total count done. If that number is high for your age and sex, have a cholesterol ratio (HDL to LDL) done. It's a hassle to do this, but it can truthfully save your life. Call the local chapter of the American Heart Association if you need to find a convenient place to be tested.

Tests at health fairs and the like: All testing used to be time-consuming, but on-the-spot testing machines are increasingly available. These "pin prick" tests are accurate and cheap, but give you only your total cholesterol count.

Your pulse. You really do have one, and it will probably slow down as you become more physically fit. Leaning to find your pulse isn't hard, either; it just takes a little practice. Try placing your fingers on your neck just under your jaw. Be very still, and you will probably feel your carotid artery pumping. (Be gentle when finding this pulse. Pressing the carotid artery too hard results in lowering the heart rate almost immediately in some people, giving a false heart-rate reading.) Or practice putting your fingers on your wrist. The key is to be very still. Count your pulses for six seconds, then add a zero to get your beats per minute. For example, eight beats in six seconds is eighty beats per minute. If it's hard to count six on your watch, count for ten seconds and multiply by six.

Your weight.   Weight can be very deceiving and in the extreme certainly depressing, but it is an accurate measure of change over time. Weigh yourself in the morning after you have gone to the bathroom and before you eat or drink. Don't weigh more than once per week, and always try to weigh on the same day of the week.

Your measurements.   Over the course of the year, the changes that will take place here will mean a lot to you. So ignore the terror the numbers may bring you now, and don't cheat when you measure. You'll probably need someone to help you. If you can, find a good blank wall to trace your outline onto and mark where each of these measurements are taken. Use the same marks every two months to chart your progress. *List your beginning stats in your notebook.*

- Height.
- Chest size, both expanded and flat.
- Stomach size, with no sucking in.
- Waist size with no sucking in.
- Thigh about midway between your hip and your knee.
- Biceps flexed and unflexed. You may or may not be interested in muscle growth this year, but you will need these measurements anyway.

Your body-fat content.   If you're really going to be gung ho this year, have yourself weighed underwater at a sports testing center, or have your fat measured by a qualified caliper user at a health club. At the very least, do a pinch test on yourself. Read about this again on page 6. *Summarize your body-fat situation in your notebook.*

What you look like on film.   If you have a Polaroid, use that; if not, use regular film. But take pictures of yourself from all angles; use a mirror if you have to, but let someone else do the snapping if you're brave enough. Wear as few clothes as your heart can stand. *Tape these pictures in the front of your spiral-ring notebook,* and look at them every morning as you think "MUD." You might want to take pictures every three months.

Your current aerobic fitness level

THE BEST TEST

How healthy is your heart and its support systems right now? If you had to make a real exertion—for instance, to run for your life from a crazed swoon walker—could your heart provide the pumping power needed to run far enough to escape? Even if you're weak right now, knowing your limitations might help you keep away from crazed swoon walkers in the first place.

You, therefore, need to know your limits right now. As noted earlier, the test which will most accurately measure your aerobic fitness and your limits is a maximal exertion stress test, usually performed on a treadmill or stationary bicycle. If you wish, have such a stress test at a really good testing center. Remember to be certain a doctor is within walking range, make sure the clinic uses at least a seven-lead EKG machine, and make sure the test is a "maximal" test (one that exercises you until you can go no further and is given by a qualified technician).

SOMETHING NEARLY AS GOOD AND A LOT CHEAPER

Dr. James Rippe and his colleagues at the University of Massachusetts, supported by the Rockport Shoe Company, have developed a walking test to measure fitness. The following test has been adapted from the larger test, which is more specific by age and heart-rate measurement, but this one is very useful for our purposes.[1]

If you're between the ages of thirty and sixty-nine, do this test before reading any further. If you have any known health problems, are greatly overweight, or a virtual slug when it comes to movement, don't do this test, however. Talk with your doctor about what's the best assessment for you and then skip to the walking section.

The walking test. Put on comfortable clothes and shoes and find a flat, smooth course one mile in length. Use a school facility if you can, or measure off one mile at any other safe place such as a large shopping center parking lot. Walk the mile as fast as you can, comfortably. Don't stroll, unless that's your true best effort, but push yourself a little. Time your walk.

How to know you're not pushing yourself too hard. You could obviously check your pulse. As we said, it should *never* go above your maximal rate. But there's an easier way to gauge your effort, and you should learn it right now. It's called the Borg Scale of Perceived Exertion, and in most cases will give you a safe understanding of your exertion level. The scale looks like this:

RATING OF PERCEIVED EXERTION

6	
7	Very, very light
8	
9	Very light
10	
11	Fairly light
12	
13	Somewhat hard [moderately hard]
14	
15	Hard
16	
17	Very hard
18	
19	Very, very hard [maximal]

Source: G. V. Borg *Medicine and Science in Sports and Exercise,* 14:377–87, 1982.

Regardless of your fitness level, consider 6 an easy stroll. Regardless of your fitness level, consider 19 an effort that feels as if it will kill you. For the purposes of your fitness test, you want to feel that your effort is about 12 to 13—somewhat hard, but a level at which you can still speak without gasping for breath.

What your one-mile walk will tell you. Right now, it's not important how long it takes you to cover the mile. Some of you might need to take a little camping gear along. Some of you might rightfully decide to stop walking after a few hundred feet. Definitely stop if you begin to feel uncomfortable. Watch out for MUD puddles. But if you make it, here is how your time stacks up against the rest of the world:[2]

WALKING FITNESS TEST

Fitness Level	Male Time	Female Time
Excellent	10 min.:12 sec.	11 min.:40 sec.
Good	10:13–11:42	11:41–13:08
High average	11:43–13:13	13:09–14:36
Low average	13:14–14:44	14:37–16:04
Fair	14:45–16:23	14:37–16:04
Poor	16:24 +	17:32 +

If you don't have any physical handicaps, and if you really did try, anything over 13 minutes for men and 14 minutes for women means you really do need to take a very serious interest in your health. And don't think your age is an excuse here, either. Being older doesn't necessarily mean you are automatically weaker in a cardiovascular sense. But don't be discouraged. When I started my remake, I made it one block walking. Within three months, I was jogging twenty minutes nonstop. *Put your results in your notebook.* You will use this result to help you decide on an aerobic activity and to help you gauge future progress.

How *ow do you rate on the overall stamina scale?*

Your aerobic fitness is obviously the most important fitness for your health, but having strength and endurance is important, too. It's nice to know things don't seem as heavy as they used to, or that you have more stamina for daily tasks and for fun. You, therefore, might want to take this sit-up test developed by the Cooper Clinic. It's a good gauge of your overall endurance and strength, and does wonders to tighten stomachs, as we'll see later. If you have back problems, or are very obese, you should do these very gently or not at all until you are in reasonable shape.

Timed sit-ups. With your knees bent and someone holding your feet, place your hands across your chest. Sit up just enough so that your lower back raises off the ground, if possible, and then lower yourself completely. Do as many repetitions as you can in sixty seconds.

How did you do? Here are the scales for both women and men:[3]

BODY WORRY

WOMEN'S SIT-UPS PER MINUTE

Category	AGE 20–29	30–39	40–49	50–59
Excellent	52+	42+	38+	37+
Good	41–51	33–41	27–37	26–36
Fair	30–40	24–32	15–26	14–25
Poor	19–29	14–23	6–14	5–13
Very poor	8–18	5–13	1–5	0–4

MEN'S SIT-UPS PER MINUTE

Category	AGE 20–29	30–39	40–49	50–59	60–69
Excellent	51+	49+	47+	44+	44+
Good	42–50	40–48	37–46	32–43	32–43
Fair	34–41	31–39	26–36	20–31	18–31
Poor	25–33	22–30	15–25	7–19	4–17
Very poor	17–24	13–21	5–14	0–6	0–3

You will be making large-scale improvements here during the year, so don't be discouraged if your results are in the "already deceased" category. *Put your results in your notebook.*

Other important things for your notebook. Feel the flesh on your upper arm. Look very honestly at your shape. Think about your energy level. *Read through the items already in your notebook, take an honest look at yourself, and then sum up your general feeling about your body and your health in a paragraph or so.* Now write a paragraph about how you got there.

And, finally, get in the habit of setting some goals for yourself in all of the areas where you plan improvement. Be specific, realistic, and patient. Set your goals after completing any base-line measurement or activity and *put them in your book at that time.* If you did ten sit-ups in a minute, your goal might be to add five more per week to that exercise. If it took you sixteen minutes to walk a mile, your goal might be to cut one minute from the mile each month for six months. Make goal-setting a part of your thinking. And while you're at it, here's one more thing to think about: *the Mantra and the blood oath.*

I forgot to tell you one other thing about the Body Worry plan, the thing that goes along with the Mantra, and it harkens back to the days of chivalry and a person's real word of honor.

We are actually about to begin your activity. So I want you to face true east (in the direction of Grand Bahama Island) and promise me you will be faithful to the plan for at least three months, regardless of any imagined laughter or amusement on the part of others and regardless of any fits of discouragement which may attack you. *Nothing can stop you for three months*—repeat that. *Moderate Up and Moderate Down*—repeat that. *You will never be too busy*—repeat that lots of times. There is nothing more important to your health and well-being than the efforts you are undertaking right now. You can now turn from the east. But keep muttering: *MUD, MUD, MUD.*

Choosing your basic aerobic activity

Later, you can mix and match these, if you like, but for now choose one.

1. Walking. If you are really sedentary (no movement other than necessary movement), really overweight, and really opposed to anything that looks like hard work, choose walking. Or if walking is simply the activity most pleasant to you, choose it for your aerobic activity.

Equipment: Good shoes designed specifically for walking and brightly colored clothes appropriate for the season. If you plan to walk in the sun, get a good wide-brimmed hat, too.

Walking is a great thing to do with others. Any ideas on the right person or persons? Incidentally, don't worry about weather. We'll tell you lots of ways to walk to avoid the temperature or humidity.

In time, if you want to, your walking program will get you ready to jog a little. Never more than twenty minutes, though. If you in your wildest dreams think you may want to try a little jogging, buy good jogging shoes rather than walking shoes.

2. Jogging. Even if jogging didn't do you any good health-wise (and it certainly does), I would recommend it for the self-satisfaction it invariably brings. Don't misunderstand me; I *hate* it when I'm doing it. But it makes you feel real good if done in moderation. If you're reasonably healthy, you can be a jogger regardless of your age, too. An eighty-seven-year-old lady really did outrun me not long ago.

Equipment: Good jogging shoes, loosely fitting clothes suitable for the season, a hat, and a runner's cassette player/radio, if you like music. These machines with their earphones also make you look very professional. Try to find a friend to begin this program with.

3. Biking.   A good stationary bike can give you a great workout, and it can fit right in front of the television or by the phone, too. Biking outside provides its own interest and seems to do a lot for your tranquillity quotient. Indoors or out, biking doesn't jar your joints, either.

Equipment: A good bike. We'll show you how to choose one later. A helmet, if you plan to bike outside or fall off your stationary bike. If you don't plan to wear a helmet outside, don't bike.

4. Water sports.   Water is about the best medium for exercise. It increases resistance, lessens impact, puts the least stress on joints, feels good, and can work your whole body. The water can be a good place to start if you have arthritis, gippy knees or ankles, or are seriously overweight. And you don't have to swim, either.

Equipment: A bathing suit, swim goggles, and a swimming pool or very large bowl.

Choosing your activity

You might want to read the section on each activity, or you might know for sure you are only going to walk or that you really like one type of activity. That's fine. But choose one activity and read that section carefully. When you have finished that section and gathered up your equipment, I'll see you back here.

The night before you begin.   Starting tomorrow, three days a week, you are going to begin to make a better heart, stronger bones, happy blood, and to build some important habits. So take your notebook, and do the following:

1. Open your notebook to a clean "spread," and put tomorrow's date on the top left corner. That date is the start of your three-month minimum commitment, and those two pages will eventually detail your aerobic, strength, and eating activities for the week.

Now, I know this is beginning to sound complicated, but it isn't going to be. Be calm.

2. Copy your aerobic program for the first week onto the left page, and put the days of the week you'll be doing that program. Be sure and have at least one day of rest between each session. Use this page for any other notes. For instance, if you're planning to be in a pool, don't forget your goggles and towel. And your bathing suit.

If you are planning to measure distance covered or to time any of your activities, you'll want to write your accomplishments for each exercise period down on this page, too. For instance, if you are beginning a walking program, you'll want to track your improvements in distance and/or time.

The first day. Start your record keeping and note taking right now. Use at least one page for each week's aerobic activities, and write some comments each week about how you are feeling. You'll enjoy these later.

Don't push yourself too hard today, either. Most people feel very plucky on Day One, overdo it, and die on Day Two. Follow the program—even if you feel as though you're in super slow motion. Remember you promised to be patient.

Every aerobic day. Try to exercise at the same time each day. Habits build easier that way. And don't forget to think about MUD as the day goes on.

Each week flip to a new page in your notebook, update your routine, take a deep breath, and go to work.

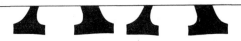

THE AEROBICS PROGRAMS

Before you begin any program

Whatever the aerobic activity you've chosen, you'll want to read the following about warming up and cooling down before taking your first step, pedal, or stroke. If you plan to exercise outdoors, be sure to read the tips for exercising in warm and cool weather, too.

Warm-up and cool-down

Especially if you are a nonexerciser, warming up and cooling down are two safety habits you must start thinking about now.

Warming up gets your blood flowing, helps you test the effects of a specific movement before you do it more strenuously, and generally gives your body some warning that weird things are about to happen. Your heart rate goes up slowly rather than dramatically; oxygen is actually distributed to your working tissues better. Each exercise section will talk about specific warm-ups, so do read them and obey them, preferably facing east toward Grand Bahama.

Cool-downs are probably more important than warm-ups. Cool-downs let your heart gradually adjust to a lighter load; they help

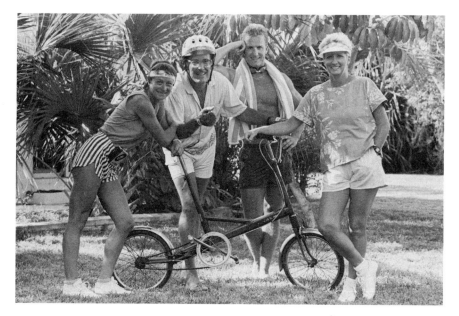

Four sports do four sports. *Marian Wilson is the jogger, "Doc" Clement the biker, Eric the swimmer, and Judy Graham the walker. Notice the museum-quality bike, complete with shock absorber. Doc says it's very old, and its brother lives in a museum in England. My friends are smiling because aerobic activity makes you healthy. They also were saying cheese. Low fat, of course.*

in the removal of metabolic wastes and prevent blood from pooling in the legs.[1] Pooled blood doesn't reach the brain and can make you faint or worse.

Cool-downs are easy to do, too. Simply do whatever you were doing at a much slower pace until your heart rate returns to normal or at least slows to below 100 beats per minute.

Exercising in the heat

Around noon each day here on the island, when the temperature is in the eighties or higher, I see a few jocks out jogging along at full pace, sweating away, looking rather proud of their ability to work out in the heat. Every time I see them, I yearn for the ambulance concession here, for sooner or later their foolishness is going to catch up with them.

For any of us, exercising in the heat and full sun puts an enormous stress on our circulatory system. Even without exercise, your body has to work hard just to cool itself down from the elements. But if you're foolish enough to add to that work by heating up your body even more, you are asking for serious health trouble.

That's why your aerobic exercise should, if at all possible, be in the morning or evening if you plan to exercise outside during the hot months. And even with that precaution, there are some other things you should do to help your body cool itself:

- Wear light clothing, both in color and material.
- If your shirt becomes soaked from sweat (what an awful thought, but it's going to happen), leave it on. A wet shirt facilitates evaporation and cool-down.
- Don't ever wear rubber or plastic weight loss suits. They are *murder* on your cooling system.
- Drink cool water before, during, and after exercise, if possible. And don't let your thirst button be the judge of your need here, either. Thirst is not a good indicator of your body's water needs. Ideally, you should drink about two cups (sixteen ounces) of water thirty minutes or so before beginning to exercise, and a cup or two every fifteen minutes during your exercise, especially if it's hot and humid.
- Pour water on your head, if you don't mind looking funny. A lot of heat is pushed off from our heads. But don't do this in lieu of drinking; it's always better to put water inside your body rather than outside.

ARE YOU PRONE TO HEAT ILLNESS?
If you are overweight, really out of shape, or not used to the outside temperature, you are probably more prone to heat illness, so take it easy and be cool.

WARNINGS OF TROUBLE AHEAD
Heat cramps, cramping and spasms in your muscles, occur when you are dehydrated and/or generally working too hard. Stop exercising immediately, seek shade (a cool place), and drink cool water.

Heat exhaustion is worse and far more dangerous. You will probably have a headache and/or dizziness, and will be sweating profusely. Stop exercising immediately, find a cool place to lie down, and drink cool water. If you have heat exhaustion, *do not* exercise for the rest of the day, and drink lots of additional water over the next twenty-four hours.

Heat stroke you won't know about when it happens, so don't ever push yourself that far. With heat stroke your sweating process shuts down; your skin becomes dry and hot immediately; you become confused and eventually pass out. A person with heat stroke can die quickly without prompt medical attention. If you see a fellow exerciser with these symptoms, *get help* and try to keep the person cool with ice packs or cold towels until medical help arrives.

Boy, all that is enough to make you want to exercise when it's cold!

Exercising in the cold

Guess what? There are things to watch out for here, too. For instance, dehydration can still occur even if you're out exercising in a blizzard.[2] Your trachea and lungs don't like the feel of cold air any more than you may. They warm that air up and moisturize it by pulling heat from your body and moisture from your tissues. This means you need to drink cool water in cold weather, too.

Wear layers of clothing.   Layers trap warm air better than one garment, and layers allow you to peel off clothes as your body warms up.

If you have any type of heart disease.   Even if your doctor has said it's okay to exercise, ask him if it's okay to exercise in really cold weather. Some studies show that breathing cold air promotes chest pain in some people with already existing heart problems.[3]

MUD applies to workout conditions, too.   You want to exercise in moderate temperatures, if possible. If you have to exercise in extreme ones, moderate your exercise.

Before going on to the specific aerobic programs, I'd like to thank Christopher Scott, *Body Worry* physiologist, for overseeing their design. His experience and insight ensured they'd be effective and interesting.

Lots of fun things to do

The specific aerobic programs follow—choose one for now.

Walking

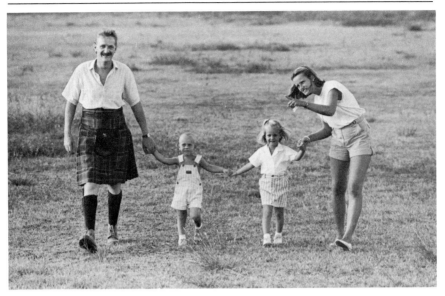

Walking is good for the soul, and good for the family, too. It's also cooler when you wear your kilt. John's dad is chieftain of the Munro Clan of Scotland. Sylvia is from Luxembourg. You can find the Munros taking long walks just about any day.

There is strolling, which you do when you are arm in arm with someone you love and time has no meaning; and there is walking for aerobic exercise, which should look a lot more as if time is on your mind.

Regardless of the type, walking is one of the best exercises you can undertake, both for your body and your mind. It's less stressful on your joints, something you can do alone or with friends, and is seldom boring. You can even do it in the rain, but watch out for the MUD.

WILL IT GIVE YOU AEROBIC FITNESS?

Yes, but you are going to have to move at more than a stroll if you plan to get your aerobic work over with in thirty minutes. Generally speaking, the faster you walk, the less you have to exercise. Any walking more than what you do now will be good for you strength- and stamina-wise, but your aerobic activity must raise your heart-beat to a higher level for at least twenty minutes—ideally to your recommended percentage of your maximal rate. Using the Borg Scale of Perceived Exertion (see page 212), that means you need to walk at 12 to 14, somewhat hard to hard. Five minutes of slow walking to warm up and five minutes of slow walking to cool down use up your thirty minutes of aerobic time nicely.

WHAT ABOUT SIMPLY WALKING LONGER AND SLOWER?

If you have more time and aren't capable of walking too fast, we are going to present you with a walking program that will eventually have you walking four miles in around an hour. Your aerobic benefits will probably be the same as a much faster pace for twenty minutes.

WHY CAN'T I JUST WALK? WHO NEEDS A PROGRAM?

You can. But go easy the first week. Find a safe place to walk, and measure your distance and time, and *put both measurements in your notebook.* If you want, measure your distance in blocks at first. As you gain strength, try to cover the same distance in a better time.

EQUIPMENT REVIEW

Be sure you have good shoes designed specifically for walking and brightly colored comfortable clothes appropriate for the season. If you plan to walk in the sun, don't forget your wide-brimmed hat, too. If your head looks like mine, wear a very wide brim.

WHERE TO WALK?

Find a route that's safe, visually interesting, and appropriate for your ability level. Here are some good bets:

- A measured track at a local school, community center, or public park. If weather's a problem, find a school or gym with an enclosed area.
- Level playing areas like football, soccer, or baseball fields. City parks are nice, too.
- If you are an urban dweller, your city may have jogging trails, walking courses, or PARS courses. PARS courses are fitness trails that have equipment and plaques along the way that suggest additional exercises for each stop. Check with your city's parks department.
- A shopping mall. Many malls are even sponsoring "mall walkers" programs that usually allow walkers in before the stores open. Malls are safe, cool in summer, warm in winter, and weatherproof.

- Pick out a good course near home. Why not pick out several, with different terrains, if possible? Measure them in blocks or use your car's odomoter.

TIME- AND BOREDOM-SAVING IDEAS

If you don't live too far from work, as you get stronger, think about walking home from work sometime. Even after an impossibly frustrating day at the prison, the walk will turn you into a decent and rested person by the time you reach your front door.

WHERE WILL IT ALL LEAD?

Hulda Crooks of Loma Linda, California, started walking seriously when she was fifty, a determined walker barely five feet tall. She decided to start walking up mountains, most particularly Mount Whitney, which she has now walked up twenty-two times.[4] Mount Whitney is 14,494 feet high.

To increase her stamina, Hulda added a little jogging to her mountain regimen at age seventy. Her last successful climb was at age ninety-one. Are there any mountains near you?

THE WALKING PROGRAM

This program was devised by Dr. Herbert deVries.[5] We've divided it into weeks. If you like, you may walk five days a week or every day; but we promised you'd only have to do it three days a week, walking every other day.

	DURATION	DISTANCE
Week 1		
Day		
1	20 min.	1 mile
2	25	1.25
3	30	1.5
Week 2		
Day		
4	35	1.75
5	40	2.0
6	45	2.25
Week 3		
Day		
7	50	2.5
8	55	2.75
9	60	3.0

	DURATION	*DISTANCE*
Week 4		
Day		
10	32	2.0
11	36	2.25
12	40	2.5
Week 5		
Day		
13	44	2.75
14	48	3.0
15	52	3.25
Week 6		
Day		
16	56	3.50
17	60	3.75
18	64	4.0

WHEN YOU FINISH THIS PROGRAM

When you have worked your way up to this point in the program, you may want simply to continue walking, gradually decreasing your times, or you can try our jogging program in the next section, or perhaps some biking and swimming. You will feel so good after Week 6, you may even want to start some serious jogging. That's great! Keep going, and keep stretching your limits.

Jogging

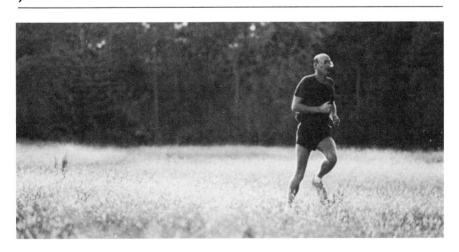

I really do hate jogging when I'm doing it, every step. But I do it because I feel so much better physically and mentally after each twenty-minute session. And that's all I jog, too. Five minutes of warm-up walking, twenty of jogging at a rather stately pace, and five of walking again.

You may remember that I couldn't exactly jog twenty minutes when I started my program, however. I walked a few steps, then jogged a few, then walked until my heart was back in my body again. At the very *most*, that's the way you should start your program, too.

Jogging, unlike walking, throws your body into overtime quickly. You, therefore, need to know your physical condition before you start (you did have that physical, didn't you?), and you need to warn your body before you begin to beat up on it.

A MEASURED WALKING-JOGGING PROGRAM TO START WITH
Herbert deVries, one of the authorities on exercise and aging, developed the program we present to you here. It is generally safe for people of about any age, if you don't have health problems that might be exacerbated by this much activity.

CAN I JUST DEVELOP MY OWN PROGRAM?
If you don't want to follow a set program, yes. But warm up for five minutes by walking briskly before you begin to jog. Start walking again when you reach your maximum exertion level. Generally speaking, you should be able to talk normally without gasping for breath. Start jogging again when you've calmed down. At first, you can measure your progress by just counting telephone poles. On Day 1, you might jog past one. You will be surprised how quickly you'll be jogging by dozens.

REMEMBER YOUR PERCEIVED EXERTION
You *never* want to push your heart rate past 85 percent of your maximal level, which is ____ percent (fill in the blank, please). Take a minute to read page 212 again on our Scale of Perceived Exertion. You want to aim for a 12 to 13. Or practice taking your pulse a time or two before you begin your first walk-jog.

THE TRANSITION TO STRAIGHT JOGGING
Depending on your condition, you may be jogging within weeks. But don't be impatient. Keep increasing the number of telephone

poles you can pass nonstop, and eventually you will be a twenty-minute jogger.

GEAR REVIEW
Good jogging shoes, loosely fitting clothes suitable for the season, a hat, and a runner's cassette player/radio, if you like music or believe that loud sound blocks pain. Incidentally, try to find a friend to suffer with.

WHERE TO JOG?
Level surfaces are important, and soft surfaces are nice. Running over uneven terrain, or over any surface with pothole potential, can lead to injuries. One turn of the ankle and your aerobic program may be over for a while.

So look for the best level surface you can find—a jogging track at a school, community center, or public park; a sports playing field; a golf course; or an indoor track, if weather's a problem at times. Many of us run on pavement because it's both convenient and level. It's not soft, however, so make sure you have good shoes if you run on the street or sidewalk.

WHAT TO DO WHEN YOU CAN JOG TWENTY MINUTES
First, accept the thanks of your heart. And then think about jogging a little further or a little faster. Once you've reached the twenty-minute level, you can start trying to beat your own record.

THE WALK-JOG PROGRAM
Set up an entire page in your booklet to keep a record of your progress here.

This program has been adapted from Dr. deVries's program.[6] As he designed it, you would have run six days a week; but I promised you only three. If you registered fair or better on the overall fitness test and find that you are not challenged at all by the first weeks program, it's okay to try starting at Week 5. But, don't overdo it. At each level you increase the sets by one each day. That means on Week 1, Day 1, you would walk fifty steps and jog fifty steps five times. On Week 1, Day 2, you would walk fifty steps and jog fifty for six times. On the last day of Week 2 you would repeat your fifty/fifty walk-jog ten times. When you reached the new level at Week 3, you'd drop back to five repetitions and work up.

WEEKS	JOG	WALK	NUMBER OF WALK-JOG SETS
1 & 2	50 steps	50 steps	5 to 10
3 & 4	50	40	5 to 10
5 & 6	50	30	5 to 10
7 & 8	50	20	5 to 10
9 & 10	50	10	5 to 10
11 & 12	75	10	5 to 10
13 & 14	100	10	5 to 10
15 & 16	125	10	5 to 10
17 & 18	150	10	5 to 10
19 & 20	175	10	5 to 10
21 & 22	200	10	5 to 10

CONTINUING JOGGING WITH THE BODY WORRY PROGRAM

At Week 23 you enter the Body Worry jogging program. At this level you will vary the intensity level of the exercise to suit yourself. On the Scale of Perceived Exertion, that might mean you want to work at a 12 to 13 for the first and last day of your three-day workout and a 13 to 14 for the middle day. You may find that taking your heart rate allows you to target your intensity level a little more accurately as well. That's not hard to do either, because you only have to know three figures—your approximate heart rate at 60, 70, and 85 percent of your maximal level. Just find your numbers on the following chart. Then it will be easy to compare them to a 10-second heart-rate count.

For example, if you are forty-three and want to work at a 60 percent intensity level, your pulse should be 18 beats in 10 seconds. It should be 20 beats for a 70 percent effort and 25 beats for an 85 percent effort.

HEART RATES FOR VARIOUS INTENSITY LEVELS

INTENSITY AND 10-SEC. COUNT

AGE	60%	10-sec. count	70%	10-sec. count	85%	10-sec. count
20	120	20	140	23	170	28
25	117	20	137	23	166	28
30	114	19	133	22	162	27
35	111	19	129	21	158	26
40	108	18	126	21	153	25

AGE	60%	10-sec. count	70%	10-sec. count	85%	10-sec. count
45	105	18	123	20	149	25
50	102	17	119	20	145	24
55	99	17	115	19	140	23
60	96	16	112	19	136	23
65	93	16	109	18	132	22
70	90	15	105	18	128	21
75	87	15	102	17	123	20
80	84	14	98	16	119	20

A NOTE OF CAUTION

If you do vary intensity levels to suit yourself, *do not push yourself too hard*. If you feel you are overexerting, slow down immediately and walk (don't stop still) until you are ready to resume jogging. If you are taking your pulse to determine intensity level, do so at the beginning of the walk periods.

Week 23
Jog for 2 minutes,
walk for 1 minute;
do this for 2 miles.

Week 24
Jog for 3 minutes,
walk for 1 minute;
do this for 2 miles.

Week 25
Jog for 4 minutes,
walk for 1 minute;
do this for 2 miles.

Week 26
Jog for 5 minutes,
walk for 1 minute;
do this for 2.5 miles.

Week 27
Jog for 5 minutes,
walk for 30 seconds;
do this for 2–2.5 miles.

Week 28
Jog for 6 minutes,
walk for 30 seconds;
do this for 2.5 miles.

Week 29
Jog for 7 minutes,
walk for 30 seconds;
do this for 2.5 miles.

Week 30
Jog for 8 minutes,
walk for 30 seconds;
do this for 2.5–3 miles.

Week 31
Jog for 9 minutes,
walk for 30 seconds;
do this for 3 miles.

Week 32
Jog for 10 minutes,
walk for 30 seconds;
do this for 3 miles.

Week 33
Jog for as long as possible,
then walk briefly if tired;
do this for 3 miles.

Week 34
Continue with this until
you can jog successfully for
the entire 3 miles.

Biking

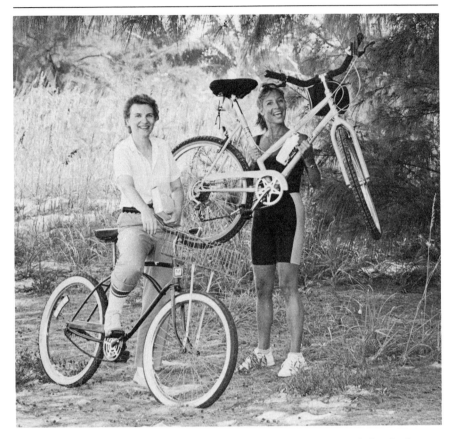

Mary Abbott bikes for fun. Kathy Bater (the "Smart Lady" of Chapter 3) bikes for serious exercise. Kathy also uses her bike occasionally for a curl or two. Don't try this unless your back insurance is paid up.

First, we're going to talk about real, all-American bikes that tour you as they make you healthy, and then we're going to talk about stationary bikes, which make you just as healthy but offer pretty boring scenery.

Biking is an *excellent* aerobic exercise. It doesn't jar you (as long as you don't fall off) and will definitely make you feel young again. When I started my remake, I hadn't been on a bike in twenty years. But the second I slung my leg over, both the nice memories and skills came back to me.

Biking takes you over a lot more territory than walking or running. Generally speaking, you need to bike four miles to get the same workout as you get with one mile of brisk walking. But that's nice, isn't it? Seeing your neighborhood from the seat of a bike is a lot better than seeing it from a car.

BUYING A BIKE

Unless you're in an extremely hilly area, you don't need to buy one with a dozen gears. You don't even need to buy a "racing" bike, either. You know—those that require you to lean down to grip those funny bars and then invariably put a crick in your neck. If you are riding simply for exercise, not competition, buy the bike that's most comfortable for you. Here on the island balloon-tired mountain bikes are the rage; they allow you to really sit up and enjoy the view.

Do think about how you will use your bike. Do you have nice mountain trails in your area? Other off-the-road-type paths? Wide tires make biking there a lot easier.

If you're worried about balancing a lot, think about a three-wheeler. But make sure the bike has a wide enough stance to give you a low center of gravity.

What size frame? While straddling the frame, the top crossbar should come within one inch of your groin. If the bike you're looking at doesn't have a crossbar, imagine one.

How much money should you spend? Until you're really sure you're going to stick with it, don't spend too much. As a matter of fact, look at used bikes. They can save you over 60 percent and, like used shovels, they aren't really that different from new ones.

The most important adjustments. Other than falling off, which I've done a few times, the only real injuries in biking come from an improperly adjusted seat and the improper use of gears. Having your seat too low places real stress on your knees. Having your gear too low (in the harder gears) does the same thing.

Adjusting the seat. We show you this in pictures, but here's how to do it: Place one pedal in the down position. Straddling the bike with your *heel* on the pedal, your leg should be completely straight. Since you should pedal with the *ball* of your foot, your leg will be slightly bent as you pedal.

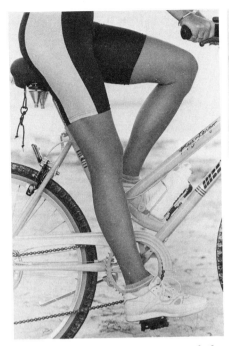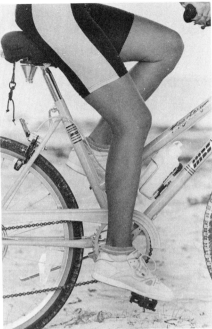

Adjusting your seat on your bike. *A well-adjusted seat is like a well-adjusted mind: it contributes to your well-being. Place one pedal in the down position. Straddle the bike and place your heel on the down pedal. Your leg should be completely straight when the seat is at the right height. Since you pedal with the* ball *of the foot, your leg will be slightly bent as you pedal. To make this adjustment without falling and breaking your neck, have a friend hold the bike for you.*

What gear to use?   The easy way to solve this is to simply have one gear. But having three or five is nice. You should choose a gear that keeps you pedaling *at all times* at your chosen speed, rather than one that has you pedaling and then coasting.

How about a speedometer?   Do get one of these. You can keep up with your miles real easily, and you'll have fun checking your speed, too. *Log your miles in your notebook.* Set up a special page for your biking.

Other doodads.   Don't forget to get a good helmet. Other than that, ride in whatever makes you feel comfortable and stylish. Also think about a basket or two. Baskets make bikes practical for errands, and are oh, so trendy.

THE BIKING PROGRAM

You can use this routine with any type of bike, whether it's with gears, two wheels, three wheels, or even one wheel if you are really coordinated. But because terrain varies so much around the country, try to find a relatively level course for your first four or six weeks of pedaling. We've designed this program with a relatively level course in mind. And at least three pedals a week, too.

How your gears affect the program. Our biking program varies the intensity within a given day's exercise. You, therefore, need to have some way to judge your intensity objective of 12 to 13 on your perceived exertion scale. For example, if you are just starting and have a single-speed bike, varying the speed between 7 and 10 miles per hour can give you that variation: 7 m.p.h. is lower intensity, 10 m.p.h. is higher. As your fitness level increases, you may use speeds of 8 to 12 miles per hour, while still working at a perceived exertion level of 12 to 13.

But speed alone won't work with a geared bicycle because the gears allow the bicycle to work harder than you are. Therefore, choose a gear that allows you to pedal continuously at your target level of intensity. If your low-intensity pace is 7 to 10 miles per hour, set your gears for continuous pedaling at that speed. When you increase your speed, set your gear for continuous pedaling at the new speed.

What about an impromptu program? If you don't want to follow our plan, fine. But remember, your goal is to keep your effort at a 12 or 13 on the Scale of Perceived Exertion. And you want to work up speed and endurance gradually; don't overdo it in the beginning.

Also think about joining a biking club. Call your local bike shops, or your local parks department for the names and numbers of clubs in your area.

THE WEEKLY PROGRAM

The program for each week should be performed at least three times on separate days.

Week 1
1–2 miles at easy
pace, 7–10 m.p.h.

Week 2
2–3 miles at easy
pace, 7–10 m.p.h.

Week 3
3 miles: 2 min. at
lower speed or lower
r.p.m. for each 1 min.
at higher r.p.m. or
speed

Week 4
3–5 miles at 7–10
m.p.h.

Week 5
4–6 miles at 7–10
m.p.h.

Week 6
5–6 miles: 1 min. at
lower speed or lower
r.p.m. for each 1 min.
at higher r.p.m. or
speed

Week 7
4–6 miles at 8–12
m.p.h.

Week 8
5–7 miles at 8–12
m.p.h.

Week 9
6–8 miles: 1 min. at
lower speed or lower
r.p.m. for each 1 min.
at higher r.p.m. or
speed

Week 10
7–10 miles at 8–12
m.p.h.

Week 11
8–10 miles at 8–12
m.p.h.

Week 12
10–12 miles at 8–12
m.p.h.

Week 13
8–12 miles: 1 min. at
lower speed or r.p.m.
for each 2 min. at
high speed or r.p.m.

Week 14
10–15 miles at 8–12
m.p.h.

Week 15
10–15 miles at 10–15
m.p.h.

Week 16
12–17 miles at 10–15
m.p.h.

Week 17
12–17 miles at 12–17
m.p.h.

Week 18
15–20 miles at 12–17
m.p.h.

Week 19
20+ miles at 15+
m.p.h.

Week 20
Individualized program combining heart-rate
percentage (70% or better) and a distance of
40–60 miles per week.

Exercising in water

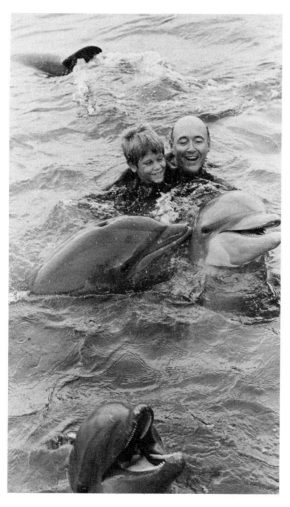

The water world is never boring. John Kruthoffer and I, for instance, do our water exercises with Uno, Stripe, and Kayla. Bimini is swimming laps in the background. He's up to fifty miles a day. John, ten, worked as an assistant trainer with the Dolphin Experience at UNEXSO.

If you have easy access to a safe body of water—a pool, a lake, or a calm cove along the shoreline—think about getting your aerobic exercise right there. Water is probably the best medium for exercise. It increases resistance, lessens stress because it's non-impact, keeps you cool, and generally strengthens your entire body.

And you don't have to be a good swimmer to exercise in water, either. We're going to present you with a good swimming program if that's your particular pleasure, but there are many good things to do in water that have nothing to do with swimming—like our Labor Day Special . . .

OUR SUPER SPECIAL EXERCISE COMBINATION, AVAILABLE FOR A SHORT TIME ONLY

If you're reasonably fit, please don't use this program in lieu of our other programs, but feel free to use it to make your pool time more productive. And once you're comfortable with our exercises here, invent some things yourself or simply duplicate the things you like to do in air while you're in the water. Like to dance? It's better for you in water. Always wanted to do hand-stands? It's doable in water, but please remember to hold your breath. We do not teach CPR here.

GEAR

If you plan to put your head underwater much, wear swimming goggles. If you want to increase the effort of a particular exercise (such as kicking while you hold on to the side of a pool), you might want to get some fins.

A COMBINED STRENGTH AND AEROBIC EXERCISE PROGRAM IN THE WATER

If you are feeling really faint at heart about all this exercise, if you are really out of shape or overweight or feel you are close to death's door from inactivity, if you are so old you remember voting for Roosevelt (Teddy), you can follow this exercise program in lieu of other strength and aerobic work. You can also do it if you simply like the water a lot. The key here is to really work (no loafing) and to eventually do each of these ten exercises for three minutes *at least three times a week*. In the beginning, do each exercise for at least fifteen to thirty seconds—for several sets, if possible.

You will be getting a real aerobic workout when your entire effort seems to be at the 12–13 perceived exertion level for a full thirty minutes, but you will be getting a good strength workout even if you are working at a lower aerobic level.

Incidentally, the first seven of the following ten exercises are based on an extensive water exercise program, *Aqua Dynamics*, developed by experts working with the President's Council on Physical Fitness. (If you'd like, you may obtain the whole program at modest cost from the U.S. Government Printing Office, Washington, D.C. 20402–9325.)

Dr. Arno Jensen developed the last three exercises.

WATER EXERCISES

Write your routine in your notebook. You can see each exercise demonstrated in the pictures below. On many of these exercises you can increase the level of difficulty by moving to slightly deeper water. To get used to the movements without taking this nonwaterproof book in the pool, I suggest you practice the *movement only* (not the level of exertion) out of the water.

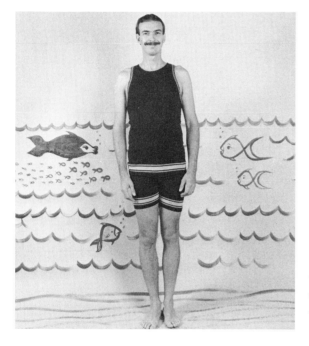

Since you can't see these exercises in the water, we thought we'd have Will McIntyre pose them for you. But we suspect he got his grandfather to do it instead.

1. Stride hops. These work your quadriceps, the front muscles of your upper leg.

Standing in water up to your waist or chest, with your hands on your hips, jump up slightly, and come down, with your left leg forward and your right leg back. Try to move your legs as far forward and back as possible. Repeat until you can do these hops for three minutes. These are great for improving your square-dancing skills, incidentally.

An alternate way to do this would be to simply walk the width of the pool with giant strides, moving faster as your strength increases.

2. Toe bounces.   Just like bouncing on the moon. These strengthen your calves. Stand in water up to your waist or chest. Hold on to the edge of the pool if you need to steady yourself, and stand on your toes. Repeat. Gradually increase your upward push until you are bouncing off the bottom. Work up to three minutes.

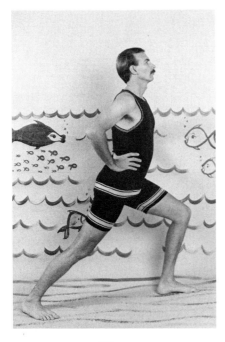 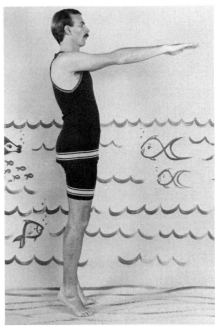

The stride hop, extended position at end of hop.   *The toe bounce, just before take-off.*

3. Walking twists.   They do this at the Carnaval in Rio a lot. In waist-deep water, with your fingers behind your neck, walk forward and twist your body, touching your left elbow to your right knee, right elbow to left knee. Repeat. Work up to three minutes, softly humming a tango as you move.

4. Standing crawl.   This is a standing version of the swimming crawl. Stand in waist- or chest-deep water. Reach out with the right hand and pull your hand through the water, as deep as possible. When your hand is by your thigh, lift it from the water; repeat this procedure with your left hand, etc. This exercise works best in chest-deep water. Work up to three minutes.

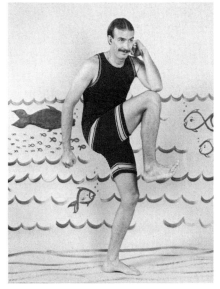 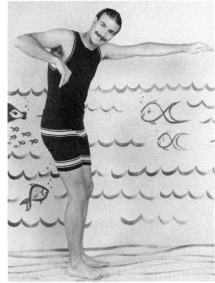

The walking twist, in mid twist. *The standing crawl. Will is just about to begin the stroke with his left arm.*

5. Leg lifts.   They strengthen your hip flexors and help flatten your lower stomach. With your back and hands against the pool wall, raise your left knee to your chest. Straighten your leg as much and as high as possible, and then drop it to the starting position. Repeat this with your right. Three minutes eventually, please.

6. Outward swings.   Do this in chest-deep water. With your back against the poolside and your hands holding on to the gutter, raise your left leg as high as possible in front of you, keeping the leg straight. Swing your leg to the left, until it touches the side of the pool (if possible). Reverse the motion, pulling your leg back through the water until it is in front of you, and then lower it. Repeat this with your other leg. Please don't use violent motions when doing this exercise. Increase your speed, which will automatically increase your effort. Three minutes . . .

7. Front flutter kick.   These are really good for firming up your buttocks. Lying with your stomach in the water, hold on to the side of the pool. With your toes pointed, flutter-kick. Churn up the pool. Keep each leg loose but straight. Work up to three minutes.

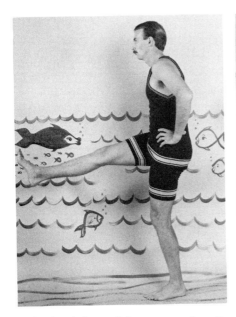

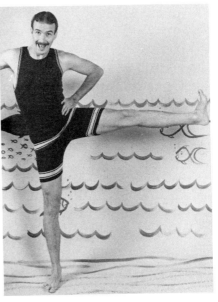

The leg lift. Will has started pulling his leg down through the water to starting position.

The outward swing. This is the position and expression to adopt as you push your leg out and start to swing it back through the water to the front position.

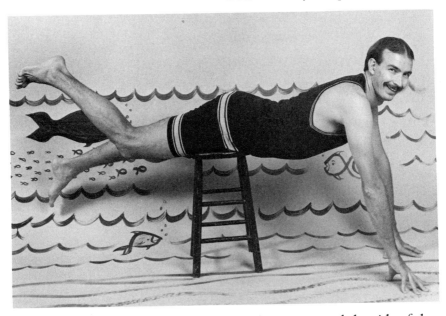

The front flutter kick. With the water for buoyancy and the side of the pool for support, you will not need the stool.

8. Front shoulder raises.   You want your shoulders under water, but your head out of water. You can do this standing or kneeling. With your arms by your side, thumbs touching your hips, raise your arms straight in front of you until they are at water level. Don't bend them much at all. Then forcefully bring them back down to your side. Repeat and build up to three minutes. At first, have your fist clinched. As you become stronger, have your hands open to increase resistance.

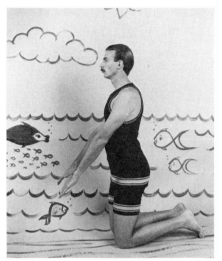 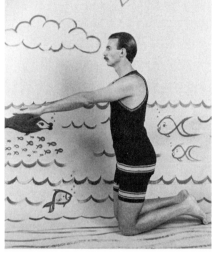

The front shoulder raise. Push up through the water (left) to the surface (right), level with your shoulders. Then pull down.

9. Side shoulder raises.   These are like exercise eight, but are done to the side. With your arms by your side, thumbs touching your hips, raise your arms to the side until they are at water level. Don't bend them much at all. Then forcefully bring them back down to your side. Repeat and build up to three minutes.

10. Underwater clapping.   Great for use at underwater concerts or Disney's Living Seas' exhibit. Stand in waist-deep water with your feet at shoulder width. Bend forward until your chest is in the water. Keep your head out of the water unless you have a snorkel. Hang your arms down as if they were the other two legs of a chair, and bring your palms together, arms straight. Then raise your arms to the side until they just break the surface of the water. Keep them as straight as possible. Repeat, and work up to three minutes. You can also increase intensity by moving faster.

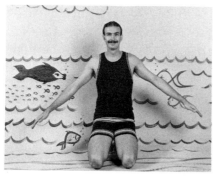 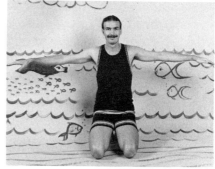

The side shoulder raise. On the way up (left). Top (right), just before pulling down.

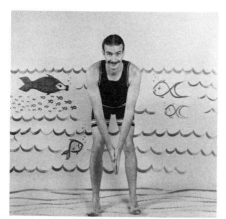 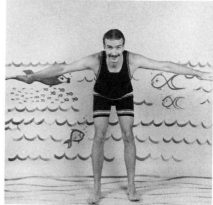

Underwater clapping. Applause, applause! Give yourself a hand for completing a vigorous workout.

AEROBIC SWIMMING PROGRAM

Swimming obviously works a lot of muscles in the entire body. But what we present here is a program primarily designed to make you aerobically fit. Which means you should do some additional strength work, if you are really going to be gung ho on the Sutton system.

Before getting in the water. Since swimming arches the back, experts suggest warming up with reach and toe-touch (knees flexed) stretches as a minimum.[7] We show you how in stretching. You may also want to use some of the water exercises in our previous Labor Day Special as warm-up, and also include a back flutter kick (face and chest to sky).

Judging your aerobic effort in the water. If you are using the Scale of Perceived Exertion to judge your aerobic intensity as you swim, you want to work at the level of 12 to 13, just as you do in other aerobic sports.

Adapting the program to your needs. This lap swimming program is designed to start you slowly and bring you along successfully. You can swim at your own speed, but remember to gradually build your endurance and sustain your aerobic intensity without over-doing it. If you wish to build up your swimming laps at your own pace, remember to use walking in the water or treading water as your rest intervals between laps. Don't just stand there. If you are swimming so far you feel the need to literally stop and rest, rather than walk or tread water, you are pushing yourself too hard on the swim laps.[8]

If you scored in the fair or better category in the general fitness test you took earlier and find the first weeks too easy here, try starting with Week 4 or so. On the other hand, if the first week pushes you and you feel you are not ready to go to Week 2, it's fine to repeat the first week's programs. Repeat any program if your body tells you it needs a little more time. MUD works here, too.

Adapting the program to your pool. God did not create all pools equal or in the same dimensions and depths. Since our program incorporates a lot of walking laps in the beginning, and since many pools with graduated bottoms will be too deep at one end and will, therefore, drown you if you try to follow our program, and since we need you to tell others about this book, here are some strategies for handling different-shaped pools. (The idea here is to keep you moving, incidentally.)

1. Use the outside lane so you can hand-walk down the side of the pool when your feet don't touch.

2. If you tread water easily, you can tread water in place to rest, for about a minute.

3. If you can't float, hold on to the side of the pool for about a minute, gently moving your legs through water.

4. In a home or uncrowded pool, you can walk the width of the shallow area and then return to swimming the length.

Amazing grace.   The definition of "grace" in our swimming program is a completed exercise, regardless of your particular swimming style. Consistent movement is what counts here.

How to read the program.   In the weekly tables that follow "1 × 25" translates into one effort for twenty-five yards. You, therefore, are going to have to know the length of your pool and adjust your program accordingly. If the pool is longer than twenty-five yards, why not leave the program as it is? You'll get a little extra workout.

The strokes.   We suggest the crawl for one of your strokes and then suggest that you alternate breast strokes, side strokes, and back strokes or choose your favorite of these. Please do not wrinkle too much.

Week 1

1 × 25 crawl
2 × 25 walk
1 × 25 crawl
2 × 25 walk
1 × 25 crawl
2 × 25 walk
1 × 25 crawl
2 × 25 walk
Total: 100 yards crawl, 200 yards walk

Week 2

1 × 25 crawl
1 × 25 walk
1 × 25 breast, side, or back stroke (b/s/b)
1 × 25 walk
1 × 25 crawl
2 × 25 walk
Repeat above.
Total: 100 crawl, 50 b/s/b, 150 walk

Week 3

1 × 25 crawl
2 × 25 walk
1 × 50 crawl
2 × 25 walk
1 × 50 crawl
2 × 25 walk
1 × 25 crawl
Total: 150 crawl, 150 walk

Week 4

1 × 25 crawl
1 × 25 b/s/b
1 × 25 walk
1 × 50 crawl
1 × 25 walk
1 × 50 crawl
1 × 25 walk
1 × 25 crawl
1 × 25 b/s/b
1 × 25 walk
Total: 150 crawl, 50 b/s/b, 125 walk

Week 5

1 × 50 crawl
1 × 25 walk
1 × 25 b/s/b
1 × 50 crawl
1 × 25 b/s/b
1 × 25 walk
1 × 50 crawl
1 × 25 walk
Total: 150 crawl, 50 b/s/b, 75 walk

Week 6

1 × 50 crawl
1 × 25 b/s/b
1 × 25 crawl
1 × 25 walk
1 × 25 crawl
1 × 25 walk
Repeat above.
Total: 200 crawl, 50 b/s/b, 100 walk

Week 7

1 × 50 crawl
1 × 25 walk
1 × 50 crawl
1 × 25 b/s/b
1 × 50 crawl
1 × 25 walk
1 × 50 crawl
1 × 25 walk
Total: 200 crawl, 25 b/s/b, 75 walk

Week 8

1 × 50 crawl
1 × 25 walk
1 × 75 crawl
1 × 25 walk
1 × 75 crawl
1 × 25 walk
1 × 50 crawl
1 × 25 walk
Total: 250 crawl, 100 walk

Week 9

1 × 75 crawl
1 × 25 walk
1 × 25 b/s/b
1 × 75 crawl
1 × 25 b/s/b
1 × 25 walk
1 × 75 crawl
1 × 25 walk
Total: 225 crawl, 50 b/s/b, 75 walk

Week 10

1 × 75 crawl
1 × 25 walk
1 × 75 crawl
1 × 25 walk
1 × 75 crawl
1 × 25 walk
1 × 75 crawl
1 × 25 walk
Total: 300 crawl, 100 walk

Intermediate program starts with Week 11.
Week 11

1 × 75 crawl
1 × 25 b/s/b
1 × 25 walk
Repeat 4 times.
Total: 300 crawl, 100 b/s/b, 100 walk

Week 12

1 × 75 crawl
1 × 50 b/s/b
1 × 25 walk
1 × 100 crawl
1 × 25 walk
1 × 50 b/s/b
1 × 75 crawl
1 × 25 walk
1 × 75 crawl
1 × 25 walk
Total: 325 crawl, 100 b/s/b, 100 walk

Week 13

1 × 75 crawl
1 × 25 b/s/b
1 × 100 crawl
1 × 50 walk
Repeat above.
Total: 350 crawl, 50 b/s/b, 100 walk

Week 14

1 × 100 crawl
1 × 50 b/s/b
1 × 100 crawl
1 × 50 b/s/b
1 × 100 crawl
1 × 50 b/s/b
1 × 100 crawl
Total: 400 crawl, 150 b/s/b

Week 15

1 × 100 crawl
1 × 50 b/s/b
1 × 125 crawl
1 × 50 b/s/b
1 × 125 crawl
1 × 50 b/s/b
1 × 100 crawl
Total: 400 crawl, 150 b/s/b

Week 16

1 × 100 crawl
1 × 75 b/s/b
1 × 150 crawl
1 × 75 b/s/b
1 × 150 crawl
1 × 75 b/s/b
1 × 100 crawl
Total: 500 crawl, 225 b/s/b

Week 17

1 × 100 crawl
1 × 50 b/s/b
Repeat above 5 times.
Total: 500 crawl, 250 b/s/b

Week 18

1 × 100 crawl
1 × 75 b/s/b
1 × 200 crawl
1 × 75 b/s/b
1 × 200 crawl
1 × 75 b/s/b
1 × 100 crawl
Total: 600 crawl, 225 b/s/b

Week 19

1 × 150 crawl
1 × 50 b/s/b
1 × 200 crawl
1 × 75 b/s/b
Repeat above.
Total: 700 crawl, 250 b/s/b

Advanced program begins with Week 20.

Week 20

1 × 150 crawl
1 × 50 b/s/b
1 × 250 crawl
1 × 75 b/s/b
1 × 250 crawl
1 × 50 b/s/b
1 × 150 crawl
Total: 800 crawl, 175 b/s/b

Week 21

1 × 200 crawl
1 × 50 b/s/b
1 × 250 crawl
1 × 100 b/s/b
1 × 250 crawl
1 × 50 b/s/b
1 × 200 crawl
Total: 900 crawl, 200 b/s/b

Week 22

1 × 200 crawl
1 × 75 b/s/b
1 × 300 crawl
1 × 75 b/s/b
1 × 300 crawl
1 × 75 b/s/b
1 × 200 crawl
Total: 1,000 crawl, 225 b/s/b

Week 23

1 × 200 crawl
1 × 50 b/s/b
Repeat 5 times.
Total: 1,000 crawl, 250 b/s/b

Week 24

1 × 200 crawl
1 × 75 b/s/b
1 × 350 crawl
1 × 75 b/s/b
1 × 350 crawl
1 × 75 b/s/b
1 × 200 crawl
Total: 1,100 crawl, 225 b/s/b

Week 25

1 × 200 crawl
1 × 50 b/s/b
1 × 250 crawl
1 × 50 b/s/b
1 × 300 crawl
1 × 50 b/s/b
1 × 250 crawl
1 × 50 b/s/b
1 × 200 crawl
Total: 1,200 crawl, 200 b/s/b

Week 26

1 × 250 crawl
1 × 50 b/s/b
1 × 400 crawl
1 × 75 b/s/b
1 × 400 crawl
1 × 50 b/s/b
1 × 250 crawl
Total: 1,300 crawl, 175 b/s/b

Week 27

1 × 250 crawl
1 × 25 b/s/b
1 × 300 crawl
1 × 25 b/s/b
1 × 350 crawl
1 × 25 b/s/b
1 × 300 crawl
1 × 25 b/s/b
1 × 250 crawl
Total: 1,450 crawl, 100 b/s/b

Week 28

1 × 300 crawl
1 × 25 b/s/b
1 × 500 crawl
1 × 25 b/s/b
1 × 500 crawl
1 × 25 b/s/b
1 × 300 crawl
Total: 1,600 crawl, 75 b/s/b

God, are you a jock (a healthy jock) by now! Why not try a one-mile (1/1,600) continuous-crawl swim next time as a celebration?

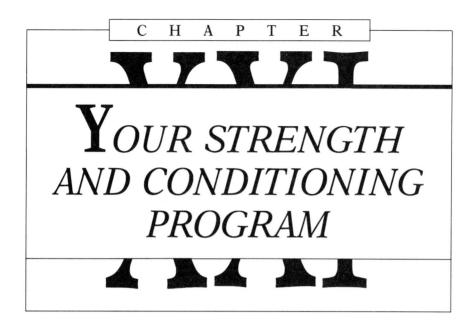

YOUR STRENGTH AND CONDITIONING PROGRAM

But wait, there's more! Your aerobic program only uses up three of the six half-hours you promised me each week, and if you are a weakling, you can stop right there. Healthwise, you'll be in pretty good shape, too. But you won't have firm flesh, and your belly won't look good and, much more importantly, as you get older, you won't be as strong or have as much stamina or flexibility as your body is capable of providing.

That's why a sensible strength program makes sense for us all. And this program is designed for you to do at home with only two sets of small hand weights. In the easiest stages, even the most out-of-shape and inactive person can do these exercises, and in the advanced stages even Mr. Universe could use them to stay tuned up.

Dr. Arno Jensen shared his expertise in developing this program.

What is the torture and what will it do?

We're going to show you and tell you how to do these in varying degrees of difficulty, but here's a little about each exercise:

Toe raises. They work your calf muscles and strengthen your Achilles tendons. Weak Achilles tendons contribute to most ankle injuries, especially as we become inactive or older.

Partial squats. They strengthen your upper thigh muscles, the quadriceps. They also make it easier to climb up and down steps. Strong muscles in your upper leg give your knee more stability, preventing injury. Having stronger legs also helps us cut down on our klutz factor as we get older. We trip and lose our balance less often.

Abdomen exercises. They will work your upper and lower abdomen and sides. The whole world wants a flat belly. These exercises will give it to you in a year, if you eat right. Abdomen exercises coupled with hamstring stretches are also the best thing you can do to prevent back pain caused by weak muscles (the cause of 80 percent of back pain).

Shoulder work. These exercises work the different areas of the shoulder and increase your upper body strength.

Chest. They help both men and women have stronger, better-looking upper bodies.

Arms. As we get older, the skin on our arms really begins to sag and feel like a sponge. These arm exercises will take that away, increase our grip strength, and increase muscle tone.

Starting up

First, call a few sporting goods stores and find one that sells dumbbells or "Heavy Hands"-type weights. If you're a man, you will want to buy a set each of five-pound and ten-pound dumbbells. If you're a woman, buy three- and five-pound sets. If you really don't want to spend any money, find some books or other household objects that weigh close to those weights and are not awkward to hold.

When you have your weights

You're going to need about thirty minutes three times a week for this. I recommend alternating days with your aerobics, but if you want, you can also strength-train on your aerobic days. You can also split the workout into morning and night sessions of fifteen minutes if that is more convenient. But decide when you're going to work out. *Flip open your notebook to the first week's spread and write your workout plan in abbreviated form on the right page. Write your schedule at the top of the page.*

And please, don't be overly enthusiastic with these movements. Though some of them sound very easy, they are not. Always start, therefore, with the easiest level for those exercises with different degrees of difficulty. In the exercises using weights, for example, you will notice that the program often suggests that you first learn the movement without weights, because the *exact* movement and your *control* of that movement provide the beneficial aspects of the exercise. You're ready to move up to the next degree of difficulty when you can do the maximum number of repetitions for the maximum number of sets.

Spreading out your workout

Many of these exercises can be done at work or while you go about your daily tasks, such as talking on the phone or standing in line at the bowling alley. Once you've learned the movements, think MUD a little, and do some extra sets during the day.

Optional work for the stout of heart

You will notice that a few of the exercises are marked "optional." Please try to skip over that word as a smoker skips over the warning label on cigarettes. But if you are really busy, or particularly afflicted with laziness, you can occasionally omit them.

Adding extra sets. You will also notice that some exercises call for only one "set." As you become stronger, feel free to increase those sets to three.

W*here all this rotten stuff can lead you*

For most people, starting a strength program is like buying your first boat: after a while, you want to go on to bigger and better things. If you really stick with this routine, for instance, you may want to go on to a more demanding one. Maybe join a local gym, or set up a small gym set at home. Your body will thank you for thinking like that.

T*he routine in picture and word*

We're going to start at your toes and work up. You might want to read the description of each exercise and then take a peek at the pictures. The good-looking people in these pictures, incidentally, aren't models. They are the people of Grand Bahama Island and other friends who have worked on this book.

GENERAL HINTS
Don't forget to start with the easiest level of difficulty, and move on only when you can do maximum repetitions for three "sets." Rest for a minute between sets. Breathe normally as you exercise, and *never hold your breath.*

LEARNING YOUR ROUTINE
Decide whether to do these beauties all at one time or partially in the morning and partially at night. *Write your routine in your notebook, charting your progress in repetitions and levels of difficulty.* You might want to have one page in your notebook to chart your progress here. Perform your routine three times per week.

1. Toe raises.   Three sets of twenty repetitions. An easy exercise to do while you're otherwise occupied. Toe raises work your calf muscles and strengthen your Achilles tendons. And I'm sure you remember what happened to Achilles when he didn't do them.
   a. With both feet flat on the floor, a hand on a table or desk for support, raise up on your toes as high as possible and then slowly lower yourself. Repeat.
   b. With both feet on a step, a hand on the wall for support, raise up on your toes as high as possible and then slowly lower yourself as low as possible. Repeat.

c. With one foot on a step, a hand on the wall for support, raise up on your toes as high as possible and then slowly lower yourself. Do this on each foot.

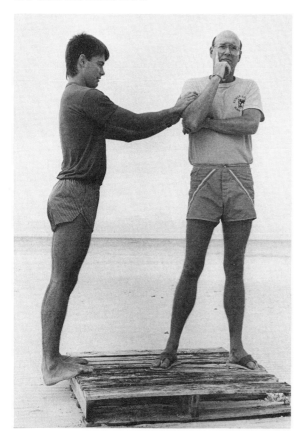

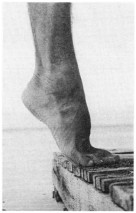

Toe raises. "Some man or other must present a wall," said Bottom in A Midsummer Night's Dream. *Russ is no Pyramus, but methinks I make an admirable wall to support him while he does toe raises.*

2. Partial squats. Work up to three sets of twenty repetitions. These exercises work your upper leg muscles.

a. At first, to do these exercises safely, you will need to support yourself between two sturdy chairs, countertops, desks, etc. With your hands on your supports, bend your legs slightly until you feel pressure on them; then straighten them completely. Repeat. *Each week, go slightly deeper as your strength increases, until your thighs are horizontal with the floor.* Important: *Stay at each level until you can do three sets of twenty repetitions.*

b. When you are nearly at the horizontal stage, you may find it easier to judge this level by finding a sturdy chair with a seat roughly at knee level. Address the chair as if you were ready to sit down. Place one hand on another chair or the wall for support.

Keeping your back straight, slowly lower yourself until your bum-bum barely touches the chair bottom and immediately go back to a standing position. Repeat. After you are able to do three sets of twenty repetitions at this level, you may increase the difficulty by adding handweights, starting with your lightest dumbbells or a couple of one-pound cans of pinto beans.

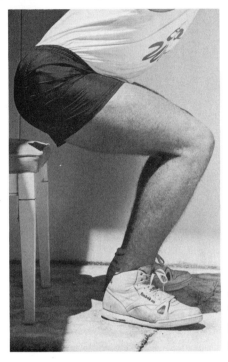

Partial squats. Using a chair will ensure that you do not take your squats below horizontal.

3. Crunches. Start with three sets of five to ten. Work up to three sets of twenty-five. Oh, God, are you going to have a good-looking stomach!

If your back hurts you after a number of repetitions, stop and rest before continuing your count. *Lie on a carpeted surface or a mat.*

Lie on your back with your arms *crossed on your chest.* Cross your legs at the ankles. Bend your legs at the knee as far as comfortable. *Slowly* raise your upper body and try to touch your elbows to your knees. *Do not jerk yourself upward.* Maintain tension in both directions, and move slowly. At first, you may want to go to the completely relaxed position between each repetition. As these get easier, raise your feet off the floor (as in the picture), and don't lower your back completely to the floor. Retain tension at all times.

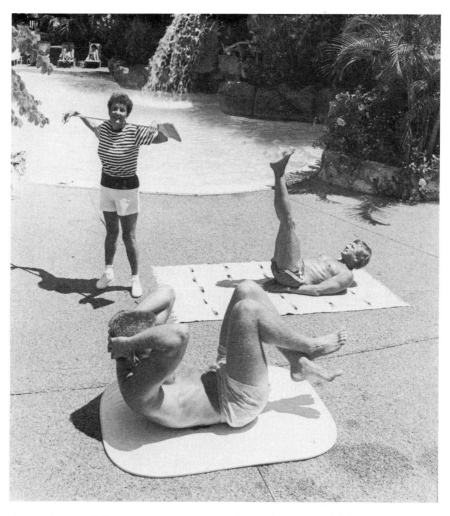

Crunches and leg raises. How would you like a pool like this to work out by? Joan, Eric, and Arnie Jensen work up a good sweat by the Bahamas Princess Country Club Pool.

At the moment, they are demonstrating some popular techniques that you should avoid. *Can you spot them? First, doing crunches, Eric has placed his hands behind his head, which can lead to neck strain or injury. Recommended position: cross your hands on your chest. Second, Arnie is lifting both legs at once, which can produce too much stress on the lower back for many people. Recommended approach: one leg at a time. Third, Joan is demonstrating the twist, which can produce strain and possible injury if you do it ballistically, bouncing your body hard to force the twist as far as possible. Recommended approach: use the twist as a stretching exercise only. See page 268.*

4. Leg raises (optional). Work up to three sets of thirty. These will really tighten the *lower* stomach, where flab likes to congregate. But if you're overweight, your good deeds aren't going to show for a while. Fat covers good-looking stomachs, so be patient.

Lie flat on your back with your hands, palm up, under your hips. Bend one leg. Raise the other leg as high as you can comfortably, keeping it as straight as possible. Lower it to the floor and rest for one second. Repeat. Alternate your legs.

When you can do three sets of thirty, raise both legs at once.

Shoulder exercises. Work up to one set of twelve as a minimum. Three sets would make me happy. These next three shoulder exercises, incidentally, are *much* harder than they look. They work all of the parts of your shoulder, and will make you much more sore than you can imagine if you try too much weight at first.

Levels of Difficulty for Each Exercise
A. Start with no weight.
B. Then use your small dumbbell or other weight.
C. Then use your heavier dumbbell or heavier other weight.

5. Military press. Work up to one set of twelve. Great for your shoulders and chest, but a little confusing to understand in words. Look at the pictures after you've read this about ten times.

Standing straight, hold your light dumbbells right under your chin, thumbs pointing out, as if the dumbbells were the shaft of a curling bar. Lift the dumbbells directly over your head, *rotating your thumbs inward as you lift*. Lower the weights, reversing the motion. When you can do one set of twelve, increase your weight.

6. Side raises. Standing straight, with your elbows nearly straight, slowly raise your arms parallel to the side, as if you were flapping your wings and became stuck in the up position. Keep your arms in line with the sides of your body; don't let them wander to the front or rear. Lower them slowly and then repeat. Work up to one set of twelve.

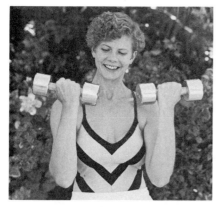

Deni demonstrates the military press. Notice the way the hands rotate during this exercise. Start by holding your dumbbells right under your chin, thumbs pointing out (top). Lift the dumbbells directly over your head, rotating (middle) your thumbs in as you lift until your arms are straight (bottom). Lower the weights, reversing the motion.

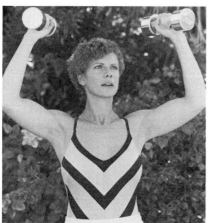

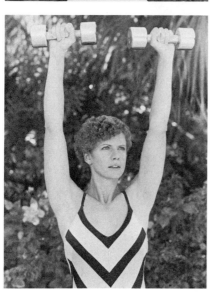

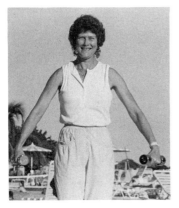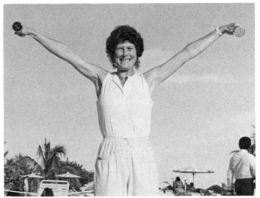

Renee Pender, friend par excellence and dynamite manager of the Tides Inn, always takes her weights with her when she stops by the Holiday Inn pool. Just past the umbrellas is the best swoon-walking beach on the island.

She demonstrates side raises. With your elbows nearly straight, slowly raise your arms parallel to the side (left) as if you were flapping your wings, and stuck in the up position (right). Keep your arms in line with the sides of your body, as Renee is doing; don't let them wander to the front or rear. Lower slowly. Repeat.

7. Front raises.   Standing straight, with your elbows nearly straight, slowly raise your arms until they are parallel in front of you (as if you were sleepwalking). Lower them slowly and repeat. Work up to three sets of twelve.

8. Bent-over raises (optional).   With your feet at shoulder width, lean forward with your back like a table top, if possible. With your elbows nearly straight, raise your arms parallel to the side—as if you were flapping your wings while bent over.

For the exercise to be effective, you must raise your arms in a straight line, which is hard to do bent over this way. The following technique may help: Imagine that your toes are touching a wall. Raise your hands along that wall, being sure not to let them wander toward your head or toward your waist. Also, use lighter weights on this exercise than you do on others. Work up to twelve repetitions.

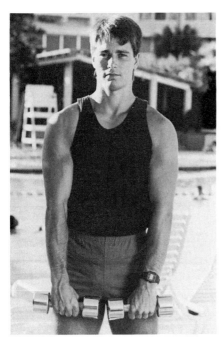 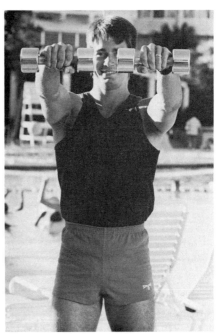

Russ does a few front raises beside the Holiday Inn pool. Standing straight, with your elbows nearly straight, slowly raise your arms to parallel in front of you (as if you're sleep walking). Lower slowly and repeat.

9. Upright rows (optional). These work your shoulders, back, *and* biceps. Very efficient, indeed. Hold your light weights in your hands, thumbs in toward you. Bring your hands up as if you were pumping on a giant bicycle pump. Lower your hands and repeat. Increase your weight as these exercises become easy. The pictures, incidentally, show this a lot better than words.

10. Flies. Work up to three sets of twelve. An exercise to strengthen your chest. If possible, use a piano bench or some other sturdy bench-type structure for this. If that's not possible, use the floor, but place a large pillow under your shoulders; the sofa cushions work pretty well. Our objective here is to have your body a little above floor level, if possible.

Take your light weights and lie on your back, with the weights resting in your hands on your chest. Extend your arms straight up. Slowly drop your arms out to the side, as if the hands of a clock at

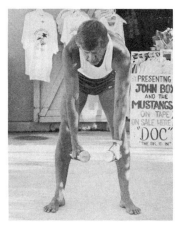 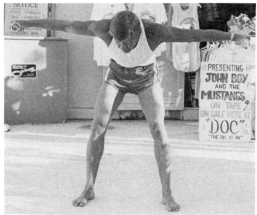

Arnie demonstrates bent-over raises by the Holiday Inn beachside snack stand. John Boy and the Mustangs, incidentally, are a wild and crazy band on the island.

With your feet at shoulder width, lean forward with your back like a table top, if possible (left). With your elbows nearly straight, raise your arms parallel to the side (right), as if you were flapping your wings while bent over. Be sure to raise your arms in a straight line.

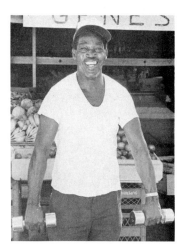 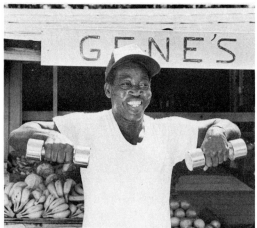

I think the best vegetables on the island are at Gene Nottage's stand at the Bahama's Market, Churchill Square. One of the best smiles is there, too.

Gene shows you how to do upright rows. Hold your weights in your hands, thumbs in toward you (left). Bring your hands up as if you were pumping on a giant bicycle pump (right). Lower and repeat.

twelve noon started going in opposite directions. *Keep your arms as straight as possible,* like the hands on that clock. Go slowly down until you feel a real stretching sensation, and then slowly go up again. Try not to bend your elbows. Your objective here is to eventually drop your arms below the level of your body. *Always go slowly, and always be in control of your weight.* If you have to bend your arms much, you are using too much weight.

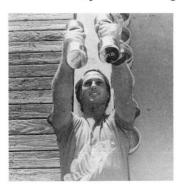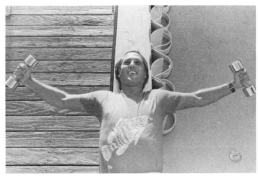

Steve Watson, diving supervisor, finds time to do a few flies on the Explorer.

Take your weights and lie on your back with the weights resting in your hands on your chest. Extend your arms straight up (left). Slowly drop your arms out to the side, as if the hands of a clock at twelve noon started going in opposite directions (right). Keep your arms as straight as possible, like the hands on that clock. Go slowly down until you feel a real stretching sensation, then slowly go up again. Keep your arms as straight as possible. Repeat.

11. Pullovers.   Work up to three sets of twelve. These help strengthen your chest and your back muscles.

Lie on your bench or on the floor with your cushion under you. Stretch both arms directly above you, palms together, fingers straight. *Without bending your elbows,* bring your arms back as far as possible or until they touch the floor. *Always practice this motion without weights before going further. Always breathe out as you go back.*

When you can do three sets of twelve motions comfortably, hold one small weight very securely in your hands and, *without bending your arms,* carefully take your arms back as far as possible, or until they touch the floor.

When you can do three sets of twelve, increase the weight.

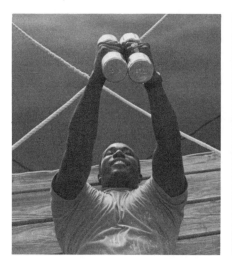
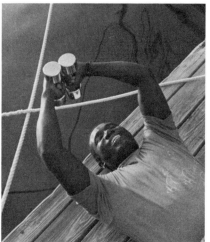

Presley Knowles says these pullovers make it easier to haul scuba tanks. Only a man of supreme strength would swing his weights over the water without fear of dropping them. Presley is Senior Dive Staff.

Lie on your bench on the floor with your cushion under you. Stretch both arms directly above you, palms together, fingers straight (left). Without bending your elbows, bring your arms back as far as possible or until they touch the floor (right). Be sure to practice this exercise without weights in the beginning.

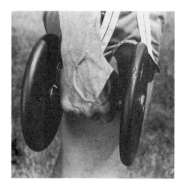
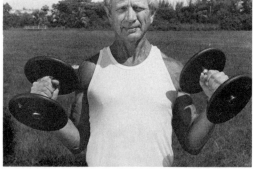

Arnie demonstrates the curl with a pair of weights from the gym. You'll notice that he holds his hands a little differently than the description in the text. Either works well.

With weights in your hands, hands at your sides (left), thumbs out, curl your arms forward at the same time until your weights are at shoulder level (right). Lower and repeat.

12. Curls.   Work up to three sets of twelve. These work the biceps. With your small weights in your hands, hands at your sides, thumbs out, curl your arms forward at the same time until your weights are at shoulder level. Lower and repeat. You may progress very quickly here to heavier weights.

13. Triceps extensions.   Work up to three sets of twelve. These work the triceps, of course. With one arm extended above your head, dumbbell in hand, bend at the elbow, holding your shoulder absolutely still. All the motion should be in the elbow. This extended arm action is like scrubbing your back with a brush or back scrubber.

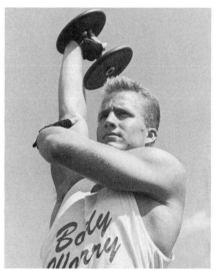 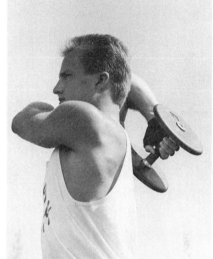

Eric shows you how to tighten up flabby triceps with triceps extensions. Notice how he supports his arm to keep the shoulder joint from moving.

With one arm extended above your head, dumbbell in hand (left), bend at the elbow, holding your shoulder absolutely still (right). All the motion should be in the elbow. This extended arm action is like scrubbing your back with a brush.

Is all this really worth doing?

You will thank me later, really. Having strength, endurance, and a tight, lean body is the best revenge in the world.

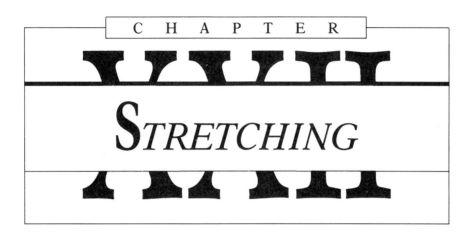

STRETCHING

To stretch or not to stretch

As we get older, we get stiff, it seems. Our range of motion becomes restricted. You, for instance, can probably remember when you could touch your toes as easily as you touch your nose. But you can't touch your toes now, I'll bet.

You can't blame your stiffness on the passage of years alone, though. For most of us, inactivity is the culprit. When you become inactive, you put your body through fewer motions, and eventually your specific parts atrophy a little.

Now, with all that said, I personally hate stretching, because it's so boring. But because it's important, and because a limber body injures itself less, we are presenting here a simple stretching program for you. You may use it simply to develop flexibility or to warm up for other activities such as aerobics or sports.

HOW QUICKLY WILL IT WORK?

For most of us, limberness comes slowly, so don't plan on quick progress. But you will see *lots* of progress if you stick with it, and you can generally do all of these things while you watch television and repeat your Mantra. MUD applies to stretching, too.

STATIC VERSUS BALLISTIC STRETCHING

When you were in school, you may have been taught "ballistic" stretching, in which you bob and jerk to place a joint through its range of motion. As science marches on, exercise physiologists are finding out that ballistic stretching can cause a lot of injuries because the motion can take you *past* your available range of motion. Injuries like these hurt a lot and make people throw away exercise books or, worse, ask for their money back.

Russell Burd, my very bright trainer, has, therefore, very wisely devised what is known as a "static" stretching routine. The principle here is based on slow and easy tension development. You stretch a muscle until tension develops, and you hold it for ten seconds—but you don't stretch to the point of true pain.

Feeling limber is nice, so think about working these ten simple stretches into your day. Three times a week would be nice, but some people like it every day. They can be particularly good as part of your warm-up and cool-down for aerobic and strength exercises. *If you plan to stretch, put your routine in abbreviated form in your notebook.*

The program

This routine hits all the major muscle groups. If something hurts *stop* immediately.

Hold positions for eight to ten seconds each; two to three reps unless otherwise indicated is adequate. If you really want to stress flexibility work, and if you love stretching, you may hold each position for twenty to thirty seconds. But remember, no bouncing.

A brief synopsis

1. Arm circles—ten to fifteen repetitions, both directions
2. Reach—each arm alternately to ceiling
3. Standing twist
4. Chest stretch
5. Standing straight-leg toe-touch
6. Pull, knee to chest
7. Seated straddle—front and both legs
8. Reverse hurdle seat—both legs
9. Standing single-leg quad stretch
10. Calf stretch

The stretches

1. Three stretches and one wall/hunk for balance. Left to right:

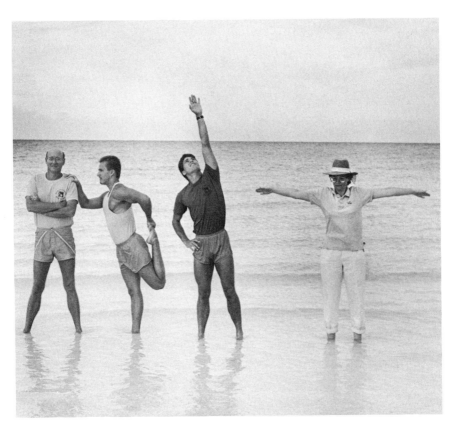

   a. *Wall.*

   b. *Standing single-leg stretch.* Also known to us as the stork. With your free hand, grasp the ankle, pull your foot toward your buttocks, and keep the knee pointing toward the floor. Hold for eight to ten seconds. This stretches your quadriceps.

   c. *The reach.* Stand with your feet apart at shoulder width. Alternate reaching to the sky with each hand. Do three repetitions, and hold each for eight to ten seconds. It's okay to bend slightly to the side and come up on your toes.

   d. *Arms circles.* How do you like Mary Abbott's hat? Holding your arms out straight, rotate them in small circles, gradually making the circles larger. Do this in both directions for ten to fifteen repetitions.

2. Why are these two guys smiling? You can do these two stretches in a doorway or against a wall, too.

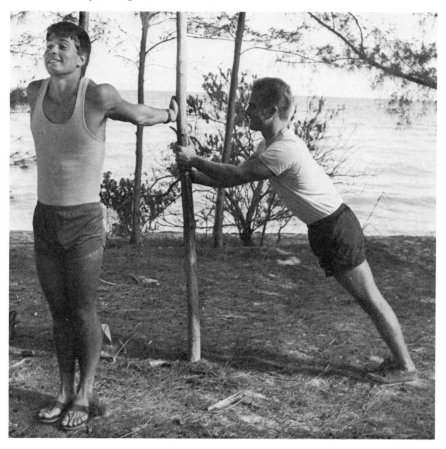

a. *Chest stretch.* Stand in the middle of a doorway or between two trees, grasp the sides of the doorway (or the trees) at shoulder height and walk on through, gently pulling your arms back. *Do not overextend your elbows.* If you need more stretch, twist slightly to the side. Hold this eight to ten seconds, and do it three times.

b. *Calf stretch.* Standing about four feet from a wall, keep your feet flat and body straight, and simply lean toward the wall, holding yourself with your hands, feeling the stretch in your Achilles tendon. Eight to ten seconds, two or three repetitions.

3. Eric, Russ, and I always stretch before swimming at Gold Rock Beach, part of the Lucayan National Park. The stretches, from left to right, are:

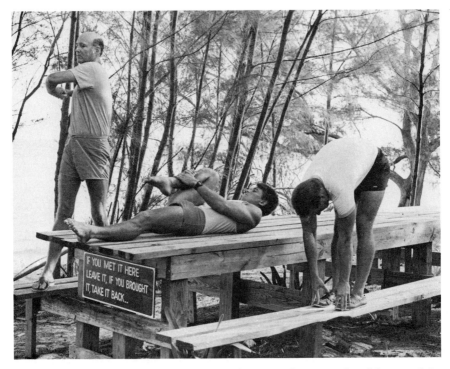

a. *Standing twist.* Standing with your feet at shoulder width, holding your feet out to the side slightly bent, twist the upper part of the torso, keeping your hips still. Twist and hold both ways eight to ten seconds for two or three reps.

b. *Leg and bum stretch—The Pull.* Lying on your back, hold the lower part of your leg, and pull the knee to the chest while keeping the other leg straight. Hold eight to ten seconds, two or three reps each leg.

c. *Toe-touch.* Stand with legs together and straight, and very carefully lean forward and touch your toes. *Don't bounce* and don't worry if you can only reach your knees. If touching your toes comes easily, then hold on to the backs of your ankles and try to touch your forehead to your knees. Or try putting your palms flat on the floor. Hold for eight to ten seconds for two or three reps.

If you have back trouble or get any twinges in your back while trying this stretch, *do not do it.* Instead, substitute this stretch: Squat slightly until you can lean forward and place your hands on the floor. (Remember the position for playing leap frog—that's it.) Then straighten your legs slowly until you look a little like a camel's hump. Hold for eight to ten seconds; then lower yourself back into a squat.

4. Good positions to practice your Mantra in.

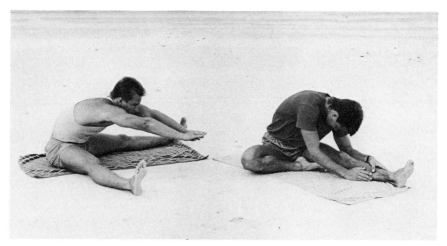

a. *Seated straddle.* Seated on the floor, spread your legs as wide as comfortable. Keeping your legs straight, lean forward, trying to touch your nose to the floor. This is also a good way to see how clean your carpets are. Hold this eight to ten seconds for three reps. You can also do this to each side, putting your nose to your knee.

b. *Reverse hurdle seat.* Sit with your legs spread and straight; then bring the bottom of one foot to the other knee, making a closed numeral four. Russ is real flexible here and can even get his foot higher than his knee. You'll be able to do this, too, later. Then lean forward, trying to touch your nose to the knee of your straight leg. Use your arms for balance. Hold for eight to ten seconds, two or three reps each leg.

A *final charge from your cosmic guru*

This is my last chance to talk with you about exercise, and, being a good guru, I would like to send you off to the kitchen with some final words about your own particular seat in the arena of human existence.

I know it would be tempting to think about accidentally dropping this book in your bedroom paper shredder right now. You're not really *that* bad off, especially compared to all those people out there who *really* deserve our concern, right? Those who no longer can make many (or any) voluntary movements—people injured in terrible accidents or struck down with terrible diseases.

My sympathy used to be reserved for those people, too, until I realized I was one of them. For most of my life, I made no voluntary movements—*none.* I lived my life with just those movements necessary to keep my life and job functioning.

That realization was not a pleasant one, but it was accurate. And it may apply to you, if you are a prisoner of minimal movement, too. The joy of living comes from doing more than life requires to exist. And as your guru, I want you to experience that joy.

So, put the aerobic and strength portions of this book to work *right now,* no excuses. I leave you with thoughts of moderation.

THE GODLY EATING PLAN IN ACTION

All good swamis give credit when it's due, and I give credit here to Mary Abbott Waite for helping to put together the expert opinions and research we gathered into the very substantial and innovative eating-modification program presented here. The swami may be speaking, but the information gathering and knowledge is that of my good friend, Mary Abbott.

M odifying your eating habits
(without making life miserable)

If you're like me, you don't really think about what you eat, you just eat. Sometimes I envision myself in my happiest state as a mindless, smiling shovel, bigger than Pac-Man and bottomless. As the preceding pages point out, however, mindless eating, like mindless sloth, takes it toll. And it takes it in a lot more ways than the lowered ego that comes with looking like a blimp.

This part of *Body Worry*, therefore, isn't about dieting (you won't find the word here), but in large part about understanding your eating habits and the implications of those habits, and then helping you modify your habits as you see fit. Modifying—or MUDifying as you should think of it—is more productive when it comes to food than to anything.

If you need to lose a lot of weight, you can design a program that will do that safely and for life, *if* you adopt your new eating habits for life. *And if* you accompany those new habits with your activity program. If you want to instill clean and godly eating habits in your family, you will be able to do that, too.

Our approach takes you from the easiest habit changes (switching from stick margarine to soft margarine, for instance) to very creative changes that will have you eventually designing your own new menus and dishes that will taste so good they will seem bad for you—the ultimate compliment you can pay a healthy dish.

$\mathbf{A}$ *preview of what's in all these pages*

---

1. FIRST, A LITTLE SELF-EVALUATION

Because so many of our food habits are as mindless as breathing, you're going to have to understand what you are really doing to your particular body with the food and drink you customarily put down the gullet. Reaching such enlightenment means you are going to have to do something very tedious for three days or so: keep a record of all your intakes. And if you don't do it accurately, you will be wasting your time in this section. (In fact, anyone in your environment—spouse, kids, friends—who is going to participate needs to keep an individual record.) This self-evaluation of your current eating habits will lead to step two—planning for change.

Keeping records like this is nearly worse than being fat and/or out of shape, but the brief effort will be worth it, and then the misery will be gone. This book is not about counting calories except for this one miserable section.

In addition to keeping a food-intake record, you'll also review what you found out about your weight and body composition when you were getting ready to exercise. This review won't be tedious, and it won't depress you, either, since you've already started your activity program—right?

2. NEXT, WE SET SOME GOALS AND PLAN THE TRANSITION TO GODLY EATING

After determining where you are, you will set goals you want to work toward and plan your personal approach to godly eating. As you probably remember, I love to scuba dive. Before I knew a lot about that sport, everything about it seemed complicated and completely foreign to me. Now, it's second nature. As you plan for godly eating, you are going to learn some concepts and tools for modifying food choices and cooking techniques that will become second nature to you very quickly.

3. AND THEN WE START TO EAT

As you put your plan into action, things get a lot better. You'll start with some simple, painless modifications of your choice. After you've got the hang of this, you get to try a couple of weeks of our menus, if you like. Very few people have died on these menus yet. Of course the book hasn't been out that long, either.

After this two-week practice session of godly eating based on our ideas, we'll show you how to modify your own favorite recipes and provide checklists and tips to simplify that task. And then we will get really creative. I know you are already a better cook than I am (I don't know if you're better than Mary Abbott, who cooks as Astaire could dance), but I think you'll like the tips and the ideas for planning imaginatively and for saving your time. And then we'll talk about eating out. There are so many nice things to do when it comes to food.

Now, that's pretty much going to be the plan, so take a break, go eat something bad, and don't come back to this part of the book until you are ready to break bread.

Evaluating your eating habits and body composition

START BY KEEPING AN ACCURATE FOOD RECORD

I have it on good authority that the devil makes you keep lots of records if you are unlucky enough to travel in that direction in the next life. (You probably will be sent there for being a bad eater.) I know for a fact that's got to be miserable, too, for I had to keep total records of my intakes for *months* when I started my remake.

But since you don't have to do it for that long, I have no pity, and expect you to do it faithfully for three days at least, and hopefully for four. (If you are a glutton for abuse or a compulsive perfectionist, you can keep a week's record for even greater accuracy.) *Do not* change your eating habits to make record keeping more convenient, or out of shame, either. Be proud of the mess you've made of yourself.

What days should I do this?   Because we eat differently during the week and on the weekend, be sure to include one weekend day and two or three weekdays. Why not start on Sunday and continue through Tuesday or Wednesday, or start on Wednesday or Thursday and go through Saturday?

What will this tell me?   You can find out if you're eating too much, if you're eating the wrong things, if you're eating too much of good things, and if you're eating at the wrong times. An accurate food record is the most important step you can take right now to ensure long-term change in your eating habits.

What do I record?   Absolutely everything other than sugarless chewing gum and snuff. Please record liquids (including water) as well.

How do I estimate portions?   Estimate portions in what are called "standard measures":

- Meats and cheeses in ounces
- Liquids and cooked vegetables in portions of a cup
- Butter, cooking oil, mayo, catsup, etc., in teaspoons and tablespoons
- Fruits, bread, whole veggies, in units (e.g., "one small apple")

How do you judge an ounce without a scale?   You are obviously going to have to do some guessing here, but you can be more accurate than you think. For instance, a three- to four-ounce piece of cooked meat is about the size of your palm. Before you eat meat, compare the portion to your palm. Make sure to wash your hand before comparing.

An ounce of cheese is about a 1½-inch cube, or one slice of presliced cheese.

If you have trouble visualizing a tablespoon of chocolate sauce or a half cup of vegetables, why not play with your food tonight? Measure a tablespoon of chocolate sauce or catsup and pour it on a plate. Measure a half cup or cup of vegetables and pour it on your plate. Measure a cup of beer or milk and pour it in your glass.

If you plan to do a good bit of your measuring at home rather than outside, why not find a set of glasses right now, find out exactly how much they hold, and use these for drinking and thus easy measuring during these next days?

How do you measure things if you're eating out? Remember the palm test for meats, but don't let anyone see you. And remember what a half cup of vegetables or a spoonful of condiments looks like from your home experiment. At fast-food restaurants, simply ask how many ounces a portion is. At very fancy restaurants, ask your waiter to have your main course weighed for your research project. Virtually all nice restaurants have scales. And finally, look on the menu. Some may have the weights, portions, and caloric content printed there for you.

What about dishes with many ingredients? Break things down into their parts. For instance, look at a roast beef sandwich, and you might see two slices of bread, enough beef to cover your palm (about three ounces), a tablespoon of mayonnaise, and one slice of tomato. Of course, record only the portion you actually eat. Looking at what you eat in restaurants may make you want to eat at home forever, but if you're going to eat out, look carefully during these few days.

What about things like casseroles or soups? If you made it at home, look at the ingredient list and divide the total portions by the number of servings you normally get from that dish. For instance, your favorite Ironman Tuna Casserole with noodles has one 1 6-ounce can of tuna, 3 cups of cooked noodles, 1 cup of garden peas, and 1 can of condensed mushroom soup. Since you're all big on this dish, you normally only get 3 servings. Your serving will be 2 ounces of tuna, 1 cup noodles, a third cup peas, and a third can of condensed mushroom soup. If all that math makes you cross-eyed, don't worry; when the time comes to figure out what's really in it our table on page 372 will help you here.

If you normally eat casserole-type dishes or soups in restaurants, you're going to have to guess the main ingredients (practice being a food critic—haven't you always thought you could do better than they anyway?) or ask your waiter for help. People don't find questions like this unusual anymore, so don't worry.

Record keeping: First, you'll want to make several copies of the daily record sheet on page 277. Either photocopy this one or make your own master and photocopy it or run something like it off on your computer printer. While you're making copies, it would be efficient to run copies of the Score Card also, which you'll need in analyzing your intakes. It's on page 279.

If you are at home, you can enter your intakes directly on this record sheet. If you are out for most of your meals, put a small pad or piece of paper in your pocket, and jot intakes down on that. When you get home, transfer the items to a copy of the record sheet.

What information do I write down? Write down the food or ingredient, its amount, the time of day, and the reason you ate it ("afternoon snack" or "afterwork drink with friends"). After your record-keeping days are over, we're going to show you how to take those tidbits of information and make them very meaningful to you. Trust me.

And while you're record-keeping, don't worry about doing anything else here in the eating section.

Evaluating what you've recorded

Until two years ago, I had never in my life thought about the ingredients—or the health implications of those ingredients—in any food. An apple was composed of apple, and a thick cut of roast beef was composed of cow. I couldn't name the four food groups. I believed that foods couldn't put on more weight than they themselves weighed.

Life isn't that nice, I found out. Our bodies need what they consider a reasonably balanced combination of foods, containing proteins, several types of fats, carbohydrates, vitamins, and minerals and, within these larger categories, cholesterol, fiber, salt (sodium), and sugar. Most of these things have calories, and all impact on our health as surely as heat follows fire.

What you need to do right now is see how your current food-intake habits stack up against the recommended intakes for a per-

DAILY FOOD RECORD

DAY: _____

NAME: _____

Food	Amount	Time	Calories	Grams Protein	Grams Fat				Grams Carb.	Sugar*	Fiber	Sodium (mgs)	Reason for Eating
					TOTAL	Sat.	Poly-un.	Mono.					

*Sugar is "simple carbohydrate" and is called such on some labels.

277

son of your age and sex. Very few of us know that, including healthy folks, so here we go. First, you'll get all the figures worked out, and then we'll discuss the whys of the recommended patterns.

1. Go to the Table of Food Nutritive Values on page 372 in the Appendix, and look up the nutrient levels of all your intakes during the past days. Fill in that amount for each item listed on your daily food intake sheet. This is almost more tedious than writing down what you eat in the first place, but don't give up now.

2. Transfer the daily totals for each category onto the Score Card and average the totals in each category. If you didn't make these copies while making the daily record sheets, take a break from figures and make some.

3. Fill out the bottom of the sheet, putting your actual totals and recommended totals in the appropriate spaces.

A NOTE ON USING THE SCORE CARD

As you can see on the model Score Card, we have filled in the recommended levels of cholesterol, sodium, and fiber. But you will have to fill in the appropriate amounts of protein, fats, and carbohydrates using the chart "Recommended Dietary Levels by Caloric Intake" on page 280.

You will notice that the Score Card has two sections of recommended levels—the first is based on your present food consumption so you can evaluate the balance of what you are eating now. The second section enables you to figure what the recommended levels would be if you need to consume fewer calories in order to lose weight.

And what about those calories? Here recommended "averages" aren't of too much use because needs differ according to sex, body size, and activity levels. So you will need to answer a few questions and do a little figuring to determine your recommended caloric intake. *Get ready to put the answers in your notebook.*

Are you maintaining your present weight or gaining? If you are not gaining weight, then you are consuming only enough calories to maintain your present weight (whether you feel your present weight is just right or too much). If you're currently gaining weight, then your caloric intake is too great to maintain your present weight, whatever it may be. You will need to determine a new target caloric intake to maintain your present weight or a lower weight.

SCORE CARD

Comparing Your Intake to Recommended Levels

Name _____

	Calories	Protein (g)	Fat (g) Total	Sat	Poly	Carbohy-drate (g)	Sugar (Simple Carbohydrate)	Cholesterol (mg)	Sodium (mg)	Fiber (g)
Your current average										
Recommended levels guidelines	╳	15–20% of total caloric intake	Fat: 30% or less of total calories Saturated fat: 10% or less of total calories			50–55% of total calories	Simple carbohydrates. See note†	Less than 300 mgs per day	Less than 3000 mgs per day	20–35 grams per day
Recommended levels at your current caloric intake	╳	Figure using table:	Figure using table:			Figure using table:	See note†	Less than 300 mgs per day	Less than 3000 mgs per day	20–35 grams per day
Recommended levels at target calorie intake							See note†	Less than 300 mgs per day	Less than 3000 mgs per day	20–35 grams per day

†Note on sugar: There is no recommended level of sugar consumption, but clearly you want to do better than the average American who consumes as much as 20 to 30% of daily caloric intake as added sugar. If your sugar intake is high, set an attainable goal for yourself. 150 to 225 calories (10–15 tsp.) may not be unreasonable. Remember this is not just the sugar you add but that found in sodas, candy, and pastries.

279

RECOMMENDED DIETARY LEVELS BY CALORIC INTAKE

Note: You may use this chart to determine more easily how many calories or grams of protein, fat, and carbohydrates equal the recommended levels for total calories eaten.

Total caloric intake	Protein 15% of total	Total fat not more than 30% of total	Saturated less than 10% of total	Polyunsat. at least 10% of total	Carbohydrate 55% of total
1,000	150 cal/37.5 g	300 cal/33 g	100 cal/11 g	100 cal/11 g	550 cal/138 g
1,100	165 cal/42 g	330 cal/37 g	110 cal/12 g	110 cal/12 g	605 cal/151 g
1,200	180 cal/45 g	360 cal/40 g	120 cal/13 g	120 cal/13 g	660 cal/165 g
1,300	195 cal/49 g	390 cal/43 g	130 cal/14 g	130 cal/14 g	715 cal/179 g
1,400	210 cal/53 g	420 cal/47 g	140 cal/16 g	140 cal/16 g	770 cal/193 g
1,500	225 cal/56 g	450 cal/50 g	150 cal/17 g	150 cal/17 g	825 cal/206 g
1,600	240 cal/60 g	480 cal/53 g	160 cal/18 g	160 cal/18 g	880 cal/220 g
1,700	255 cal/64 g	510 cal/57 g	170 cal/19 g	170 cal/19 g	935 cal/234 g
1,800	270 cal/68 g	540 cal/60 g	180 cal/20 g	180 cal/20 g	990 cal/248 g
1,900	285 cal/71 g	570 cal/63 g	190 cal/21 g	190 cal/21 g	1,045 cal/261 g
2,000	300 cal/75 g	600 cal/67 g	200 cal/22 g	200 cal/22 g	1,100 cal/275 g
2,100	315 cal/79 g	630 cal/70 g	210 cal/23 g	210 cal/23 g	1,155 cal/289 g
2,200	330 cal/83 g	660 cal/73 g	220 cal/24 g	220 cal/24 g	1,210 cal/303 g
2,300	345 cal/86 g	690 cal/77 g	230 cal/26 g	230 cal/26 g	1,265 cal/316 g
2,400	360 cal/90 g	720 cal/80 g	240 cal/27 g	240 cal/27 g	1,320 cal/330 g
2,500	375 cal/94 g	750 cal/83 g	250 cal/28 g	250 cal/28 g	1,375 cal/344 g
2,600	390 cal/98 g	780 cal/87 g	260 cal/29 g	260 cal/29 g	1,430 cal/358 g
2,700	405 cal/101 g	810 cal/90 g	270 cal/30 g	270 cal/30 g	1,485 cal/371 g
2,800	420 cal/105 g	840 cal/93 g	280 cal/31 g	280 cal/31 g	1,540 cal/385 g
2,900	435 cal/109 g	870 cal/97 g	290 cal/32 g	290 cal/32 g	1,595 cal/399 g
3,000	450 cal/113 g	900 cal/100 g	300 cal/33 g	300 cal/33 g	1,650 cal/413 g
3,100	465 cal/116 g	930 cal/103 g	310 cal/34 g	310 cal/34 g	1,705 cal/426 g
3,200	480 cal/120 g	960 cal/107 g	320 cal/36 g	320 cal/36 g	1,760 cal/440 g
3,300	495 cal/124 g	990 cal/110 g	330 cal/37 g	330 cal/37 g	1,815 cal/454 g
3,400	510 cal/128 g	1,020 cal/113 g	340 cal/38 g	340 cal/38 g	1,870 cal/468 g
3,500	525 cal/131 g	1,050 cal/117 g	350 cal/39 g	350 cal/39 g	1,925 cal/481 g
3,600	540 cal/135 g	1,080 cal/120 g	360 cal/40 g	360 cal/40 g	1,980 cal/495 g
3,700	555 cal/139 g	1,110 cal/120 g	370 cal/41 g	370 cal/41 g	2,035 cal/509 g
3,800	570 cal/143 g	1,140 cal/127 g	380 cal/42 g	380 cal/42 g	2,090 cal/523 g
3,900	585 cal/146 g	1,170 cal/130 g	390 cal/43 g	390 cal/43 g	2,145 cal/536 g
4,000	600 cal/150 g	1,200 cal/133 g	400 cal/44 g	400 cal/44 g	2,200 cal/550 g

Is your current weight okay, or are you overweight or under-weight? The pinch test and/or body-fat content test that you took earlier gave you a general answer to this question. But you need a more specific answer now in order to judge your food intake accurately and to set goals for MUDification.

To determine whether or not you are within a desirable weight range, find your Body Mass Index on the table on page 282.[1] (This device is a bit more accurate and lots more fun to use than height-weight tables.) To use it, take a ruler or piece of paper and place the edge at your height in inches on the left and at your weight in pounds on the right. Where the edge of the ruler or paper falls on the grid in the middle of the chart indicates your current weight situation. For example, a 5'10" man (i.e., 70 inches tall) who weighs 165 pounds is in the middle of the desirable weight range, but would be overweight at 185. A 5'10" woman would be in the middle of the desirable weight range at 150 but overweight at 175.

You can place your body within the desirable weight ranges more specifically by taking your frame size into account. The edge of the ruler or sheet of paper should fall into the top of the block for large frames, the middle for medium frames, and the bottom for small frames. These divisions are roughly marked on the chart. To determine your frame size, just use your common sense; there are no good, simple criteria for this.

How much do you need to lose or gain to reach a desirable weight?
To determine this, simply slide the edge of the ruler or paper up or down until it falls into the proper desirable range. Note the weight on the right-hand column. Subtract that new target weight from your present weight to see how much you need to lose. Or vice versa, if you need to gain. For example, an average 5'5" woman who weighs 155 might set a target of 125 to 130; she needs to lose 25 to 30 pounds.

How much do you need to eat to maintain this desirable weight?
You can make a quick estimate of how much caloric intake it will take to maintain your desirable weight by multiplying that weight by 13 calories per pound if you are sedentary, 15 calories a pound if you are lightly to moderately active, and 18 to 20 calories a pound if you're strenuously active.[2] Beware of that last category; 13 to 15 is right for most of us. For example, if your ideal weight is 145 and you're moderately active (what our program makes you), 145 times

BODY MASS INDEX

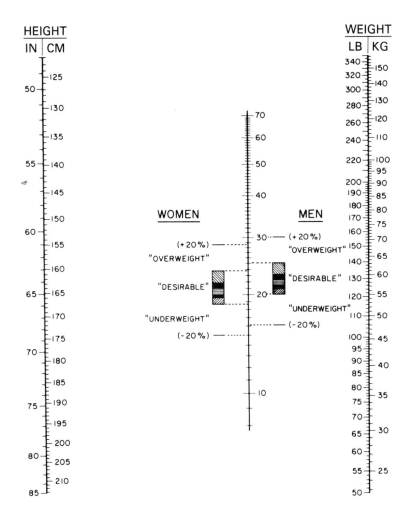

Note: Be sure to read your level on the *central scale.* To tell if or where your weight falls in the "desirable" range, mentally impose the men's or women's scale (pictured as shaded boxes to either side) on this grid as the dotted lines indicate. Do *not* read from the shaded boxes in their present position. The solid black sections in the shaded boxes represent the overlap of categories.

Source: Anthony E. Thomas, Ph.D., David A. McKay, M.D., and Michael B. Cutlip, Ph.D. "A nomograph method for assessing body weight." *The American Journal of Clinical Nutrition,* 29:303, 1976.

15 equals 2,175 calories per day. *Figure your caloric intake for maintaining your desired weight. Put this figure in the appropriate blank on your Score Card.*

Caution: this is the intake for maintaining a desirable weight. If you wish to lose weight a little more quickly, you might subtract 200 to 400 calories from that. But remember that *any modification for the better is useful. Think MUD.* (Do not go below 1,200 because it is difficult to obtain adequate amounts of all nutrients below this level. Also, isn't that too much like a diet? Slow, gradual loss stays off more permanently than quick loss.)

Now that you've figured this out, let's consider where you are now.

Smoking guns

Down the road, when doctors tell you bad news about your health, or compliment you on your good health, many of their words will be traced to their knowledge of the kind of information you've recorded on your Score Card, a line of evidence pointing more specifically to cause than any prosecutor could dream for. You, therefore, need to compare your totals in each of these categories to the recommended levels carefully and without the least flippancy. And if you are like me, expect to be confused and disturbed a little. No one other than a weirdo, for instance, could ever really keep up with the percentages of different things actually considered ideal. But you do need to have a general feel for proportion in what you eat. You do need to know what you are eating too much of now and what you are slighting so that you can modify your intakes for the better. I, for instance, used to feel uncomfortable if my breakfast didn't consist of eggs, a meat, and coffee. That sense of rightness over the years had become subliminal. When I first began to eat a lighter, more balanced breakfast, my mornings didn't seem complete for a while. Now, they seem a little out of kilter when I occasionally eat my old breakfast.

Just as scuba diving has become second nature to me, a sense of the rightness of eating balanced meals will come to you. For instance, if your sheet shows you eat virtually no fiber, don't worry about percentages right now, just file away the name of a few good foods with fiber in them. What you want to do now is get an overall picture.

COMPARING YOUR INTAKES TO RECOMMENDED LEVELS

Earlier in *Body Worry*, we talked about the basic nutritional concepts important to healthy eating and discussed briefly how the body uses such components as protein, carbohydrates, and fats. So here I'll repeat only enough to be clear and to remind you why these concepts are important.

These recommended levels were not dragged out of a magician's hat, either, but are based on "The Dietary Guidelines for Americans" developed by the government and the specific recommendations of such expert bodies as the American Heart Association, the National Heart, Lung and Blood Institute, and the National Cancer Institute.[3] What you want to do now is compare your actual levels to the recommended levels with an eye toward setting some goals for improvement. Don't worry at this stage about *how* to cut fat or increase carbohydrates or fiber, for instance, but about whether or not you *need* to do so. In the next step, we'll show you how to do this with checklists and specific examples.

TOTAL CALORIES

If your total caloric intake is more than that recommended for a person your age, activity level, and sex, you can no longer blame extra pounds on your pet crystal. You are taking in more calories than your body needs to spend right now. And the weight you will gain from that is simple to calculate: every 3,500 calories will put a pound on you, all things being equal. If you take in 120 calories a day more than your body needs to maintain its equilibrium (about one nondiet soft drink), you will put on roughly a pound every month. Creeping fat. The more extra calories, obviously, the quicker the weight gain. *How many calories are you over your body's requirements? Calculate how many days it will take your body to gain a pound.* Scary, isn't it? Put the answer in your notebook.

PROTEIN

Protein provides the amino acids essential to maintaining the body's enzymes and structural protein. Proteins are found in both animal and plant products, but while any meat or animal product such as cheese or an egg contains all "essential" amino acids, no one vegetable or plant product does. Though protein is essential to our well-being, most Americans exceed the daily requirements. Protein intake should be about 15 percent of your total calories. If your protein is over 20 percent of your total intake, you are probably also taking in too many fats and not enough carbohydrates. *Do you need to modify your protein intake? Put the answer in your notebook.*

FATS

We need all the types of fats—saturated, polyunsaturated, and monosaturated—to be healthy, because they supply essential fatty acids. But most of us seem to crave more fat than we really need to be healthy; in many industrialized countries such as ours, fats account for about 40 percent of total intake.[4] And that fat is calorically high, too, since it has nine calories per gram compared to four calories per gram for protein and carbohydrates.

For adults, the recommended level for total fat intake is 30 percent or less. No restriction in fats should be made for very young children (those under two) because fats are necessary for proper growth and development. Experts such as the American Heart Association and the American Pediatric Association differ about recommendations for children over two, but all agree that teaching healthy patterns of eating, of which this guideline is part, is important.

Do you need to lower your total fat intake?   As we now know, too much saturated fat can lead to increased cholesterol in the blood and increased heart disease. Animal fats, hydrogenated vegetable fat such as that in vegetable shortening or stick margarine, and the fats in coconut oil, palm oil, and cocoa butter are all saturated fats. Your saturated fat intake should be less than *10 percent* of your total calories. If your saturated fat level is 20 percent of your intake (most Americans average 15 to 20 percent of intake as saturated fat), you are going to need to cut your meat lust in half. *How much do you need to change?*

Polyunsaturated fats and monosaturated fats, on the other hand, are not associated with an increase in cholesterol levels and heart disease. Substituting polyunsaturated fats for saturated fats while keeping total fat consumption below 30 percent, therefore, can work to lower cholesterol levels. Your polyunsaturated fat level should be 10 percent of your total calories. *Do you need to increase your use of polyunsaturates?*

CARBOHYDRATES

Carbohydrates broken down into their simplest form, glucose, fuel our bodies. Found in fruits, vegetables, grains, and cereals, carbohydrates are both "simple" and "complex." A simple carbohydrate is merely sugar—whether that in honey or maple syrup, or refined corn syrups or table sugars—the "empty" calories. Complex carbohydrates, which are found in fruits and vegetables and whole-grain products, are what we want to emphasize. They have fewer calories, plenty of vitamins and minerals, and more fiber.

Most Americans, however, consume only about 40 to 45 percent of their calories as carbohydrates, and of that, one third to one half are simple carbohydrates, or sugar.[5] *How do you measure up?* About 50 to 55 percent of your total calories should be in carbohydrates, and most of that should come from vegetables, fruits, and grains— not from cakes and candies and soda pop.

SUGARS

As we just said, sugars are simple carbohydrates, which add to our daily total allotment of calories without doing us any good. Most of the carbohydrates in our chart are not broken down into complex and simple carbohydrates, but the major culprits, such as soft drinks and sweets, generally are. We've put this category in primarily so you can get a better idea of just how much of your caloric allotment you use up in this manner. *Note your answer.*

CHOLESTEROL

Cholesterol is found in animal products—meats, eggs, dairy products. It's so vital to the body's well-being that virtually every one of our cells also manufactures it at times. But we increase the level of cholesterol in our blood dangerously by eating too much saturated fat and too many foods which contain cholesterol. Excess cholesterol in the bloodstream, as discussed earlier, clogs the system and contributes to damage to the arteries and consequently to heart disease.

If your cholesterol levels are above the norm, you have probably begun the clogging process. It's a silent, progressive process, and the longer you wait to correct your excess here, the more drastic your dietary changes must be down the road. The changes will need to be drastic then because your health problems will in all likelihood be drastic then. Now, flip back in your notebook and look at your cholesterol levels (you did have that done, didn't you?). If your level is high, the reason is partially here in the amount of saturated fat and of cholesterol-rich foods you eat. *What are the main choles-*

terol-rich foods in your diet? Do you need to lower your intake of cholesterol? Note the answers.

SODIUM

Sodium, a major element in salt, occurs naturally in many foods and is important to our bodies because it attracts water into the blood vessels, helping maintain the right volume of blood and the right blood pressure among other functions. Salt also appeals to our taste buds, so we add even more to our food in processing or cooking and at the table. Extra salt can, over time, lead to high blood pressure and other very unpleasant realities.

The key here again is moderation. Modest changes in your salt intake now may prevent you from doing without salt completely later. Your taste buds will get used to the change, too. Friends who have had to restrict their salt intake have told me that their taste buds adjusted to the lower salt content fairly quickly, in about three or four weeks.

Many experts recommend limiting sodium intake to 1 gram (1,000 milligrams) for each 1,000 calories you eat, or less than 3 grams (3,000 mg.) per day. Remember that one teaspoon of salt has 2,000 mg. *How much sodium are you consuming?* Note your answer. Average consumption by Americans is estimated at 5,000 to 7,000 mg. per day.[6]

FIBER

Fiber is an indigestible carbohydrate. Dietary fiber has gotten a lot of press lately because eating adequate amounts of fiber seems to help lower our risks of getting certain kinds of cancer. In addition, some types of fiber, such as those in oatmeal and beans, have been associated with lowered cholesterol in the blood. So experts are recommending that we get between 20 and 35 grams of dietary fiber in our diets each day. *How many grams of fiber are you currently consuming? Note your answer.*

LIQUID INTAKE

This category is not on your Score Card, but you may want to take a moment to look over your food intake records and see about how much liquid you consume daily—a rough count.

You need lots of liquids each day, and there are lots of liquids in many forms to choose from. Water is the best in many ways.

Liquids such as real fruit juices, which contain healthy nutrients, are good, though they may contain a good number of calories as well. Pop is tasty, but it honestly doesn't do much for you. How much pop is reflected in your sugar total? Switching to diet pop can save you virtually all of those calories. Alcoholic beverages aren't necessarily bad, either, but they, like soda pop, add non-productive calories to your calorie count, a number fixed for your particular weight or target weight. Alcohol can eventually cause health problems, as we know, too. But modest reductions here can help a lot.

And speaking of moderation when it comes to alcohol, you might want to turn back to page 58 and read what the definitions of light to heavy drinking are. My personal definition of "moderation" used to qualify me for the heavy drinker category. *How much alcohol in calories are you consuming on an average day? What percentage of your total caloric intake is alcohol? Remember this percentage has no food value. Put this figure in your notebook.*

WHEN AND WHY YOU EAT

Now that you've compared what you are really eating to the recommended patterns, you've got an idea about where you've sinned and where you can do better. As you work toward setting some goals for change, you need to look at when and why you eat to see if these patterns may also in some way contribute to how healthily you eat. For instance, how often do you snack? Constant nibbling is a wicked calorie builder, and very few nibblers know the extent of their sin. You might want to reflect on the number of times you nibble each day. Or do you skip breakfast or grab a cup of coffee and a single piece of toast, only to snack on sugar-rich treats at mid-morning, when you get hungry? Do you tend to eat very big dinners after skimping on lunch? Does relaxing with friends after work mean you are having a couple of drinks a day and loading up on "happy hour" snacks?

Other evidence of crimes committed

Earlier I asked you to make some tests and record the results in your notebook. Several are related to the smoking guns above, and a brief review may add a little perspective to the next part of *Body Worry:* "Planning Your Transition to Godly Living."

1. *What's your weight?*

2. *Compared to your ideal weight range, as determined by the Body Mass Index above, approximately how many pounds are you overweight?* Of course, an "ideal" weight is a lot like an "ideal" lover— hard to define, seldom achieved, but nice to think about. Though your weight by itself doesn't necessarily tell the tale, the range given on the Body Mass Index (as opposed to standard height/weight tables), taken together with a pinch test or a test for body-fat percentage, can give you a good idea of what you need to aim for.

3. *So how much fat can you pinch? Or what percent of your body is actually fat, if you have had a skinfold or underwater test?* You'll recall that a pinch of over an inch indicates that you are probably overblubbered. You may want to keep track of your thickest area as time goes by, for it will get smaller if you remain determined to seek godly living.

4. *What are your measurements?* These, like the pinch test, can serve as a baseline for your progress over time. Your measurements, pinch-test results, and actual weight together will give you an accurate record of progress in attacking fat and reshaping your body.

WELL, THAT'S ENOUGH OF THAT

All this self-evaluation probably isn't good for your disposition or general outlook on life at the moment, but that's okay. Now that we understand where we are with our eating habits and shape, it's time to set some goals and learn how to start some changes.

Planning *your transition to godly eating*

SETTING SOME GOALS—GENERAL AND SPECIFIC

If a hard look at your weight, your Score Card, your blood pressure, and your cholesterol levels pronounces you a clean and godly person already, you can skip the rest of the food section and go take a hike. One of the things recommended in the activity section.

But if your intake habits need some adjusting, and your habits are well ingrained, you need to set some goals for improvement; you need a plan to help you achieve those goals *and* some tools to help you form the plan and then carry it out.

Earlier you set some specific goals for achievement in aerobic activity and strength building. Now it's time to get out your notebook and open it to a clean page up front, ready to set some goals for *mouth control*, remembering at all times that mouth control is only part of our total plan for health, hunkiness, and beauty.

You can shove the end of the rainbow even farther off if you don't accept that we can't separate the factors that impact on our health—everything must work in concert to some degree. Simply losing weight doesn't make you healthy; simply eating "good" foods doesn't make you healthy; running five miles a day and then rewarding yourself with a fat burger doesn't make you healthy, either. Our problem, of course, is having enough information and discipline and patience to think about long-range change in the first place.

First, then, the goal setting. Earlier, I asked you to commit your activity program to at least a three-month trial. Though the changes brought about by modifying what you eat can also start in just a few weeks, long-term change requires long-term modifications—you will be learning some new healthy habits that will last a lifetime. You'll also be starting slowly and gradually, taking things at your speed and your pleasure—the idea is enjoyable change, not deprivation. So if you set too short a trial period, you may not see the change you like.

I, therefore, want you to commit yourself to trying these ideas for at least six months, preferably a year. Yes, I know you'd rather this was the "Revolutionary Plan to Eat Your Way to a Lifetime of Better Health in Ten Days." But it's not. Those schemes improve only the health of the writer's wallet, as we've often said.

So pick up your pen and get ready to write your goals in your notebook. Please, be very specific with your own personal goal setting.

Your goals should include:

- A renewed commitment to moderation—in your intakes and in your activity patterns.
- A commitment to patience. You've spent all your life getting the way you are, and neither your habits, your shape, nor your health is going to change by the morning.
- A commitment to real honesty when it comes to what you're doing to your body. For instance, look at your food intake sheet. If you are taking in too many calories for your body, or too many fats, or

too much salt or alcohol, this book is a complete waste of time unless you accept that these factors are within your control. Remember that virtually the only weight loss and health improvement that is permanent takes place in people who *take control of their own lives.*

Your more specific goals should include:

- A commitment to changing your eating habits over time until they generally fit within accepted definitions of healthy eating. Look very carefully at your food intake Score Card and pinpoint your problem eating areas. *Write the problem areas in your notebook, and,* again, be specific: "I need to cut down my fats by half; I need to increase my fiber by a third. I need to cut down on Twinkies and beers." For now, don't worry if you can't tell a fat from a fiber; we'll show you how to do that soon. Just focus on your particular problem areas.
- A commitment to a certain weight loss, if necessary. I put this last, because it is a result of your other commitments. If you adjust your eating habits (and work a little on your activity), the weight loss will happen as a by-product of your other achievements.

I*f you're in the boat with the rest of us—planning to achieve your goals*

Though it may seem as if we've got the donkey pushing the wagon rather than pulling it, we are going to stop here and talk about some of those concepts and tools you will need before you can make your final *Lifetime Eating Adjustment Plan.*

First, we're going to resurrect an old concept that's been gathering cobwebs in the recesses of your mental attic at least since the seventh grade—a simple way of understanding a balanced diet when you see it. Second, we're going to explore the concept of modification in some detail. And then we'll plan. Really.

BACK TO THE FUTURE—REMEMBERING AND
USING THE FOUR FOOD GROUPS

I once had a chance to buy a Tiffany lampshade at a junk store, and I didn't because I did not understand what was in front of me. Most of us are like that when it comes to recognizing a balanced meal.

That's why a while ago some very knowledgeable nutrition experts at the Department of Agriculture developed the concept of the Four Food Groups. They designed a scientifically valid but easily understandable way to help nonexperts recognize and organize a balanced meal and eat more of them. By eating from each group each day, the average person would come closer to a balanced intake than by just choosing foods based on habit and taste buds.

The Food Group concept is not flawless, but you must understand it and then we'll show you how to use the concept of modification to make it a little better. So take a look at this basic road map. (You'll notice that a fifth group has been added, but it's there simply to help you become aware of the "extras" which aren't basic to nutritional balance but do contribute to our caloric intake.)

THE FOUR FOOD GROUPS

1. Vegetable and fruit group.

4 servings a day
1 serving = ½ cup or a typical portion such as 1 banana
Be sure to include one good source of vitamin C such as citrus fruit each day and to eat deep yellow and dark green vegetables frequently for vitamin A.

2. Bread and cereal group.

4 servings a day
1 serving = 1 slice bread; ½ to ¾ cup of cooked cereal, rice, macaroni, or noodles; 1 oz. ready-to-eat cereal (though this varies by cereal, generally one serving; the boxes have exact amounts on the label).
Eat mainly whole-grain bread or cereal; cereals and grains not made from whole grains should be enriched.

3. Milk and cheese group.

The number of servings a day varies by age:
    Children under nine: 2 to 3 servings
    Children nine to twelve: 3 servings
    Teens: 4 servings
    Adults: 2 servings
    Pregnant women: 3 servings; nursing mothers: 4 servings

1 serving = 1 cup (8 oz.) of milk or yogurt, 1 oz. cheddar or Swiss cheese, ½ cup cottage cheese (these portions are about equal in calcium but not in calories or fat)

4. Meat, poultry, fish, and bean group.

2 servings a day
1 serving = 2 to 3 oz. of lean meat, poultry, fish, 1 egg, ¾ to 1½ cups beans

The latest guide from the USDA has a fifth group—all those extras: the fats, sweets, and alcohol group. It includes butter, margarine, mayonnaise, salad dressing, candy, sugar, jam, jelly, soft drinks, alcoholic beverages, tea, coffee. It's not part of the basic four because it's not *basic* to nutritional balance. So you should start with the basic four groups and supplement from the foods in this fifth category. Some things in the fifth category are "bad"—empty sugar calories, excess fat; others are essentially "free"—coffee or tea without sugar, diet soft drinks.[7]

As you can see, the Four Food Groups chart can be a helpful guide or reminder of the variety of foods and proportion of foods we need to eat for healthy living. For instance, the vegetable/fruit and bread/cereal groups come at the top of the chart—they represent the bulk of carbohydrates, fiber, essential vitamins, and minerals in our food supply. Remember that our guidelines emphasize making carbohydrates 50 to 55 percent of your intake.

Milk products and meat supply protein and most of the fat in our food. Since protein should represent only 15 percent of our intake, and fat less than 30 percent, these categories come after the carbohydrates on the chart. As you see, this is not a rigid pattern but a helpfully suggestive one about how your "plate" should balance—remember our earlier advice about making the vegetables *the main course* and the meat the "side" dish? The Four Food Groups are given in an order to help you do that.

Think before you bite

Because it is a brief "sketch" map to all foods, the Food Group Plan doesn't give some of the more specific guidelines we need to achieve our goals. For instance, it doesn't distinguish between low-fat and whole-milk dairy products or between a leaner meat and a fattier meat. These distinctions are important if you are trying to lower saturated fat and cholesterol intake. Nor does it recognize that a "serving" of two different items in one food group may not have the same caloric value. This fact can be important if you are trying to lose or maintain weight.

So, while the Four Food Groups help us to get a variety of basic important nutrients, we need something to help make choices *within* a given group simple—here's where MUD arrives again.

W*hen MUD is fun*

Moderately increasing the good things and moderately decreasing the bad things, our MUD principle, is the essence of sensible eating. And four basic principles will help you internalize that modification:

First, in the foods you like, learn to substitute ingredients which will help you reach your goals for those which will not. Think skim milk rather than whole milk on your cereal, for example.

Second, learn to shift the balance of what you eat toward the recommended ratios. For instance, eat more chicken and less beef and pork, or eat smaller portions of red meat with larger portions of vegetables.

Third, lessen the frequency with which you enjoy sinful favorites. For instance, if you eat red meats three times a week, cut down to slightly smaller portions twice a week. If you eat chocolate cake for dessert every night (my kind of person), switch to fruit every other day, or to a diet fudge bar sometimes.

Fourth, gradually try new dishes. For instance, grill a salmon steak rather than a T-bone for that Friday night barbecue.

P*utting principles into action: aids to modification*

Thinking about these high-minded principles may make you feel good, but unless you put them into action they are useless. To do that you need to know more specifically what and how to modify. And here there are two stumbling blocks: (1) most of us can spot the obvious changes, but don't know where the hidden dangers lie.

(2) We run out of ideas or are too busy to think of all the ways we can modify.

A *scavenger hunt*

Tackling the first problem calls for a party—a scavenger hunt, to be exact. The jungle preserve is the family pantry (and later the grocery store), the prizes to be bagged are hidden fats, sodiums, cholesterol, and other dangers, and the weapons are a keen eye and lightning-quick label reading. Fun, as those old ads say, for the whole family.

Things that are more than meet the eye.   It isn't hard to know what constitutes a piece of steak, or to know that small red peppers bought from roadside stands in Mexico will charcoal your tongue. But it is a lot harder to know what we are really eating when we eat commercially prepared foods—which can be generally defined as anything God didn't make whole. He, for instance, made cows, peanuts, and hot peppers (those last probably on a bad day), but He didn't make cereal, Spam, or Twinkies.

These prepared products can have hidden fats, sodium, sugar, and cholesterol. But not all similar products have similar ingredients. Knowing where these hidden ingredients are in your favorite foods (the foods in your pantry) and comparing similar products to find a better one can help you modify painlessly. Label reading is, therefore, as important to your health consciousness as airplanes are to airlines.

KITCHEN DEMONS

If you live alone, are the staid type, and have a rainy afternoon to kill, you can hunt by simply idly looking through your cupboard. But if you have a family, why not turn something boring into something fun? A scavenger hunt through the larder can help all of you better understand about fats, cholesterol, sodium, and empty sugar calories and your daily eating. It can help label reading become second nature. It can also be a real eye opener and mouth closer, and thus a great motivator.

The target areas.   Pantry and cabinet shelves, refrigerator, freezer.

Target ingredients to hunt. (1) Fats. Bad: saturated fats. Good (within guidelines): polyunsaturated and monounsaturated fats. (2) Cholesterol. (3) Sodium. (4) Sugar, particularly hidden sugar.

Information you'll need for the hunt. *Labels.* All products have ingredient lists, and many now have nutritional information labels which give a breakdown of ingredients, usually by serving size.

Let's look at a sample label for one of the kinds of products you may find in your cupboard, in this case a baking mix:

NUTRITION INFORMATION PER PORTION

Portion size	2 oz. (about ½ cup)
Portions per package	20
Calories	240
Protein, grams	4
Carbohydrate, grams	37
Fat, grams	8
Sodium, mg.	700

PERCENTAGE OF U.S. RECOMMENDED
DAILY ALLOWANCES (U.S. R.D.A.)

Protein	6
Vitamin A	*
Vitamin C	*
Thiamine	20
Riboflavin	15
Niacin	10
Calcium	10
Iron	8

INGREDIENTS: Enriched flour, bleached [wheat flour, niacin (a B vitamin), iron, thiamine mononitrate (vitamin B_1), and riboflavin (vitamin B_{12}], animal and/or vegetable shortening (contains one or more of the following partially hydrogenated fats: soybean oil, cottonseed oil, beef fat, and/or nonhydrogenated lard) with leavening (baking soda, sodium aluminum phosphate, monocalcium phosphate), whey, salt, dried buttermilk.

LOOK AT PROPORTIONS OF INGREDIENTS
The nutrition label gives you a quick look at what's in a portion of the food. In this case, you can see that carbohydrates predominate, but there is a sizable amount of fat as well. How much relatively

speaking? If you eat 2,200 calories a day (remember your Score Card), then you want to consume no more than 73 grams of fat a day (about 30 percent of total calories). Eight grams is more than a tenth of that. And what kind of fat is it? A glance down at the ingredient list shows you that some of it, perhaps most of it, will be saturated fat. Why? Animal fat (the beef fat and lard) and hydrogenated vegetable shortenings (the soybean oil and cottonseed oil) are high in saturated fat. There may be some hidden cholesterol here too, depending on whether or not any animal fat was used. Manufacturers are allowed to list such alternative ingredients so that on a given day they can use whatever is the most economical and available shortening without having to change the label constantly.[8]

That doesn't help you know exactly what's in this box, for instance, but knowing this about ingredients could help you choose a baking mix made with all vegetable shortening (no cholesterol) and choose one with "nonhydrogenated" or "partially hydrogenated" vegetable shortening over one labeled "hydrogenated."

The other thing quick math with the nutrition label can tell you is that fat supplies about 30 percent of the calories in the mix (8 grams fat × 9 calories per grams). Okay, you say, that's about on the guidelines, and hey, it's only part of my meal. Correct, but that means when you make biscuits or pancakes with the mix, you'll want to use skim milk and two egg whites instead of an egg.

And what if you were planning to have a treat of bacon or sausage (9 to 16 grams of fat) with your biscuits or pancakes, and slather on a little margarine (11 g. fat per tablespoon)? Suddenly the total calories from fat in your breakfast comes to 60 or 70 percent, lots of it saturated. And you've eaten 28 to 49 grams of fat, or anywhere from 40 to 70 percent of your recommended daily intake of 73 grams of fat, if your caloric intake is 2,200 calories.

LOTS OF SALT

What about other target ingredients? Well, there's lots of salt. One portion here has 700 mg.? That's almost a quarter of your recommended levels, and you still haven't eaten that salty bacon or sausage. And all the sodium in this mix is not immediately evident, either. Two of the leavening agents, baking soda and sodium aluminum phospate, have sodium in them. Hidden sodium is the reason the front of a package may read "salt-free," but the product may not be sodium-free. Always check the detailed label.

HOW'S THE SUGAR CONTENT?

High marks for this product. No hidden sugar that we can see. But for practice, here's a label with some hidden sugar. Can you spot them?

> INGREDIENTS: Bleached flour, sugar, partially hydrogenated vegetable shortening, dextrose, water, corn syrup, carob, whey blend, corn starch, salt, sodium bicarbonate, lecithin, artificial flavorings, artificial colors.

Right. The hidden sugars are dextrose and corn syrup.

INTERPRETING THE INGREDIENTS LABEL

As you can see from our sample runthrough, you need to use all of the label, not just part. The nutritional breakdown can give you the proportion of one ingredient to another and can allow you to tell just how much of some ingredients are in the product. The list of ingredients names the items *in order of weight.* So if corn syrup is the first ingredient listed for a product, it has more corn syrup (sugar) in it by weight than any other product. In our biscuit mix, there is more flour than any thing else and less dried buttermilk.

In addition to telling you the amounts, the ingredient list can often provide a clue as to what types of fat or sugar are in the product when the nutrition label does not.

Labels don't tell the whole story, by any means, but you can use them to help you do a better job of selection.

Terms which mean sodium.   If a label doesn't tell you how much sodium is in a product, look for the following terms or items in the ingredients list:

Baking soda or sodium bicarbonate
Baking powder
Brine (salt and water)
Broth (usually high in sodium)
Bouillon (same as broth)
MSG (monosodium glutamate)
Any other compound with the word sodium in it.

Sugar by any name tastes as sweet.   The following ingredients are all sugar. If you see a lot of these in the ingredients list up near the top, then you can bet that a number of the carbohydrate grams on the nutrition label are simple carbohydrates—empty calories:

corn syrup, brown sugar, honey, invert sugar, maple syrup, molasses, cane syrup, any term ending in "-ose" (sucrose, fructose, dextrose, glucose, lactose), sorbitol (the alcohol form of glucose), mannitol, xylitol.

What to do on your scavenger hunt. First, divide up the categories among participants. If you are doing this solo, practice using your schizoid personality. Divide any way that works for your house and kitchen, but these suggestions may help: (1) cereals, dry mixes, and prepackaged convenience foods such as boxed macaroni dinners or soup mixes; (2) frozen convenience foods (entrées, dinners, pizza), vegetables, ice cream; (3) condiments or the stuff in the refrigerator door—catsup, mayonnaise, mustard, relishes, pickles, spreads, jellies, peanut butter, etc; (4) canned goods; (5) cookies and snacks.

Second, get busy and have fun looking. All participants might like to make notes on what they found—which products seemed particularly good and which seemed most misleading, which most surprised them (went against their idea of what was in it).

An informal evaluation. Your objective is not to write a thesis on your larder but to have some entertaining education. So evaluate your discoveries informally. Some questions which come to mind include:

- Where did you find hidden target ingredients that surprised you?
- In similar products such as cereals, did you find differences between two similar ingredients (sodium, fat, or sugar) that surprised you or might lead you to choose one product as more healthful?
- How does your larder stack up in various areas—for instance, snacks? Do you have lots of potato chips, snack crackers, cookies and candy bars (high in fats, salt, and empty calories) or do you go for more fruit, plain popcorn, etc.?
- How do the claims on the front of the package such as "lite," "no salt," "low in fat," "no cholesterol," etc. compare with your overall evaluation of the product? Are some misleading? In what way?
- With just what you have on your shelves, do you see some modifications you might easily make? *Write your modifications in your notebook.*

Taking the search a step further: storming the supermarket.   We've all got our favorite foods and brands, so comparing ingredients between similar products may not be possible within the limits of your kitchen. Here's where a trip to the supermarket can help.

Most of us, I think, tend to look at similar prepared foods as more or less the same and as singular entities. One can of chili, other than minor taste differences, is like any other can of chili. No-cholesterol vegetable margarines are all alike. One bottle of buttermilk salad dressing is like another.

That thinking is wrong and dangerous. Just as two twins can be as different as salt and pepper, the particular ingredients of similar processed food can be radically different, too. And becoming aware of those differences is what your trip to the supermarket is about.

Using the label-analyzing skills you learned in the pantry scavenger hunt, make a hit list of family favorites to take to the grocery store. You are going to look at different brands of the same product to see if one would be a better choice than another from a health standpoint. Target ingredients are the same: fats, sodium, sugar, cholesterol.

Here are some product possibilities for your hit list:

Peanut butters	Breaded fish fillets
Pickles	Mayonnaises
Brownie mixes	Catsups
Cookies	Salad dressings
Cake and muffin mixes	Canned baked beans
Snack crackers	Canned peaches
Cereals	Canned chilis
Margarines	Canned tunas
Yogurts	(compare water pack to oil)
Cottage cheeses	Prepared spaghetti sauces
Frozen chicken dinners	Luncheon meats
Frozen pizza	Juices vs. juice drinks:
Frozen lasagna entrées	canned, frozen, and dairy case

A word of caution here. Reading all these labels on boxes and cans and jars, may make you want to flee the supermarket for more "natural" foods. But wait a minute. As we said much earlier, *prepared and processed foods are not necessarily bad for you*. Indeed, most of the items in any store—supermarket and health-food store alike—are "prepared" and "processed." Anything that isn't fresh produce or meat could fit that definition. Grocery store brands are a lot cheaper and certainly are as healthy as any health-food brands—at times a lot safer, too. Generally speaking, you can count on the word "natural" to mean only one thing when it comes to food: a higher price.

MUD lists: tips for dietary modification

Now that your hunt through the pantry and grocery store has raised your eyebrows and shut your mouth, we're going to give you lots of help in opening it safely and pleasurably once again. The checklists at the end of this section are arranged by goal. Each list summarizes where the items you want to modify are found and gives you lots of ideas about how to MUD—Modify Up and Down. Our tips are not exhaustive, but they'll give you a good start and keep you going for months.[9]

If you didn't browse through them already, you might want to do so now before you draw up your personal plan.

AT LAST, THE ATTACK PLAN!

Get out your notebook and turn to the page where you wrote down your personal goals. You might lay your Score Card in front of you, too, since it shows exactly how far you have to go in various areas.

Decide which goal or goals you wish to tackle first. If you are methodical, you may want to tackle one thing at a time. Do you eat all the peas on your plate first, and then all the potatoes? Others like variety and might want to tackle a couple of goals at once. Whatever your preference, remember that these goals tend to work together. If you need to lower your fat intake, for instance, many of the substitutions will tend also to lower calories and raise carbohydrates.

Put your goals for the week in your notebook. Then, using the checklists, identify three to five modifications which you will try this week. During the week, judge how you like the changes and substitutions. Give everything several chances; make minor modifications in what you are doing; experiment. If you don't like one tub of margarine, for instance, try another. At the end of the week identify two or three more modifications and add them.

Every two weeks review your goals and add new ones until you are working on all your goals. If this schedule of change goes too fast or too slow for you, slow it down or speed it up a little, but always be conscious of making progress.

EVALUATING YOUR PROGRESS

One of the beauties of the Godly Eating Plan is that you don't have to worry constantly about how much this and how little that. But if you are comforted and encouraged by playing with numbers, you can get a rough estimate of what you've gained and lost in your goal areas by taking your modifications of the week and playing around a bit with the charts in the back and your daily food records to see how much saturated fat you've knocked out and how many carbos you've added, and so on. Truth be told, however, this is fairly meaningless data, since it is progress over the long run that counts in the Godly Eating Plan.

I recommend waiting until you start your third month on the plan to do any evaluation. Then you might want to keep a food record for a couple of days to see how you are doing. You might also want to have a blood test to check your cholesterol levels and triglycerides. I must caution you, however, that if you began your changes very gradually you may not see too much progress in three months. In my case, I had made good progress in four months, but even better progress by the end of the year. Individual bodies are not as exact as a calculator, so be patient.

If losing weight is one of your goals, you've probably been on and off the scales three times a day. Even once a day is too much. Under the Godly Eating Plan, your goal should be gradual, long-term loss, no more than one or two pounds a week. Try not to weigh more than once a week, the same day and time each week if possible.

OPEN THE MOUTH

With your plan in place, you have your swami's permission to eat. And he will not desert you yet, either. Lots of other nice things are in these pages.

After the checklists, you'll find three more eating helpers. First, to show you what all these principles and techniques we've been talking about look like in action, we've included a two-week cycle of menus. You may follow the whole thing if you like or just borrow ideas from it. Recipes featured in the menus are in the back of the book.

Second, since modifying dishes to make them healthier is an

important part of the Godly Eating technique, we'll give you some examples of how to do it. How about a party dip that's as tasty as one made with sour cream but which has almost no fat and only ten calories a tablespoon (enough to dunk two cauliflower buds, two carrot sticks, and a shrimp)? How about a beef stroganoff that's sinfully tasty but good for you?

And remember, the real world is full of temptations, not the least of which are restaurants, both fast and fancy. Some tips for dining out will help.

But *first, tips on just about anything you could imagine, including what your favorite movie star eats for breakfast*

These next pages really will teach you lots of interesting things about food. If you'd like, skim through them now and go on to the menu section on page 326, or the eating-out tips section on page 339. *And then for sure read your swami's super-whammy close to this entire book on page 342.*

But during the next weeks, do become very familiar with the following pages. Read them many times, and expand your awareness of the many good and bad things out there in the world of food.

Tips *on lowering total fats and particularly saturated fats*

GOALS:
(1) To lower total fat intake to approximately 30 percent of total calories and (2) to lower saturated fat to 10 percent and to raise polyunsaturates to about 10 percent. (Monounsaturated fats will make up the remaining percentage.)

WHERE FATS ARE FOUND
Polyunsaturated fats.   The good guys, these are found in:

- Safflower, sunflower, corn, soybean, and cottonseed oils contain a high proportion of polyunsaturated fatty acids.
- Some fish such as salmon, mackerel, herring, sardines, and fresh tuna.

Monounsaturated fats.   They're pretty good, too. Olive and peanut oils are high in monounsaturated fatty acids, as are olives and peanuts themselves. Most nuts are high in monounsaturated fat, as are avocados and avocado oil.

Saturated fats.   Here are the really bad guys. *Watch out for these sources of saturated fat:*

- All fats that are solid at room temperature.
- All animal fat. The fat surrounding red meats or in chicken skin is obvious, but even greater amounts can be hidden in processed meat products: Salamis, hot dogs, luncheon meats, and sausage get as much as 75 percent or more of their calories from fat, most of it saturated.
- Butterfat, an animal fat, is present in cream and whole milk and in whole milk products, including butter, cheese, cream cheese and cottage cheese made with whole milk, and ice cream.
- Some vegetable fats—coconut, palm, and palm kernel oil—are saturated. They are often used in prepared mixes and foods (cookies, cake mixes, bakery goods) because the fat is stable and has a long shelf life. Cocoa butter is also a saturated vegetable fat.
- Hydrogenated vegetable oil. Hydrogenating, a process which hardens vegetable oil, makes it saturated. Some examples are solid vegetable shortening and stick margarine. A number of prepared products such as some peanut butters and baking mixes have significant amounts of hydrogenated oil.
- Fried and processed foods. Not all the fat is saturated, but lots of these foods, such as potato chips or frozen TV dinners, are often high in total fat—you've got to read the label.
- Look out for these terms on labels which indicate saturated fat: animal fat, hardened fat or oil, hydrogenated, lard, meat fat, milk chocolate, shortening, vegetable fat or oil (this will often be coconut or palm oil), coconut, vegetable shortening, whole milk solids.

TIPS FOR SUBSTITUTION AND MODIFICATION

Meat modifications.

- Eat chicken and fish more frequently, beef and pork less frequently. If you usually eat meat three or four times a week, eat it twice a week and in smaller portions.

- Skin chicken before cooking if possible, but certainly before eating.
- Trim all visible fat from beef, pork, and other meats.
- Choose roasted, broiled, baked, and braised meat dishes over fried dishes or dishes in cream sauces.
- Grill your steaks or hamburgers on a charcoal grill or oven grill pan so that the rendered fat drops away from the meat. Make sure you choose a lean steak and trim it well and that you select the leanest hamburger.
- Many stores are now labeling the percentage of fat in their ground hamburger—choose the leanest available. Did you know that ordinary ground meat may have up to 30 percent fat?
- When making a dish or sauce with browned ground meat, brown the meat thoroughly in a separate pan and discard all the rendered fat before continuing with the recipe.
- Substitute ground turkey, available in many groceries, for any dish calling for ground meat.
- Substitute skinned chicken breasts in any veal cutlet recipe.
- When you eat fried meats, take off the batter, or part of it. Don't scarf down all the gravy.
- When you choose fish or shellfish more frequently, don't undo the good by frying it. There are scads of good broiled, grilled, braised, and baked methods of preparation.
- If you eat luncheon meats, select sliced whole turkey or chicken, lean roast beef, or even lean ham over processed meats such as salami, bologna, olive or pickle loaf, or liverwurst, which are all high in fat. Save the salami for a treat. Don't choose overstuffed sandwiches with gobs of meat.
- Place only 1 or 2 slices of meat (1 to 2 oz.) in your sandwich rather than a mound. Add lettuce, tomato, sprouts, green or red peppers, or watercress to give the sandwich added flavor and that overstuffed look you love.
- Eat more combination dishes that give you smaller portions of meat per serving than a meat dish by itself—provided those dishes are made without lots of other added fat. Examples: ground beef casseroles, almost any Chinese stir-fry meat dish (mooshu pork, moogoo-gai-pan, subgum chicken), sukiyaki, beef or pork stew (made with less meat and more vegetables), stuffed cabbage or eggplant, chicken or seafood jambalaya, pepper steak.
- When making meat or chicken broth, or soup or stew, skim the fat off the surface. There are several inexpensive separators which can make the job easy. If you've time, it's best to pop the dish in the refrigerator to chill (perhaps overnight), then spoon or lift the congealed fat from the surface.
- When making a favorite dish which calls for seasoning with bacon

or fatback, substitute a small quantity of very lean ham and the dish will be just as flavorful but much lower in fat.

Milk and butter modifications.

- If you now drink whole milk, 3.3 to 4 percent fat, switch to lower-fat milks—2 to 1 percent to skim milk. Make the switch as quickly as you can and in as many uses as you can.
- Even if you feel you can't drink anything less than 2 percent try using skim milk in cooking or on cereal.
- Replace butter with soft margarine. Work your way down the saturated fat scale: butter to soft tub margarine, liquid margarine, "diet" margarine. Check the ratio of polyunsaturated fat to saturated fat on the labels and choose the product with more polyunsaturates.
- If you must have a buttery taste on your vegetables, try liquid margarine or even a butter/margarine substitute such as Butter Buds.
- Try dressing vegetables with something other than a fat. For example, lemon juice is good on broccoli, cauliflower, green beans, parsleyed new potatoes, asparagus, steamed carrots, and many other vegetables. A sprinkle of dill weed or mixed herb seasoning such as Mrs. Dash or The Original Herb Seasoning goes nicely with the lemon juice. Vinegar picks up cabbage, collards, and mustard and turnip greens. Experiment with other favorites—thyme, sage, oregano, basil, marjoram.
- Choose a cheese made with skim milk over whole milk—for instance, mozzarella made with part skim milk instead of cheddar.
- Many groceries are now offering a number of traditional cheeses made with skim milk and low sodium. Try some, but read the nutritional label carefully; don't go only by front-of-the-package claims.
- Where appropriate, choose a small portion of a cheese with lots of flavor rather than a large serving of a mild cheese. For instance, using four tablespoons of bold-flavored grated Parmesan in your casserole rather than ½ cup (3 oz.) of swiss or mozzarella will save you approximately 12 to 18 grams of fat and more than 100 calories.
- Sour cream substitutes include the following. You may also use them in place of mayonnaise in some recipes such as chicken or tuna salad:
  - plain low-fat yogurt—good in sauces and recipes and on baked potatoes, and a good dip base, too.
  - blender-whipped low-fat cottage cheese.

- 2 parts blended cottage cheese to 1 part yogurt and lemon juice, to taste, is very good in place of sour cream in recipes and dips.
- buttermilk—good in sauces and in making mashed potatoes.
- Instead of nondairy sour cream, which often is made with coconut or palm kernel oil high in saturated fats, substitute one of our suggestions listed above.
- Instead of nondairy coffee creamers, whether powdered, liquid, or frozen, try skim milk. If you need nonrefrigerated convenience, try powdered dry skim milk. Experiment with brands until you get one you like. Or try drinking your coffee or tea black.
- Nondairy whipped toppings also usually contain saturated fats in the form of coconut and palm kernel oils. Moderate the frequency and amount you use.
- Instead of ice cream, choose ice milk or frozen yogurt or sherbet, but *read the label* to be sure your new choice is better and doesn't have too much sugar. Avoid the various "gourmet" ice creams, which are high in butterfat and calories.
- Instead of ice cream, pop into the food processor frozen unsalted and unsweetened black raspberries, blackberries, or red raspberries
- with a dollop of yogurt till just blended (about the consistency of soft churned homemade ice cream). Yum.

Sauces, gravies, and salad dressings.

- Try some of the new low-calorie low-fat/low-calorie commercial salad dressings. Some are very tasty and have as little as one gram of fat per tablespoon (which will dress a good-size salad) and most of that gram is often polyunsaturated. Many of these dressings have much less fat than plain oil and vinegar. *One caution:* the sodium content can be high, so check the label.
- Dress a salad with a little fancy mustard and dill weed whisked into lemon juice.
- When you choose an ordinary dressing, use only half of what you normally use.
- Instead of mayonnaise on your sandwich, try a little mustard. There are many types with different flavors and different "bites," so you'll probably find one you like.
- Instead of mayonnaise to dress your potato salad, chicken salad, or coleslaw, try a low-fat buttermilk dressing or one of the sour cream substitutes listed under "milk modifications."
- Avoid frozen vegetables which come with "butter sauce"; they are usually high in fat and sodium. Select plain vegetables and dress them yourself.

- Thicken a soup or sauce by using cornstarch or flour, rather than starting with a butter and flour roux (paste). To thicken 2 cups of liquid with cornstarch, mix 1 tablespoon of cornstarch with about ⅓ cup of water until smooth; then stir gradually into the sauce. Stir the sauce constantly until it thickens or the cornstarch will lump. To thicken 2 cups of liquid with flour alone, gradually sift 1 to 2 tablespoons of flour into the sauce, stirring constantly to prevent lumping.
- When making a special dish, perhaps a favorite ethnic dish which calls for bacon fat or chicken fat, cut the amount in half. If that leaves you with too little fat (it usually won't) and adding a little stock to make up the liquid difference won't work, use half the bacon or chicken fat and then add enough polyunsaturated oil to finish the job.

Snack modifications.

- Instead of a yeast doughnut or a danish, select a bran or fruit muffin for a typical savings of 40 to 50 percent on fat. Better yet, choose a piece of fruit for a snack.
- Choose plain popcorn over potato chips. Air popped or microwaved is best. Dress it very lightly with salt or seasoned salt if you like. Some folks like to give it a dusting of chili powder or curry powder. Some even like Butter Buds or a light squirt of butter-flavored cooking spray (but don't forget that the vegetable cooking spray is still fat).
- Choose dry-roasted nuts rather than oil-roasted. Nuts get from 70 to 95 percent of their calories from fats, mostly monounsaturated and polyunsaturated fats, loaded with calories, but awfully good.

Baking and bread modifications.

- When making biscuits, rolls, bread, or cookies use soft margarine instead of butter or shortening. When possible use polyunsaturated oil—for instance, you can make a decent pie crust using oil.

Tips on increasing intake of polyunsaturated fats

GOAL

To increase intake of polyunsaturated fats to about 10 percent of total caloric intake. And now, a caution: This checklist applies only if you are working on lowering your total fat intake and only if you need to increase your intake of polyunsaturates.

WHERE POLYUNSATURATED FATS ARE FOUND

- Polyunsaturated fats and monosaturated fats are both fats that are liquid at room temperature. Both have been associated with a decrease in cholesterol in the blood, but the effect is greater with polyunsaturates.
- Most polyunsaturated fats come from vegetable sources, but the fat from fish is also polyunsaturated.
- Vegetable oils that have high amounts of polyunsaturated fats compared to saturated fats include (in order of highest to lowest ratio of polyunsaturates): safflower, sunflower seed, corn and soybean oils.
- Soft tub margarines, either regular or diet, and liquid margarines are high in polyunsaturated oils. But even all soft margarines are not equal; be sure to check the labels.
- Fish high in polyunsaturates (the omega-3 fatty acids of much recent fame and publicity) include salmon, mackerel, herring, sardines, sablefish, lake trout, fresh tuna, whitefish, and anchovies. Halibut, bluefish, rockfish, rainbow and sea trout, ocean perch, bass, hake, pollock, smelt, and mullet are moderately high in fat. Oysters also have fairly high amounts of this fat.[10]

TIPS ON MODIFICATION

Many of the substitutions you will make to lower your saturated fat intake will boost your intake of polyunsaturates. Below are some of the more specific suggestions.

- When you use a vegetable oil in cooking or in dressing a salad, choose an oil high in polyunsaturates, as noted above.
- Choose soft margarines with a high ratio of polyunsaturated oil to saturated.
- Choose a broiled, poached, or grilled fish dish at least two or three times a week and let it replace meats which are high in saturated fats—a grilled salmon or tuna steak in place of a T-bone beef steak or a pork chop.
- Choose a salmon salad for lunch instead of a hamburger. A small serving of canned red salmon dressed with freshly squeezed lemon juice, dill weed, and freshly ground pepper is delicious and high in protein as well.

Tips on modifying cholesterol intake

GOAL

To limit dietary cholesterol intake to 300 mg. per day or less.

WHERE DIETARY CHOLESTEROL IS FOUND

Watch out for the following sources of high cholesterol:

- Egg yolks. One yolk contains 274 mg., nearly all of your recommended daily intake of 300 mg., making the egg about the most concentrated source of cholesterol in the American diet.
- Organ meats. Beef liver, for instance, has 410 mg. in a 3-oz. slice (about 6½ × 2⅜ × ⅜). One chicken liver has 125 mg. Other organ meats include brains, sweetbreads, gizzards, heart, kidney.

Cholesterol is also significantly found in:

- All animal tissue. Interestingly, cholesterol is associated with *lean* tissue. Cutting off the visible fat does not appreciably lower cholesterol—it lowers the saturated fat, which also helps raise blood cholesterol.

  The cholesterol content of all meat is one reason we recommend only two servings (3 oz. = a serving) of meat or poultry each day.
- Whole milk products. A tablespoon of butter has 31 mg.; a cup of whole milk has 33 mg. compared to skim milk's 4 mg. per cup.

Foods without cholesterol, or with low levels.

- All plant products—vegetables, fruits, grains—have no cholesterol.
- Skim milk products. Low-fat (1 percent) milk products such as cottage cheese or buttermilk have very, very low cholesterol levels per serving.
- All fresh- and saltwater fish are low in cholesterol. Most shellfish are also low, though many experts caution against eating too much shrimp (approximately 43 mg. per ounce). Beware caviars—they contain about 48 mg. per tablespoon.

Note: If you are going to try to lower the cholesterol levels in your blood, you *must* lower saturated fats in your diet as well as your intake of dietary cholesterol.

SUBSTITUTIONS AND MODIFICATIONS

Egg modifications.

- In scrambled eggs, use only one yolk per serving. For most folks that would be one yolk for two whites.
- Try substituting egg whites in recipes calling for whole eggs: two egg whites equal one whole egg. This works for muffins, pancakes, cookies, and puddings. It also works in recipes where you use the egg as a binder—for instance, if your favorite salmon-loaf recipe calls for an egg to hold it together, the egg whites will work fine and save you a lot of cholesterol.

Meat modifications.

- Trim all meat of as much fat as possible before cooking. Skin chicken before cooking. Even though there is not too much dietary cholesterol in the fat, such trimming lowers saturated fat and, therefore, helps lower the cholesterol level in the blood.
- Choose fish as the "meat" in your meal at least twice a week—even more if you really like fish.
- At least once a week enjoy a no-meat, low-cholesterol, and low-fat meal. Some suggestions:
  - Vegetarian spaghetti—see our dynamite recipe.
  - Red beans and rice—go New Orleans (prepare with olive oil rather than bacon fat).
  - Pinto bean tostadas—go Mexican.
  - Vegetable curry with dhal—for an Indian evening.
  - Minestrone soup—make it thick as a stew for a satisfying feast and serve with corn bread.

Tips on sugar

GOAL

To reduce the number of empty calories consumed.

WHERE SUGAR IS FOUND

We know where the obvious sugar is—in sweet things: soft drinks, candy, jam, desserts, pies, cookies, cakes, sweet pastries. But sugar is hidden in lots of places we don't expect to find it—look at the label on the jar of peanut butter on your shelf, for instance.

The following terms on labels indicate that sugar has been used. Sugar in this sense is also called "nutritive sweetener" because it has calories (and how!):

- Words ending in "-ose" usually refer to forms of sugar—sucrose, fructose, dextrose, glucose, lactose, maltose.
- Look out for these chemical-sounding words which also indicate sugars: sorbitol (the alcohol form of glucose), mannitol, xylitol.
- And these forms which you may not think of as "sugar": corn syrup, brown sugar, honey, invert sugar, maple syrup, molasses, cane syrup.

TIPS FOR MODIFICATION

Drinks.

- Try out various artificial sweeteners for your tea or coffee. If you want to stay with sugar, try gradually decreasing the amount you use, until you're using about half of what you now use.
- If you've never tried to drink your coffee or tea black without sugar, experiment. Lots of folks find they like it even better.
- Instead of regular soft drinks, experiment with diet varieties.
- Substitute fruit juice for soft drinks. Juices may have almost as many calories in some cases, but they've lots more nutrients.
- If you like the fizziness of soft drinks, make your own with one part fruit juice to one part soda water or seltzer. Pineapple-grapefruit or orange juice with soda water is particularly good.
- Take a tip from the Far East and refresh yourself with a *nimbu pani*—a lime water. Put the juice of one-fourth to one-half of a lime (or lemon) in a tall glass with ice and fill 'er up with plain or soda water. No sugar or sweetener needed. Give this a couple of tries. It's not really bitter, and the refreshing bite grows on you.

Alcoholic beverages.

- The easiest way is to drink fewer drinks when you do drink and savor those. For example, have one gin-and-tonic and then switch to only tonic.
- If you don't gulp them like lemonade, spritzers can be light and enjoyable—a little white or red wine, seltzer, and a twist of lemon or lime peel.
- Experiment with "light" beers till you find one you like, and trim the number you drink. Ditto for "light" wine coolers.
- Always use a jigger when pouring mixed drinks.

Spreads for breads.

- Gradually trim the amount you spread on toast or a biscuit. I found that 1 to 1½ teaspoons of jam worked as well as 2 to 3.
- Preserves made with fruit only and no sugar are surging onto the market these days. Though they are lower in calories, they are not as low as you might think—from about forty-two calories per tablespoon for "no-sugar" preserves or fifty-five for regular preserves.
- Try spreading a little unsweetened applesauce, sprinkled with cinnamon (or another favorite spice) on your toast, muffin, waffle or pancakes.
- Some "light" syrups have less sugar and are tasty. Try them in moderation.
- Invent your own pancake or waffle syrup. Or try ours: Mash one banana in a small saucepan with enough orange juice to give it the desired consistency. Add cinnamon to taste and heat until well blended and bubbly hot. Mary Abbott and Chris like it just like this; I like to add a little artificial sweetener.

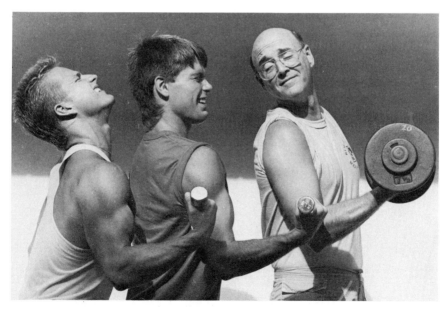

I hope you notice who has the heavy weight. I always humiliate the guys with my superhuman strength.

In recipes.

- Decrease sugar in recipes (particularly breads, muffins, cookies) until you've decreased it by about a third.

Sweet treats.

- Choose fresh fruit when possible and unsweetened frozen fruit next. Select fruit canned in juice or water rather than in syrup. A half cup of frozen sweetened fruit has six teaspoons of added sugar; a half cup of canned fruit in heavy syrup has four teaspoons of added sugar and in light syrup, two teaspoons.
- Make your own Popsicles by freezing fruit juice.
- Pop frozen unsweetened raspberries, blackberries, or strawberries into the food processor with a dollop of yogurt. Blend to a soft ice cream consistency but still stiff enough to sit up on a cone.
- Work toward having one of these fruit treats for dessert on most nights or every other night. Enjoy your regular favorites on other nights—cake or pie—but make your serving smaller.

Tips on salt (sodium)

GOAL

Limit sodium intake to 3,000 mg. a day or less.

For most of the readers of *Body Worry*, unless you have high blood pressure and/or have been told to watch your salt intake, this goal will be of less importance than getting your intakes of saturated fats, carbohydrates, and cholesterol right. But even minor modifications here can help the overall picture.

LOOKING FOR HIDDEN SODIUM

When the food label says "salt," the presence of sodium is easy to spot. More and more foods are putting the amount of sodium on the label too in milligrams, so check that first. But a lot of salt still masquerades in compound ingredients or under highfalutin chemical monikers we mentioned earlier. The key to spotting most of them is the word "sodium."

Some of the terms or compounds:

baking soda or sodium bicarbonate

baking powder
brine (salt and water)
broth (usually high in sodium)
bouillon (same as broth)
MSG (monosodium glutamate)
sodium chloride
sodium ascorbate
sodium caseinate
sodium tripolyphosphate

TIPS FOR LOWERING SODIUM INTAKE

Added salt.

- Consciously use salt less as you cook; use herbs and spices instead.
- Try reducing by half the amount of salt a recipe calls for. After you season the pot, wait a minute or two before tasting to give the salt flavor a chance to meld with the ingredients.
- Experiment with prepared herb mixtures such as Mrs. Dash. You can save a lot by this one step, since experts estimate that about one-third of our average daily intake of sodium comes from adding salt to our food in cooking or at the table.[11]
- Leave the salt shaker on the shelf, not the table.
- Taste your food before you salt it. If you must have a little more salt, try one shake rather than two or three.

Salt in prepared foods. The overall rule here is to be aware that sodium is often added in large quantities to prepared food, so check labels and where possible choose the lower-sodium version of similar foods. A number of specifics are spelled out in the following:

- Choose fresh vegetables and foods when possible—these have the least sodium, since none is added in processing.
- Choose frozen and canned vegetables prepared without salt.
- Many condiments are high in sodium. Many now are available in sodium-reduced versions. Check the labels. Here's a partial list:
  - Onion salt—substitute onion powder.
  - Garlic salt—substitute garlic powder.
  - Celery salt—substitute celery seed.
  - Meat tenderizers—marinate meat overnight in wine or other low-sodium, acidic marinade.
  - Bouillon—reduced sodium bouillon cubes are available, but making your own low-sodium stock is tastier.

- Soy sauce—a reduced-sodium version is available; experiment with using less than the recipe calls for.
- Steak sauce.
- Barbecue sauce—it doesn't take long to make your own, but watch ingredients such as catsup and mustard, which have plenty of sodium themselves.
- Worcestershire sauce.
- Mustard—we recommend using mustard instead of mayo to dress sandwiches because a little mustard goes a long way, and at about 63 mg. of sodium per teaspoon or packet, this seems a better trade off than 11 grams of fat and 80 mg. of sodium per tablespoon of mayo—both about average servings.
- Salad dressings.
- Pickles.
- Relishes.
- Olives.
- Eat fewer pickles and foods preserved in brine, such as sauerkraut. When you do eat sauerkraut, for instance, rinsing it well will remove some of the brine.
- Check the label on your ready-to-eat cereal. Some types and brands are much higher in sodium than others. (You can look for hidden sugar at the same time.)
- Do you need crunchy munchies and don't like vegetable sticks? Treat yourself in moderation to unsalted dry roasted peanuts, plain popcorn, unsalted pretzels, the occasional pack of unsalted potato chips.
- Convenience foods often contain high amounts of sodium. Check the labels on the following:
  - Frozen dinners and combination dishes. Avoid those that are high in sodium (a number are also high in fat as well).
  - Canned condensed soups are often high in sodium. Check the labels and look for reduced-sodium versions which are available.
  - Dehydrated mixes for soups, sauces, and salad dressings usually have lots of sodium. You can avoid these by making your own and checking for reduced-sodium products. Making your own salad dressing or soup really takes very little time and can taste lots better than the mix.
- Cured and smoked meats such as ham, bacon, and smoked fish are often high in sodium, so you may want to check on your favorites and eat them less frequently. Such processed meats as salami, hot dogs, sausage, and luncheon meats are even higher in sodium as well as high in fat.
- When you eat a dish relatively high in sodium, such as ham, balance

it by serving lower-sodium foods such as vegetables cooked without added salt.

- Frozen vegetables with sauce—the kind that usually come in a little plastic pouch—are usually high in sodium. Check the label to be sure. Select fresh vegetables or those frozen without salt and dress them with a little lemon juice and herbs instead of lots of salt.
- Fast-food places serve lots of food high in sodium, and it's hard to know just which items those are. In one analysis at one restaurant the regular order of french fries, salted, had less sodium than the hamburger.[12] But many fast-food chains are now supplying lists of the nutrition ingredients in their dishes; ask your favorite if they have such a list.
- Natural cheeses vary widely in how much sodium they have per 1½-oz. serving; sodium can range from 110–450 mg. for this amount. So check the labels of your favorites and choose the brand or variety lower in sodium. (You can look for lower fat at the same time.) As a general rule, processed cheese foods and spreads have the most sodium per serving, and cottage cheese falls between processed cheeses and natural cheeses.

Tips on fiber

GOAL
To include adequate fiber in what you eat, about twenty to thirty-five grams a day.

WHERE FIBER IS FOUND
Dietary fiber is the parts of plants our human digestive system cannot break down. Different kinds of plants have different kinds and amounts of fiber such as cellulose, pectin, lignin, and gum, which function differently in our bodies. Therefore, it's a good idea to eat a range of plant foods with fiber.

Good sources of various types of fiber include:

- Whole grains and products made from whole grains. Whole grains include whole wheat, cracked wheat, bulgur, oatmeal, whole corn-meal, popcorn, brown rice, whole rye, whole barley. Products made of whole grains can include breads, cereals, tortillas, grains in soup, pastas.

- Vegetables are good sources of fiber, particularly those with edible skins, seeds, and stems. Among those with more amounts of fiber are beets; vegetable greens such as beet, turnip, collard, and mustard greens; corn; broccoli; fresh beans and peas; winter squash; sweet potatoes.
- Dried beans and peas. These are also good sources of fiber. Think beans: lima beans, pinto beans, great northern beans, black beans, kidney beans, soybeans. Also think peas: black-eyed peas, split peas, chickpeas, cow peas. Think lentils.
- Fruits. Again those with edible skins, seeds, and stems are good sources. Fresh apples, pears, and berries probably head the list. Prunes, dried figs, dates, oranges, and grapefruit are also good.
- Nuts and seeds. Pecans, filberts, sunflower seeds, peanuts, and so on. A caution, though: nuts are high in fats (monounsaturated and polyunsaturated), so too many can send your fat and calorie intake soaring.

TIPS TO HELP YOU GET ADEQUATE FIBER

- Choose whole grain breads and cereals rather than breads and cereals made totally from white flour or refined grains. The variety and texture in these whole-grain products is enormous these days, so experiment to find ones you like.
- Many breads, cereals, and pastries are made with a mixture of whole-grain and refined flours. These can give you more fiber, too. Check the ingredients list to see how high up on it the whole-grain flours are.
- Look for whole-grain pastas. Whole wheat and buckwheat products are available in a wide range of types.
- When you bake, try substituting whole-grain flour for half of the white flour called for in the recipe. This goes well in muffins, pancakes, waffles, biscuits. Many cookbooks also have recipes for using whole grain flours.
- Breakfast is a good time to get fiber by picking cereals, bread, and muffins made with whole grains and/or bran.
- When you need a second helping at dinner, eat more vegetables and fruit, not more meat. It's okay to have that other new potato if you eat the skin.
- Eat the skins of vegetables, when possible. Don't peel the tomato, for example.
- When you need a snack, reach for a fresh, unpeeled apple, pear, plum, peach, or nectarine. Or eat a tangerine or orange. Avoid sugary candy bars and pastry or even cheese crackers from the vending machine.

- Choose two or three vegetables for dinner and serve one raw—perhaps as the salad (carrot-and-apple salad, for instance) or in the green salad (cucumbers, cauliflower, broccoli, carrots, tomatoes, tiny green peas, and summer squash work well).
- To eat more dried peas and beans, make one night a week international festival night and go around the world (or just this country) via some classic bean and pea dishes:

From the U.S.

Hopping john—the South
Red beans and rice—New Orleans
Chili with beans—the West
Boston-baked beans—the East
Senate Bean Soup—Washington, D.C.
Split-pea soup
Three-bean salad

From around the world

Black beans and rice or feijoadas—Brazil
Bean burritos and tostadas—Mexico
Cuban black bean soup—Cuba
Pigeon peas and rice—the Bahamas and the West Indies
Cassoulet—France
Beans and cabbage—the Mediterranean
Minestrone soup—Italy
Falafel—the Middle East
Beans bretonne—France
Dhal and pappadoms—India
Miso soup—Japan

When making a dip for an appetizer, include a bean dip or two. Dips made from pinto beans or chickpeas are very tasty.

Tips for eating enough carbohydrates

GOAL

To achieve a carbohydrate intake that is about 50 to 55 percent of total caloric intake. To emphasize complex carbohydrates and limit simple carbohydrates (sugar, "empty" calories).

ABOUT CARBOHYDRATES

Carbohydrates can be either complex carbohydrates or simple carbohydrates. The complex carbohydrates provide energy for our bodies, and fiber, vitamins, and minerals. Complex carbohydrates are found in vegetables, fruits, grains, and cereals. Simple carbohydrates are sugar, providing empty calories. They are found in sweets, candies, all refined sugar, corn syrup, honey, etc.

A note of good cheer: If you have been working on modifying other aspects of your eating patterns, such as lowering your consumption of total fat and saturated fat, chances are you have already boosted your carbohydrate intake. So these tips will probably just reinforce ideas you've already adopted.

TIPS FOR MODIFICATION

Vegetables. For fun and to increase your range, try some vegetables you rarely eat or have never tried. Also explore in your cookbooks and find some new ways of fixing old favorites. Don't expect to like everything (parsnips do nothing for me, I find), but be prepared to add some new tastes and to find that something you hated in your childhood you may now like (M.A. now finds beets tolerable about once a month).

To spur your imagination here is a list:

Alfalfa sprouts
Artichokes
Asparagus
Bamboo shoots
Bean sprouts
Beets
Beet greens
Black-eyed peas
Bok choy
Broccoli
Brussels sprouts
Butterbeans and butterpeas
Cabbage—green, red, savoy, Chinese
Carrots
Cauliflower
Celeriac
Celery
Collard greens
Corn
Cowpeas
Crowder peas
Cucumbers
Daikon (mild radish used in oriental cuisine)
Dandelion greens
Eggplant
Endive
Fava beans
Green beans—snap beans, pole beans
Jerusalem artichoke
Jicama (crisp tuber used in Mexican and Chinese cuisine)
Kale
Kidney beans
Kohlrabi
Lettuce—iceberg, Boston, Bibb, butter, romaine, leaf
Lima beans
Mushrooms—regular, Chinese black, cloudear, straw, chanterel

Mustard greens
Okra
Onions
Parsley
Parsnips
Peas, green garden
Peppers, sweet and hot, red,
  green, and yellow
Potatoes
Pumpkin
Radishes—white, red, black;
  round and fat, long and skinny
Rutabagas
Sauerkraut (cabbage)

Seaweed—kelp, nori, etc.
Spinach
Squash—summer squash, yellow
  crookneck, matapan, etc.
Squash—winter squash such as
  acorn, butternut, turban, hubbard
Sweet potatoes
Tomatoes
Turnips
Turnip greens
Water chestnuts
Watercress
Yams
Zucchini

Fruits. Substitute fruit for a sweet snack or dessert full of empty calories. Here's a list of fruit to stimulate your imagination:

Apples—fresh, juice, applesauce
Apricots—fresh and dried, nectar
Avocados
Bananas
Blackberries
Blueberries
Cantaloupes
Cranberries—fresh, frozen, juice
  (watch for lots of added sugar
  in most cranberry drinks, but
  artificially sweetened versions
  are available)
Dates
Figs—fresh and dried
Gooseberries
Grapefruit—whole, juice
Grapes—fresh and juice
Kiwi fruits
Lemons
Limes
Mangoes

Melons—honeydew, Crenshaw,
  Persian
Nectarines
Oranges—whole, juice
Papayas
Peaches—fresh, frozen, dried
Pears—Bartlett, Bosc, Anjou, and
  lots of varieties
Pineapples
Plantains
Plums—lots of varieties
Pomegranates
Prunes—fresh prune plums and
  dried, juice
Raisins
Raspberries—black and red
Rhubarb
Strawberries
Tangerines—fresh and juice
Watermelons

Bread. Remember, "it's not the bread, it's the spread" which has the calories we tend commonly to associate with starchy carbohydrates such as breads, cereals, potatoes, rice, and pasta. Cut way back on (or omit) the margarine you spread on your bread, the margarine and sour cream you dump on your baked potato, the cream sauce you put over pasta, and the gravy over rice. Remember the substitutions you learned on the checklist for lowering fats.

Breakfast is a good time to stoke your furnace with carbohydrates to get the day off to a good start. Concentrate on fruit, cereal (hot or ready-to-eat), and bread (toast, muffins, even pancakes) rather than meat or eggs. Two sausage patties have 200 calories, 16 grams of fat and 12 grams of protein; 1 cup of oatmeal with ½ cup of skim milk has only 187 calories, 2 grams of fat, and 10 grams of protein. Oatmeal with milk, though, has 31 grams of carbohydrate whereas sausage has only a trace. And which would fill you up more? A cup and a half of milk and cereal, or two sausage patties?

"Bread" need not be just a slice of loaf bread or a dinner roll. Here are some ideas to give you an idea of variety. (We've left out items such as croissants, which are made with lots of butter or fat, but we've left in some things, such as biscuits, which can have moderately high amounts. So remember your other guidelines.)

- Loaf breads—whole wheat, rye, pumpernickel, cracked wheat, oatmeal bread, Irish soda, multigrains of various sorts. Lots of bakeries are beginning to make unsliced loaves of a variety of breads that not only taste great but look great with your meal, too.
- Quick breads—applesauce bread, banana bread, walnut bread, datenut bread, squash bread, pumpkin bread.
- Muffins—bran muffins with fruit such as apples, dates, blueberries, apricots, cherries, bananas; corn muffins; oatmeal muffins; graham muffins (whole wheat).
- Biscuits—graham and regular.
- English muffins—whole wheat, rye, raisin.
- Rolls—all shapes and sorts, from small dinner rolls to large poppy seed and onion rolls.
- Crackers—graham crackers, whole wheat crackers (watch fat content), melba toast.
- Coffee cake—if made at home, it can be low in fat and not too high in sugar either. Avoid commercial products drenched in sugar.
- Bagels.
- Rice cakes.

Cereal, pasta, and rice.

- Ready-to-eat cereals can not only taste good, but be good for you. Most cereal companies are now providing complete carbohydrate information on the label so that you can tell how much sugar is in the cereal and choose those who get most of their calories from complex carbohydrates.

- To avoid extra sugar in hot cereals, pick the plain products and add your own fruit, milk, and (if you must) sweetener so that you can keep track of the amount.
- Pasta comes in more shapes than you can remember. Experimenting can be fun and no two dinners need look alike.
- Rice goes great under lots of things besides gravy. In the South we like to eat our butterbeans or black-eyed peas on top of rice. In fact, beans and rice dishes are eaten the world over. Rice is also great under stewed tomatoes, or okra and tomatoes. Try it under entrées in place of pasta for variety. Brown rice, especially, can add variety and can be used in most instances where you would use white rice.

Two weeks of menus on the Godly Eating Plan

We've looked at lots of menu plans from various sources as we did the research for this section, and one observation came up over and over: Too many of the menu cycles were too ideal. They ignored life as it is lived. Lots of them seemed to be based on the idea that we singlemindedly fix and eat all our meals at home. But many of us are busy working as we eat lunch. Sometimes we brown-bag it, sometimes we go out or send out for a quick lunch, and other times we have to take someone to a business luncheon. The *Body Worry* cycle takes this into account—of the five working days, we allow for two brown-bag lunches, two "fast-food" meals, and one business luncheon. We do assume you will eat breakfast and dinner at home, but if you don't, you can follow most of the breakfast menus when eating out and can come close with many of the dinners at restaurants.

Speaking of breakfast, every day was different on many of the plans we read. Yet for most of us breakfast is something of a ritual— we tend (our very informal survey shows) to eat about the same thing every morning. This two-week cycle offers more patterns than you might choose—both to give you an idea of what variety is possible and to show you how what you eat at breakfast can affect the balance of food choices for the rest of your day. For example, if you don't eat a dairy product with breakfast, you might include it at both lunch and dinner or as a snack.

Dinner comes closest to real life (as we see it) in the ideal cycles, because most people dine most nights at home and do give some attention to making a substantial, balanced meal. We continue pretty much in this style.

Snacks. Lots of ideal menus pretend these don't exist and imply a slapped wrist if we reach for one, or at least for more than one in a day. Since there are no snacks, the three meals on these ideal cycles often seem really big, particularly lunch. The Body Worriers working on this book (like most folks) like snacks—we get to feeling a little peckish at about 10:30 A.M. and 3:30 P.M. (coffee break times) and sometimes want a little something to go with the movie or ballgame on TV. Our menus recognize the urge to snack and provide some tasty but healthy tidbits. And we include the snacks in the day's balanced intake.

Treats. This book is about modifying lifestyle habits, not deprivation and suffering for life. So the occasional treat is okay, as we've said many times previously. Most of the treats built into this menu are not of the "smaller piece of chocolate cake less frequently" type recommended earlier. Why not? Well, you can do that yourself. Our desserts are an attempt to show you ways you might not have thought of to satisfy your sin-loving sweet tooth while eating like a saint.

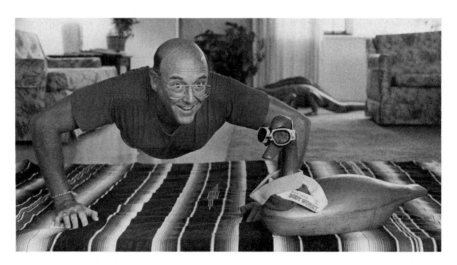

I like push-ups. Howie prefers swimming (and would like to have shotguns covered under gun control laws). Rex, my watch lizard (background), just "crawls on his belly like a reptile."

Nutritional aims of the menus

We've tried to incorporate the goals and guidelines presented earlier into these menus, just as you might do it if you were planning your own. Each day's menu is based on the plan illustrated by the Four Food Groups and on the modifications presented in the checklists. For example, fish and chicken are eaten more often than red meat, and the recipes feature dishes modified to keep fats and saturated fats low. Each day emphasizes lots of fruits and vegetables, not meat.

HOW MUCH SHOULD YOU EAT?

Every individual reading this will have different needs and goals. Each of you will need to eat different amounts to maintain your weight or to lose weight. That's one reason why we haven't stuck quantities on some of the items (mostly the vegetables). You have set your goals and know approximately how much you must eat to reach them.

If you eat the portions as presented in the menus and eat the vegetables in half-cup servings, the menus without snacks average 1,500 to 1,600 calories a day—a level at which most people will lose weight in the gradual manner recommended. If you include the snacks the menus include 1,800 to 2,000 calories. If you need more to maintain your weight, eat more vegetables, a bigger bowl of cereal, another whole grain roll. Those of you who need this are mostly men, and you are mostly used to eating these larger servings anyway. The trick is to make sure that you have another ear of corn-on-the-cob (watch the margarine), not another piece of steak.

SOME TIPS ABOUT LUNCH

Even if you brown-bag your lunch only two days a week and go out for a quick lunch on two days and a more leisurely lunch on one day, you can MUD along easily.

Brown-bagging is easy. Good sandwiches prepared in healthy ways are a mainstay because they are so easy to pack. But there are lots of good dishes that are too liquid to put in a sack. A snap-lid plastic container (flat, 2" tall, about 6" × 8" or so) can hold these types of foods and fit in a briefcase. Some nifty flat compartmentalized containers are available, too. These can be a good investment, producing nonboring lunches without damaging your executive image.

Quick lunch out. The sandwich shop or deli that makes sandwiches and other dishes to order is usually a better bet than the fast-food joint because you can get them to make exactly the sandwich you want with the fixings you desire. They often also have fresh fruit and fruit cups, yogurt, and salad plates.

But fast food is not impossible, as we'll show in a later section. If you're trying to avoid sodium, though, stay out of fast-food places. Even those fast foods that have lower-fat contents usually are full of salt.

The menus

*See our recipe section, page 347.

MONDAY, DAY 1

Breakfast
½ grapefruit
1 cup oatmeal
1 cup skim milk (put part on the oatmeal and drink the rest as you like)
1 slice whole-grain toast with 1 tsp. margarine or 1 tsp. jelly

Lunch
Brown bag:
Lean ham sandwich
   2 slices lean ham (2 oz.), 2 slices whole-grain bread, mustard, lettuce,
   tomato
Carrot and cucumber sticks
Apple or pear
1 cup skim milk

Dinner
Shirley's Baked Chicken*
Baked potato with 1 or 2 tbs. of yogurt or Mock Sour Cream*
Steamed broccoli seasoned with lemon juice
Spinach Salad*
Whole-grain roll with 1 tsp. margarine
Dessert: oatmeal cookie

Snacks
Orange or tangerine
2 cups plain popcorn (air-popped or microwaved)
1 banana (the banana in calories equals the other two put together)

TUESDAY, DAY 2
Breakfast
⅔ to 1 cup orange juice
1 oz. nutritious ready-to-eat cereal with ½ cup skim milk (for example, about 1 cup of bran flakes, shredded wheat, or oat circles)
1 or 2 slices whole-grain toast with 1 tsp. margarine per slice or 1 tsp. jelly

Lunch
Fast food:
1 or 2 slices of 12-inch cheese pizza. Add green pepper, onions, and/or mushrooms as desired.
Large green salad (see our tips about the salad bar, page 341) with 1 tbs. dressing, low-calorie if available
Iced tea (artificially sweetened) or diet soda

Dinner
Fish with Caper Sauce*
Rice with Wild Rice and Herbs*
Green beans seasoned with lemon juice and dash of garlic powder
Green salad (include tomatoes and carrots, for sure) with 1 tbs. low-calorie, low-fat dressing
Whole-grain roll with 1 tsp. margarine
Dessert: Fresh Fruit Cup*

Snacks
Pear or apple
2 graham crackers (2½-inch-square)
2 cups plain popcorn (air-popped or microwaved)

WEDNESDAY, DAY 3
Breakfast
Grapefruit juice (6 oz. to 1 cup)
Whole-grain English muffin with ½ cup applesauce
1 cup skim milk
Coffee or tea

Lunch
Brown bag:
1 cup Hunky Chicken Salad (made with apples and grapes)*
   1 cup with whole-grain roll on the side
   or as a sandwich with 2 slices of bread
1 cup low-fat yogurt with fresh fruit (preferable to yogurt with preserves)
Choice of noncaloric drink

Dinner
Braised Pork Tenderloin Medallions with Caraway*
Braised Red Cabbage*
Green salad with 1 tbs. low-fat dressing
Corn muffin
1 5-oz. glass red wine (optional—have another muffin if you have a non-caloric drink)
Dessert: melon cup with cantaloupe, honeydew, and watermelon

Snacks
1 cup Cereal Snack Mix*
Orange or pear
1 small packet raisins (1½ tbs.)

THURSDAY, DAY 4
Breakfast
¼ cantaloupe
1 cup hot cereal
1 cup skim milk
1 slice whole-grain toast with 1 tsp. margarine or 1 tsp. jelly
Coffee or tea

Lunch
Business lunch:
Cup of clear vegetable soup
Crab Louis with sauce on the side
Green salad (In most restaurants the Crab Louis comes surrounded by the salad. If the salad has a hard-boiled egg, eat only the white. Use only about 1½ tbs. of the dressing, unless it is low-calorie, low-fat. A squeeze of lemon on the crab is also tasty in place of the dressing.)
1 or 2 rolls or slices of bread
Choice of noncaloric drink

Dinner
Chicken Paprika* (sauce made with mock sour cream)
²/₃ to 1 cup rice or noodles
Whole spinach braised with lemon juice
Artichoke Salad*
Dessert: ½ cup sherbet

Snacks
Banana
2 cups plain popcorn
1 handful pretzel sticks (about 30 sticks, 2½ inches long)
  Look for unsalted sticks if you're watching sodium.

FRIDAY, DAY 5
Breakfast
Orange or grapefruit juice
Eggs (1 yolk, 2 whites) scrambled with ½ cup cottage cheese
2 slices of whole-grain toast with 1 tsp. margarine or 1 tsp. jelly each
Coffee or tea

Lunch
Fast food:
Turkey submarine, 6-inch variety
  Whole-grain bun with sliced turkey, lettuce, tomato, green pepper, on-
  ions, mustard and a splash of oil (1 tsp.) and vinegar, NO mayo.
Apple or orange
Skim milk

Dinner
Remar's Vegetarian Spaghetti*
Green salad with 1 tbs. low-fat dressing
1 slice of Italian bread
Glass of red wine (Optional. If you're watching your weight and choose
  the wine, skip the peanuts [see below] as a snack. Have fruit instead.)
Dessert: Baked Apples with Cinnamon and Raisins*

Snacks
2 plums
1 oz. dry-roasted peanuts
1 cup plain popcorn (air-popped or microwaved)

SATURDAY, DAY 6
<u>Breakfast</u>
½ grapefruit or 1 cup of fruit cup
Homemade Muffins* with applesauce, jelly, or honey
1 cup skim milk
Coffee or tea

<u>Lunch</u>
Avocado Surprise* (low-fat cottage cheese, avocado, green peppers, olives)
Green salad with 1 tbs. low-calorie, low-fat dressing
Whole-grain small roll or slice of bread
Choice of noncaloric drink

<u>Dinner</u>
Watercress Soup*
Shrimp curry with 1 tbs. mango chutney
½ to 1 cup rice
Lemony Brussels Sprouts*
Dilled Carrots*
Green salad (if desired)
Dessert: fresh strawberries with 2 plain small cookies (such as vanilla or tea wafers)

<u>Snacks</u>
1 cup cereal snack mix
Apple or orange
2 cheese crackers (¼ inch of 1-inch-square cheese on whole-wheat cracker)

SUNDAY, DAY 7
<u>Breakfast</u>
Orange or apple juice
Pancakes with Orange Banana Sauce*
Fruit cup
1 cup skim milk
Coffee or tea

Lunch
Corn Chowder*
½ chicken sandwich
Carrot and celery sticks, radishes, and dill pickles (if pickles fit your sodium
    plan)
Choice of noncaloric drink

Dinner
Beef Stroganoff*
¾ cup noodles
Green Beans with Pimento*
Green salad with Belgian endive, dress with low-calorie Italian or vinai-
    grette dressing
1 glass of red wine (optional)
Dessert: Baked Pear with Chocolate Sauce*

Snacks
2 cups plain popcorn (air-popped or microwaved)
½ cup grapes

MONDAY, DAY 8
Breakfast
Orange juice
1 cup low-fat yogurt with frozen or fresh fruit (blueberries, strawberries,
    and/or peaches)
2 slices whole-grain toast with 1 tsp. margarine or 1 tsp. jelly each
Coffee or tea

Lunch
Brown bag:
Tuna Salad* sandwich on whole-grain bread with lettuce and tomato
Melon slice or melon chunks
1 cup skim milk

Dinner
A Chinese treat:
Hot and Sour Soup*
Chicken with Asparagus*
½ to 1 cup rice
Gingery Chinese Cabbage*
Hot tea
Dessert: Sliced Oranges with Raspberry Delight*

<u>Snacks</u>
Apple
2 cups plain popcorn
1 packet (½ oz.) raisins or 4 dried apricots

TUESDAY, DAY 9
<u>Breakfast</u>
½ grapefruit
1 cup hot oatmeal
1 or 2 slices whole-grain toast with 1 tsp. each margarine or jelly
1 cup skim milk
Coffee or tea

<u>Lunch</u>
Business lunch:

Pasta with clam sauce (*not* a cream sauce)
Green salad with 1 tbs. dressing
Choice of noncaloric drink

or

Grilled chicken dish
Boiled new potatoes (2 or 3 small)
Green vegetable (green beans, spinach, zucchini)
Green salad with 1 tbs. dressing
Choice of noncaloric drink

<u>Dinner</u>
Beans with Cabbage, a Mediterranean dish*
Corn on the cob, with 1 tsp. margarine
Green salad with low-calorie dressing
Whole-grain Garlic Toast*
Choice of noncaloric drink
Dessert: fruit cup with melon, strawberries, apples, oranges, cherries

<u>Snacks</u>
1 cup of skim milk and 1 graham cracker with ½ tbs. peanut butter
Orange, pear, or tangerine

WEDNESDAY, DAY 10
<u>Breakfast</u>
Orange or grapefruit juice
2 muffins (from the freezer, where you put them Saturday) with applesauce
1 cup skim milk or 6 oz. nonfat yogurt
Coffee or tea

<u>Lunch</u>
Fast food:
Chef salad from salad bar
   (See hints on how to select in discussion of fast-food section, page 341.)
1 whole-grain roll or slice of bread
Skim milk
Apple or pear

<u>Dinner</u>
Shepherd's Pie* (casserole with ground beef, vegetables, and a mashed-
   potato top)
Green salad with low-calorie dressing
Whole-grain roll
Choice of noncaloric drink (or drink your milk here instead of at lunch)
Dessert: 1 2-inch slice of cantaloupe with 1 scoop ($\frac{1}{3}$ cup) sherbet

<u>Snacks</u>
Apple
Popcorn (as before)
2 graham crackers

THURSDAY, DAY 11
<u>Breakfast</u>
Orange, apple, or tomato juice
1 oz. nutritious ready-to-eat cereal with $\frac{1}{2}$ banana and $\frac{1}{2}$ cup skim milk
1 slice whole-grain toast with 1 tsp. margarine or jelly
Coffee or tea

<u>Lunch</u>
Brown bag:
Pita Pocket*
Apple
1 cup skim milk

Dinner
Marinated Baked Fish, Bahamian Style*
Brussels sprouts dressed with lemon juice, 1 tsp. margarine
Stuffed Yellow Squash* (2 halves)
1 slice bread from whole-grain loaf (buy a treat at the bakery)
Choice of noncaloric drink
Dessert: Treat yourself to ½ piece chocolate cake or 1½-inch slice of apple pie.

Snacks
4 dried apricots
1 cup Cereal Mix*
Apple or pear

FRIDAY, DAY 12
Breakfast
Grapefruit juice
Melon slice
1 cup oatmeal (whole-grain hot cereal) with ½ cup skim milk
1 slice whole-grain toast with 1 tsp. margarine or jelly
Coffee or tea

Lunch
Fast food:
Chili with beans (as at Wendy's)
4 saltine crackers
Green salad (greens, tomatoes, cukes, green peppers, mushrooms, radishes, carrots, only) with 1 tbs. dressing
Skim milk

Dinner
Chicken and Broccoli Casserole*
Baked sweet potato with 1 tsp. margarine
Green salad with low-calorie dressing
Whole-grain roll with 1 tsp. margarine
Choice of noncaloric drink
Dessert: ½ cup fresh pineapple with 1 cookie

Snacks
Peanut butter pocketbook (1 slice whole-grain bread spread with 1 tbs. peanut butter and 1 tsp. jelly, then folded over and cut to make two little "pocketbooks")
Apple or orange

SUNDAY, DAY 14
Breakfast
Orange or apple juice
2 scrambled eggs (1 yolk, 2 whites)
1 slice lean Canadian bacon (1 oz.)
Grilled Tomatoes*
1 or 2 slices of whole-grain toast with 1 tsp. margarine, jelly, or honey
Coffee or tea

Lunch
Quick Fish Chowder*
Green salad with 1 tbs. low-calorie dressing
Corn muffin
Choice of noncaloric drink

Dinner
Pepper Steak* (or a grilled lamb chop, if you prefer)
Yellow rice (1 tsp. turmeric per cup rice in cooking water colors it a lovely yellow)
Green peas
Baby carrots with dill weed and lemon juice
Dessert: Peach Delight*

Snacks
Skim milk with 1 graham cracker spread with ½ tbs. peanut butter
Apple
Small packet (½ oz.) of raisins (1½ tbs.)

Adapting *your favorite recipes*

As you can tell from the recipes included in the menus, we've adapted a lot of old favorites—beef stroganoff, spaghetti, french toast—to the Godly Eating Plan. I hope you agree, given your experience with these recipes, that thinking and eating in a MUDly frame of mind can be refreshing and tasty as well as healthy.

You can MUD about in your own kitchen with your own favorite recipes, too. And I'm going to show you how to go about it by using a few examples in a moment. But first, a few principles to help bolster your self-confidence:

1. Experiment.   Don't be afraid to fail on the first try. You may produce something truly awful, but nobody said you have to eat it. Also, in all my experimenting, I've produced some mediocre dishes I wouldn't try again just that way, but only one inedible disaster: I don't seem to have the right touch with chicken necks.

Instead, go to school on your mistake. What to your tastebuds seemed wrong with the dish? What specific changes could you try that might improve it? A favorite African proverb of mine reads: "To fail is to fall forward faster." Post it on your refrigerator door.

2. Stimulate your imagination with some outside input from time to time.   None of us is chock full of new ideas all the time. For new ideas, I recommend a little outside reading. Dust off those cookbooks, browse through that food magazine in the dentist's office, or clip a tasty-sounding recipe from the newspaper. Try a different cuisine—the library has good cookbooks on various international cuisines: Chinese, Italian, Scandinavian, Greek, and on and on. At the beginning, look for dishes that contain ingredients you like; then progress to dishes that have you trying something new but interesting-sounding. Of course, the dishes you choose should meet MUD guidelines. Take Japanese food, for example. You know you'll probably like chicken teriyaki, so try it first. You'll probably then be ready to try "Yakidofu To Toriniku No Nimono"—simmered chicken and bean curd. And that brings me to a final comment: don't be put off by a strange-sounding name. Read the ingredients. You might be a bit shy of "dolmades," but most folk love "stuffed grape leaves." The same goes for "moo-goo-gai-pan"—stir-fried chicken with vegetables.

3. Use your common sense.   Most times if something sounds like a terrible taste combination (not just strange; lots of strange things are good), it probably is. Go ahead and try if you like, but be prepared to throw it away. See principle 1.

4. Be patient.   Don't expect to turn into a wiz in a week or two if you're new to cooking experimentation. But don't quit. Take a tip from Daniel Boone, whose greatest pleasure in life was lighting out for unexplored territory. "Nope," he is reported to have said, "I've never been lost, but I have been bewildered for up to six weeks at a time."

M*UD in the kitchen: lesson one*

Let's start with something easy. It's Friday night and the gang is coming to your house for a little relaxation. You grab that old munchies standby: chips and sour-cream onion dip. Tasty but full of calories, saturated fat, and salt. How can you easily modify it?

Original dip recipe: 1 pint sour cream and 1 package onion soup mix.

The biggest culprit is the sour cream. One pint of sour cream has 990 calories, and 864 or 87 percent of them are fat. The onion soup mix is high in sodium (900 mg. or more).

How can you modify the recipe? You can substitute something for the sour cream. Yogurt would work, but it may be a little liquid and a little sour for your taste. What if you put a little nonfat yogurt with some low-fat cottage cheese? That would be about the right taste, but a bit lumpy. Take care of the lumps by blending the mixture in a blender or food processor.

Modified dip recipe: 1 12-ounce carton of low-fat cottage cheese; ½ cup of yogurt (or to taste). Blend until smooth. If too thick, add 1 tablespoon of skim milk. Complete with soup mix (if salt is no problem) or with an herb mixture of your own devising. See the recipe section for some ideas.

The new dip has only 260 calories for the pint, and of those only 14 (5 percent) are fat. For further MUD, you could substitute raw vegetables for chips or put both out.

A *little more ambitious: lesson two*

Now things get a little more complex, but not really tougher. Beef stroganoff has long been a favorite dish for a special meal, one that is rich in deadly things. But you can make it a much healthier dish with just a few changes. (Since most folks usually make stroganoff with ground beef to save a few pennies, we'll start with that recipe.)

Here's a pretty standard recipe:

1 pound ground beef
1 tbs. butter
1 small onion, minced
1 tbs. butter
½ pound fresh mushrooms, sliced
Salt, white pepper, nutmeg
1 cup sour cream

Sauté the onion in 1 tablespoon of butter until yellow; then add the ground beef and brown. In another pan, sauté the mushrooms until tender. When the beef has browned, pour off the excess fat, and season with salt, pepper, and nutmeg. Add sautéed mushrooms and sour cream, heat through, and serve over noodles.

Very tasty, and very bad for you! At a rough estimate, one serving of this dish (one-quarter of the above recipe, including noodles) would have about 600 calories and 38 grams of fat. But whoever stopped with just one-quarter of the above recipe?

MUD to the rescue! First, you could improve the dish by going back to the original, substitute one pound of very lean trimmed beef steak cut across the grain in strips about 2 inches long, 1 inch wide, and ⅛ inch thick. (Round steak is probably the leanest, though you may need to add a little water after the next step and simmer about twenty minutes till the meat is tender.) Next, sauté the onions and beef in a nonstick pan. Try a nonstick spray or as little vegetable oil or soft margarine as possible (try 2 teaspoons). Sauté the mushrooms in a nonstick pan, sprayed very lightly with nonstick spray if necessary. The mushrooms will soon exude enough moisture to keep them from sticking. Finally, substitute 1 cup of yogurt or 1 cup of mock sour cream for the sour cream. This version, also with noodles, has only about 400 calories per serving and only 12 grams of fat (27 percent of calories), which comes mainly from the meat.

If you want to stick with ground beef, try to find the leanest in the market. Some stores are now offering ground beef that is 85 and 90 percent lean. Ordinary ground beef is only about 70 percent lean. You could also make the dish with ground turkey or sliced, skinless chicken breast. Of course, that wouldn't be "beef" stroganoff, but it would still be good.

The final lesson

These examples ought to give you a good idea about how to put MUD to work as you cook. The final lessons will come from experimenting.

Tips for dining out

You can track MUD into your favorite restaurant, too. The tips and substitutions you've learned at home, through putting the checklists to work and experimenting, will work when you eat out, too. But here are a few additional suggestions.

Choose a restaurant that will help you.   First, choose a restaurant that you know has dishes to fit your objectives; and second, choose a restaurant that is willing to adjust to help you. For example, you might choose a restaurant offering an ethnic cuisine which features lots of low-fat dishes: Chinese, Japanese, Thai, Korean, and Indian all come to mind as having lots of low-fat dishes on the menu. Or, if you want to eat seafood, you might choose a seafood restaurant you know serves broiled and sautéed dishes, not just fried ones.

Choose dishes that will help; skip those that won't.   In an Italian restaurant, for example, you might choose a pasta with a marinara (tomato) sauce—not fettucine alfredo, with all that cream, cheese, and butter. You might choose chicken cacciatore rather than lasagna.

In that seafood restaurant, you might decide you just have to have fried oysters anyway. Pull off most of the batter. Order a baked potato rather than french fries. Go easy on the hushpuppies and have a big salad with a light dressing.

Avoid sugary desserts piled with whipped cream and sweet sauce. Try fresh fruit or a single scoop of sherbet or sorbet.

Make special requests. Most folks have gotten used to saying "NO MSG, please" in Chinese restaurants. If you ask courteously for help with your MUD goals, you'll usually get a courteous response.

You might request, for example, that the chef not use added butter when he broils your fish or that he take one yolk out of your order of two scrambled eggs.

Ask for the sauce on the side for entrées, salads, vegetables.

Request a lemon wedge or a little yogurt to dress your salad. Ask if they have low-calorie/low-fat dressing available.

But *what about fast-food restaurants?*

Remembering your Mantra is not impossible in fast-food establishments, but the sound of frying foods can tend to overpower its effectiveness in your mental ear. If you eat infrequently at these restaurants and as carefully as possible, however, you can do all right.

First, avoid those fried foods as much as possible. A single hamburger with lettuce and tomato, no special sauce or mayonnaise, is usually better than something which is battered and fried such as a chicken fillet sandwich.

Next, stay away from highly caloric treats, such as milkshakes, regular sodas, and fried pies or other desserts. And beware of foods that look as if they'd be better for you, but may not be: Take for example, a stuffed baked potato. The plain potato is great, but most stuffings such as cheese and bacon, chili and cheese, and even cheese and a vegetable may give the potato more fat and calories than a single cheeseburger.

Third, here too you can choose a restaurant which will help you. For example, some chicken places now offer a baked chicken dinner; some seafood joints may have a shrimp or seafood salad that comes with the sauce on the side; and some hamburger joints offer chili or a salad bar, for example.

If you are trying to cut down on sodium, you might as well stay out of fast-food places. As a general rule, most items on the menu, whether the hamburger or the fries or the salad dressing, are high in sodium.

Finally, on the good side, some fast-food restaurants are now offering nutritional information about their offerings. Consulting this carefully, with your guidelines in mind, could help you make wiser choices.

MAKING THE MOST OF THE SALAD BAR

These guidelines have probably left you thinking that the thing to do is to skip the burger counter and go directly to the salad bar. That may not be a bad idea, if you know how to build a healthy salad. If you dip too deeply into some of the bowls, though, you might just as well have ordered a triple-decker burger with double cheese and mayo. So, herewith are some tips on building the best salad:

- Start green: lettuce, spinach, green peppers, cabbage, alfalfa sprouts, cucumbers.
- Add a little red: tomatoes, radishes, sweet red peppers, red onions, red cabbage.
- A touch of light and white: mushrooms and, if it's clearly low-fat, some cottage cheese.
- A few beans: 1 tablespoon of garbanzas (chick-peas) and red kidney beans can be very good if they are not floating in an oil-based marinade.
- On the side: fresh fruit, if available.

Avoid or go very easy on the items high in fat and calories. You might choose to have a little bit of one or two, but no more:

- Cheese, bacon bits, ham, salami
- Eggs
- Olives, avocados, nuts, seeds
- Croutons
- Slaws or mixed salads with creamy or oily dressings
- Fruit in syrup
- The dressing: Avoid creamy dressings. Instead, drizzle lemon juice and/or vinegar and just a touch of oil, or if the restaurant offers a low-calorie, low-fat dressing, help yourself to about 1 to 1½ tablespoons. (Most salad-bar ladles hold about 2 to 3 tablespoons.)

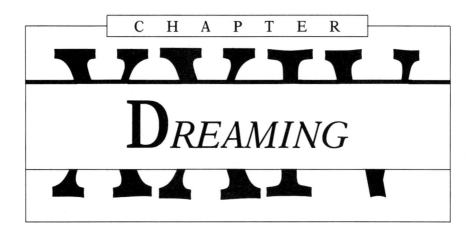

CHAPTER

Dreaming

23 Months Later

<u>*Grand Bahama Island*</u>

In 1979, a Massachusetts man named Steve Silva started walking slowly up and down one flight of stairs to lose weight and gain strength. Mr. Silva weighed 430 pounds, and had been told by his doctor that he would not live to see his one-year-old child's sixth birthday if he did not make changes in his lifestyle.

Eight years later, he celebrated the health benefits and weight loss brought on by his program (he lost 245 pounds) by running up and down the Eiffel Tower seven and a half times in two hours. I'm sure he was cheered on by his nine-year-old, too.

Steve Silva's accomplishments make my weight loss and health improvements during the last months seem pretty insignificant. But do you know what really impresses me? The man, at 430 pounds, simply decided that moderate changes in his lifestyle would change his life completely in time. It took *eight years*, but he was right, and right here I award him my hunk mantle as a man who has tackled the demons in his life head-on and won.

I don't know this for a fact, but I'll bet you two things helped Mr. Silva win: He wasn't afraid to set what must have seemed like

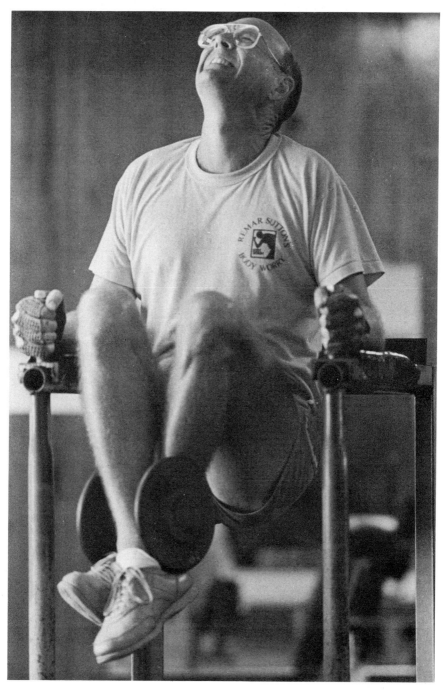

Guess what? When you can do all your exercises at home without effort, this is what awaits you at the gym.

an impossible goal at first (many people are afraid to even ride the elevator up the Eiffel Tower), and he had people who cared about him, encouraged his effort, and comforted him in moments of despondency.

I told my friend Kathy Bater about Mr. Silva's accomplishments, and she told me about *her* dream and the moral support that got her there. Kathy, some of you may remember, was the first beautiful woman on this island really to give me moral support as my remake began. She would pull her car over as I jogged and yell, "Hey, Remar, you're looking *great*! Keep going!" I, of course, knew I didn't really look great, but, boy, did her thoughtfulness make my steps lighter from then on.

Kathy is trim, tight, and beautiful. She looks like a born jock (see for yourself: her picture introduces the biking section), but she is not. Seven years ago Kathy was completely inactive. She smoked two packs of cigarettes a day; she drank more, ate more, and weighed more than she wanted to, and had been doing those things for ten years.

Then a friend talked Kathy, at thirty-one, into training for the Bahamas Air-Sea Rescue two-mile ocean swim. The first day, Kathy swam less than 200 feet in the choppy ocean before giving up. "I thought, 'This just isn't going to work,' and crawled onto the beach ready to quit. I couldn't swim two hundred feet and I needed to swim ten thousand feet!"

Standing there was Bernie Butler, veteran from the race. "Bernie told me *he* couldn't swim very far the first day he trained, either," Kathy said. "He convinced me that, though I couldn't do it that day, *I could do it.*" She continued to swim. In five months, she not only swam in the race, but won in her age group.

That victory—and I'm speaking of finishing the race, not even winning—began to change Kathy. She started to cut back on her smoking to improve her stamina; she ate less and drank less without thinking about it. Staying in shape for the race became her goal.

"I started asking myself questions," Kathy says. "Before I would overeat, or have an extra drink, I'd always ask, 'What will I get out of it and what will it cost me?' "

And then, five years after her first swim, she decided to quit smoking completely. "A friend talked me into using nicotine gum, and for a year rooted for me as I weaned myself off cigarettes and finally weaned myself pretty much off the gum."

Kathy Bater doesn't smoke now and, at thirty-eight, looks like thirty. She's won eleven open-ocean races, including one first place in the overall women's division. She spends a lot of time now working on our island's Conch Man mini-triathlon (swim one mile, bike ten miles, run four miles). The lady who encouraged *me* to keep on running is out there encouraging other people to train for the Conch Man.

Dante David, fifty-three, general manager of the Princess Hotel properties on Grand Bahama, won't need much prompting. Dante started running ten years ago in Korea when his body "started getting sloppy." He ran his first race in Mexico, his first marathon in Miami, and just completed his seventh New York Marathon in the Big Apple.

Dante founded the Princess Hotel's 10K race in 1985, and runs in the race every January. He also jogs every morning at 5:30 A.M., and if you'd like to come down here and train with him, Mr. David will always cheer you on.

Well, you may be saying, Steve Silva, fat though he was, started to change at thirty-one. Kathy Bater became active at thirty-one. Dante David started running at forty-three. None of them were "old" when they started to change. There's therefore no hope for the aged in body or spirit, right?

That's why Hulda Crooks continues to amaze me. Hulda's the lady I told you about earlier who has now climbed Mount Whitney, 14,494 feet tall, twenty-two times. And in 1987 she went to Japan and climbed Mount Fuji, 12,385 feet tall. Hulda was ninety-one then.

It starts with the left foot: Is there a stairwell close to you? How many steps are there between floors in your building? How many steps to the top of the Washington Monument or the Statue of Liberty? Have you ever wondered what it would be like to run in a six-mile race? Wanted to climb a mountain, or maybe even rappel down a mountain?

Or have you wistfully thought about taking up snow skiing this year? Or ice skating? Or ballroom dancing? How about sky diving? That may not be aerobic but, boy, will it set your heart to racing.

Life is a lot more fun when you dream and push the limits some. And you will never know your limits if you don't push yourself. I personally am running in my first race in January right here on the island—the Princess 10K (6.2-mile) run—and would like nothing better than to have some of you running with me.

And now that we're dreaming, why don't you start training right now for a Grand Bahama Conch Man triathlon on some Thanksgiving weekend? *You can do it.* As a matter of fact, I'll make you a deal: If you will write me right now with your commitment to do it, I'll provide us the celebration dinner at my house, about two miles from where the Conch Man ends.

It doesn't matter if you come in last. I will probably take that honor. What matters is the triumph of *doing it.* Anybody out there interested in a really good meal of conch salad, broiled lobster, and baked grouper?

Remar Sutton
P.O. Box 77033
Atlanta, GA 30357

RECIPES FOR *BODY WORRY*

APPETIZERS AND DIPS

Mock Sour Cream
Not only is this mock sour cream a good dip base but it can be used almost anywhere you would use sour cream.

> 1% fat or nonfat cottage cheese
> low-fat or nonfat plain yogurt
> lemon juice

You may vary the proportions of this mixture as you like, but we like 1 part yogurt to 3 parts cottage cheese, with just a squeeze of lemon juice. For 2 cups of mock sour cream, use one 12-ounce carton of cottage cheese and ½ cup of yogurt.

Place cottage cheese in food processor or blender and whirl until smooth. Add yogurt and mix. Season to taste with lemon juice or a touch more yogurt. If the mixture is too thick, thin slightly with skim milk.

Use as a base for your favorite dip or in recipes calling for sour cream.

Curry Dip

For each cup of mock sour cream, stir in ½ tsp. onion powder, 2 tsp. curry powder, ½ tsp. paprika, and ½ tsp. salt. Let sit for ½ hour, then sample and adjust flavorings.

Scallion Dip

For each cup of mock sour cream, stir in 2 finely minced scallions, including green tops, and ½ tsp. seasoned salt.

Green Goddess Dip

For each cup of mock sour cream, stir in 2 tsp. finely minced chives, ½ to 1 tsp. dill weed, ½ medium cucumber seeded and chopped very fine, and ½ tsp. seasoned salt.

Marinated Mushrooms

Though not technically marinated, these low-calorie mushrooms taste like it. In a noncorrosive bowl, mix ½ cup red wine vinegar, 2 tbsp. water, 1 tbsp. dried parsley, ½ tsp. salt, and ¾ tsp. garlic powder. Let sit for at least 20 minutes. Clean and trim 1 pound mushrooms. Place mushrooms upside down in a flat baking dish or a quiche dish. When marinade has melded properly, pour over mushrooms until buttons around stems fill up. Cook on high in a microwave oven until mushrooms begin to shrink in size. Serve hot.

SOUPS

Corn Chowder

    1 tsp. margarine
    1 small onion, chopped
    2 cups chicken broth, preferably homemade or low-
        sodium
    3 medium potatoes, peeled and finely diced
    1 bay leaf
    3 tbsp. flour
    2 cups skim milk
    1½ cups fresh or frozen corn (or 12-oz. can)
    Salt, Tabasco sauce, or white pepper to taste
    Dill weed or chives

Melt margarine in a saucepan and sauté onion until translucent, about 3 minutes. Add broth, potatoes, and bay leaf. Simmer until potatoes are soft, about 30 minutes. Make a thin paste of flour and a little milk. Add to saucepan, stirring constantly until thickened. Scald the rest of the milk (I heat it in a microwave oven) and add it and corn. Stir until thickened. Taste and adjust salt. Add a touch of Tabasco sauce or white pepper, if you like. Serve with a sprinkle of dill weed or chives on top. Serves 4.

Quick Fish Chowder

> 1 tbsp. margarine
> 1 medium onion, chopped
> ½ to ¾ lb. firm while fish fillets, such as cod, catfish, whiting
> 3 medium potatoes, peeled and finely diced
> 2½ cups water
> 1 bay leaf
> 3 tbs. flour
> 2 cups skim milk
> Salt to taste
> Chives, parsley, or paprika

Melt margarine in a saucepan and sauté onion until translucent, about 3 minutes. Add fish, potatoes, water, and bay leaf. Simmer until potatoes are tender and fish falls apart, about 30 minutes. Make a thin paste of flour and a little milk. Add to saucepan and stir constantly until thickened. Add scalded milk and keep stirring until thickened. If too thick, add a touch more milk. Taste and adjust salt. Serve garnished with chives, parsley, or a dusting of paprika. Serves 4.

Watercress Soup

> 3 cups chicken broth
> 2 cups watercress, roughly chopped, loosely packed
> 2 to 3 tbsp. cornstarch
> 2 to 3 tbsp. water

A nicely flavored homemade chicken broth is preferable, but if you don't have some on hand, the reduced-sodium canned variety does well. Heat the broth in a saucepan. While it is heating, rinse watercress, pick off any large or tough stems, chop cress roughly into approximately 1″ lengths. Mix cornstarch with equal amount of water to make a thin paste. Pour into simmering broth, stirring constantly. Continue to stir until broth thickens slightly. Then add chopped watercress all at once. Cook just until watercress is wilted, about 2 minutes, and serve. Serves 4.

Hot and Sour Soup

        4 dried black mushrooms
        Water
        1 chicken breast
        ¼ lb. lean fresh pork
        1 small can bamboo shoots
        3 cups chicken broth
        1 cake bean curd (tofu)
        3 tbsp. white vinegar
        1 tsp. ground black pepper
        1 tsp. soy sauce
        Scallions

A note on ingredients: Most supermarkets now carry bean curd (tofu); look in the produce or the health food sections first. If you can't find tofu, you may omit it. Dried black mushrooms may be harder to find; check with a specialty market or an Asian market if your supermarket does not have them. You may substitute ordinary mushrooms (about 12), but the flavor is very different. You may also use leftover chicken and pork (perhaps a few tenderloin medallions or a chop).

Advance preparation: Soak the dried mushrooms in water to cover at least 20 minutes and reserve the liquid. Slice chicken, pork, soaked mushrooms, and bamboo shoots into matchstick strips. Cut bean curd into 1″ slices, about ⅓″ to ½″ thick.

Cooking: Place chicken, pork, and black mushrooms in chicken broth, add mushroom soaking liquid, and bring to a boil in a covered saucepan. Lower heat immediately and simmer for about 10 minutes if meat is raw, about 5 minutes if already cooked. Add bamboo shoots and tofu (and ordinary mushrooms, if you substituted them). Simmer for 5 more minutes. Add white vinegar, ground black pepper, and soy sauce. Simmer for 1 more minute. Serve garnished with minced green scallion. Serves 4 to 5.

Note: This version of hot and sour soup has not been thickened.

If you prefer a thick, velvety soup, mix 2 tbsp. cornstarch with an equal amount of water and add to soup after the meat is cooked. You will need to stir constantly until the soup thickens and then add bamboo shoots and bean curd.

LUNCH DISHES

Avocado Surprise

> 1 avocado, diced
> 2 cups low-fat cottage cheese
> 2 medium green peppers, diced
> 20 medium ripe olives, sliced
> Pepper
> Lettuce, spinach, or tomato

Gently mix avocado pieces, cottage cheese, diced green peppers, and olives together. Season with dash of black pepper if desired. (Cottage cheese is usually already salty, so no extra salt is needed.) Serve on lettuce or spinach leaf or in the center of a sectioned tomato. Serves 4.

Ham Rolls

These are simple but attractive. Use your imagination to vary the ingredients.

Select a very lean packaged sliced ham. If the slices are large, cut in half. Spread a little mustard on the center of each ham slice and roll it up around a sliver of dill pickle. If you're watching sodium intake, roll the slice around a cooked asparagus spear.

Tuna Salad

> 1 6½-oz. can tuna, water packed, drained
> 1 rib celery, finely minced
> 1 small apple, finely minced (optional)
> 2 tsp. dill pickle cubes
> 1 tbsp. diet mayonnaise (low-fat and low-calorie)
> Mustard and/or garlic or onion powder

Mix the above ingredients together. Season with a little mustard and/or garlic or onion powder.

Pita Pocket

You may stuff a number of good things into pita bread, but we suggest that, if you prepare your lunch in the morning, you carry the bread and stuffing separately and stuff the bread just before eating so that the sandwich is not soggy. Do slice over the end to make the pocket before leaving home, since the sharp knives are all in the kitchen, not the office.

Dress the sandwich with mustard, 1 tbsp. diet mayonnaise, or a little mock sour cream seasoned with garlic or onion powder. You can mix the dressing with the stuffing if that is easier.

Stuffing:

> 2 oz. leftover lean chicken, turkey, ham, or roast beef
> Cucumber, halved and sliced
> Alfalfa sprouts
> Grated carrot
> Diced tomato or cherry tomato halves

MAIN DISHES

Mediterranean Beans and Cabbage

> ½ large head of savoy cabbage, about 1½ pounds
> 3 oz. very lean ham
> 2 tbsp. tomato paste
> 1 cup water
> 1 tbsp. olive oil
> 1 small onion, chopped
> 3 to 4 cloves garlic, minced
> 1 can Great Northern white beans, rinsed and drained
> Tabasco sauce
> Salt to taste

Preparation: Quarter the cabbage, core, and cut into thin strips. (Don't chop into small pieces.) Cut ham into julienne strips (matchsticks). Mix tomato paste in a measuring cup with 1 cup water.

Cooking: Heat oil in a large skillet with lid, add onion and garlic, and sauté until onion is translucent, about 5 minutes. Add the cabbage to the skillet and mix the onions in well. Then pour tomato paste and water over the mix. Cover the pan, reduce the heat, and simmer until the cabbage is nearly tender, about 30 minutes. Add the beans and stir everything together. Add about 4 to 5 drops of Tabasco sauce. Continue simmering until cabbage is done and beans are hot, about 15 more minutes. Check seasoning and add a touch more Tabasco sauce or a dash of salt if the dish needs it. If too much liquid remains, uncover and raise heat to boil off excess, but be sure not to scorch the food. Serves 3 to 4 as a main dish.

Remar's Vegetarian Spaghetti Sauce

This is the large, feed-the-gang recipe I use for entertaining. You can cut the proportions down and adjust the ingredients to your taste. Spaghetti sauce is *very* adaptable.

> 2 large cans crushed plum tomatoes
> 1 large can tomato puree
> 1 can tomato paste
> 2 large onions, chopped
> 8 to 10 cloves garlic, minced
> Basil, oregano, marjoram, black pepper
> Hot sauce
> 3 large bell peppers, chopped
> 1 large bunch of broccoli (if the bunches are small, get 2)
>   (Separate into flowerets and stems; peel and chop stems.)
> 1 pound mushrooms, sliced

In a large soup kettle, put all the tomato products and stir well. Add the onion and garlic. Add about 1 tsp. each of dried basil and oregano and ½ tsp. of marjoram and black pepper. Bring to a boil and reduce immediately to a simmer; cover and let simmer for 45 minutes to an hour. (This simmering cooks the onion and garlic and releases their flavors, in contrast to sautéing in oil.) Taste. Add a little more oregano, basil, and garlic if needed. Add hot sauce to taste—I like a lot. Add green peppers and broccoli stems. Simmer another half hour or so. Taste. Adjust seasonings. Add broccoli flowerets and mushrooms. Cook until flowerets and mushrooms are tender but not mushy. Serve with grated Parmesan cheese.

You may also use cauliflower or carrots or other crunchy vegetables if you like. Serves 6 to 8.

Shirley's Baked Chicken

>   2 tbsp. seasoning salt
>   1 tbsp. oregano leaves
>   1 tbsp. garlic powder
>   1 tbsp. freshly ground black pepper
>   1 tbsp. liquid hickory smoke
>   2 tbsp. water
>   2 whole frying chickens cut into serving pieces or 3 to 5
>   pounds of drumsticks, thighs, or breasts, skinned

Mix dry seasonings with liquid smoke and water in a small container. Place chicken in a baking dish. Pour the seasoning mixture over the skinless chicken pieces and use both hands to rub it evenly over all the chicken pieces. Bake in a preheated oven at 375° until chicken is tender when pricked with a fork, about 40 minutes to 1 hour. This is a double recipe that serves 4 to 6 for one meal, the remainder to be used for a salad or another dish.

Hunky Chicken Salad

>   1 cup celery, chunked
>   2 cups apples, chunked
>   2 cups seedless whole white grapes
>   1/2 cup toasted slivered almonds
>   4 cups cooked chicken (see baked chicken recipe, above)
>   3/4 cup buttermilk salad dressing
>   1/2 tsp. dill weed
>   1/2 tsp. lemon juice
>   1/2 tsp. freshly ground black pepper

We like to make this with Shirley's Baked Chicken recipe because the chicken is so flavorful. You could make it with stewed or steamed chicken if you prefer. (See note on stewing, next page.)

Put celery, apples, grapes, and toasted slivered almonds in a large bowl. Pull cooled baked chicken from bones in chunks and mix with chunked fruit and celery. Add buttermilk dressing, dill weed, lemon juice, and pepper and mix together just until ingredients are coated. Serve immediately or chill in refrigerator first. Serves 6 as a main course for lunch or dinner.

Almonds can be quickly toasted by putting them in a flat baking pan under the broiler for a few minutes. But watch them like hawks watch prey.

Note on stewing chicken: Stewing a chicken can give you not only chicken for salads or casseroles but also good homemade stock to use in soups or other dishes. To stew 1 chicken, skin the chicken, place in heavy pot with lid, add ½ carrot and 1 stalk celery cut into 2″ pieces and 1 bay leaf. Add water to cover about ⅔ of chicken. Bring to a boil and reduce heat immediately to simmer. Simmer until chicken is done, about 1 hour. Remove chicken from broth and pick off meat for use in salads or other dishes. Use soon or store in freezer. Remove carrots, celery, and bay leaf from broth, skim or strain any residue, and then chill broth and later remove any fat that congeals. Use broth in any recipe calling for it.

Chicken Broccoli Casserole

>2 to 3 cups broccoli, flowerets, steamed
>2 cups cooked chicken, roughly shredded or chopped
>2 tsp. soft margarine
>1 cup skim milk
>1 cup chicken broth
>2 tbsp. flour
>1½ tbsp. grated Parmesan cheese
>Salt to taste
>Tabasco sauce
>Paprika

You may use leftover broiled or baked chicken for this recipe, but steamed or stewed is best. Broccoli flowerets should be bite size; steam them for 3 to 5 minutes until cooked but still crunchy. If you are using frozen broccoli, simply thaw and drain the package; no additional cooking is necessary.

Place the chicken and broccoli mixed together in a casserole dish.

To prepare the sauce: Melt the margarine in a saucepan and stir in 1 cup skim milk. Heat slowly, stirring; do not let boil. Stir in broth and heat. When mixture is hot, slowly sift 2 tbsp. flour into the liquid, stirring constantly to prevent lumps. When sauce begins to thicken, in 2 to 4 minutes, slowly add grated Parmesan cheese. Stir until cheese melts. Taste sauce and adjust seasonings. You may need to add a smidgen of salt or a dash of Tabasco sauce. Pour sauce over chicken-and-broccoli mixture. Dust heavily with paprika. Bake about 30 minutes in a preheated 350° oven. Serves 4.

Chicken Paprika

    2 tsp. polyunsaturated oil
    1 medium onion, halved and sliced thinly
    2 cloves garlic, crushed
    4 chicken breasts or thighs, skinned
    1 tbsp. paprika
    1 cup chicken broth
    3/4 cup mock sour cream
    1 tbsp. flour

Heat oil in a nonstick skillet with tight-fitting lid. Sauté onion and garlic over low heat until translucent, about 3 minutes. Add chicken, brown on both sides, about 2 minutes each side. Remove chicken to a plate or a platter. Mix paprika thoroughly with onion and garlic; stir in chicken broth. Return chicken to pan, cover tightly, and simmer for 20 to 30 minutes, until chicken is done (when pricked with fork, chicken juices will run clear). Be sure to turn pieces once so that paprika coloring sinks into both sides (leave the side you will serve up in the sauce the longest).

When chicken is done, remove to a platter. Pour mock sour cream into pan; sift flour over top; stir mixture continuously as it heats. Because the mock sour cream is blended from cottage cheese and yogurt, it will appear to separate initially (it will look a little stringy). But as the sauce cooks, the flour will bind it together. It may never look as smooth as a true sour cream sauce, but it will taste as good. When sauce is hot and smooth, return chicken (and accumulated juices) to pan and heat 3 or 4 minutes. Serves 4.

Chicken with Asparagus

    3 boneless, skinned chicken breasts (about 3 oz. each)
    1/2 lb. asparagus
    Water
    1 tbsp. polyunsaturated oil
    1 scallion, minced
    1 cup chicken stock
    1 tbsp. cornstarch

Slice chicken across the grain into thin strips. Trim and clean asparagus and cut into 1 1/2″ lengths. Drop asparagus into boiling water and blanch for 2 minutes. Then drain and put aside.

In a wok or a large nonstick skillet, heat the oil until hot. Drop in half the scallion and stir for 30 seconds, then add chicken and quickly stir-fry until done, about 3 minutes. You will need to stir constantly and turn chicken to keep it from sticking and scorching. When it is done, remove to a platter. Add blanched asparagus to pan (there should be an adequate coating of oil left) and stir-fry for about a minute, then add chicken stock. Cook until asparagus is tender but still crunchy, about 3 minutes. Mix cornstarch with an equal amount of water and add to stock and asparagus, stirring continually. When stock thickens, return chicken to pan, heat through, and serve. Serves 4.

Braised Pork Medallions

   1 lb. lean pork tenderloin
   1 tsp. olive oil
   3 cloves garlic, crushed
   ½ cup dry white wine
   ½ cup water or chicken stock
   ½ tsp. salt
   1 tsp. caraway seeds
   Parsley or watercress

Buying pork tenderloin: A whole pork tenderloin, about 2 lbs., is usually sold in a vacuum plastic package. (Don't confuse it with the trimmed boneless loin, also sold in this fashion.) It looks expensive, but because it is boneless and well trimmed, it can cost little more per pound of edible meat than cuts with lots of fat and bone. Pick out the leanest tenderloin you can. Cut it in half (freeze the part you won't need) and trim any visible fat. Cut the tenderloin into medallions ¼" thick. Their diameter will range from 2" to 1" as the tenderloin tapers down.

Preparation: Heat 1 tsp. olive oil in a nonstick pan with tight-fitting lid; sauté crushed garlic for 1 to 2 minutes. Place pork medallions in pan with garlic and brown quickly on both sides. Lower heat as necessary to keep meat from sticking or scorching or add 1 tbsp. water.

When meat has browned, 1 to 2 minutes each side, add wine and water or chicken stock. Sprinkle salt and caraway seeds over medallions. Put lid on skillet and simmer until pork is tender, about 30 minutes. Check periodically to see that the meat is not drying out. Add a little more water and lower heat if the liquid is cooking off quickly.

When the meat is tender, you should have a few tablespoons of sauce in the pan. To serve, arrange the medallions on a platter, spoon the sauce over them, and garnish with parsley or watercress. Serves 4.

Pepper Steak

      1 lb. lean flank or round steak
      ½ tsp. soft margarine
      1 to 1½ cups beef broth
      2 tsp. soy sauce
      2 medium green peppers
      1 tbsp. flour
      Salt and pepper to taste

Cut steak into thin strips across the grain. Melt margarine in a nonstick skillet with lid. Add meat strips and sauté over medium heat for 3 minutes or until browned. Add beef broth and soy sauce, cover, and simmer until meat is almost tender (about 15 to 30 minutes—time will vary depending on the type of steak used). Add green peppers and cook until tender but still crisp, 3 to 5 minutes. Sift flour over sauce and stir continually to thicken, if desired. Taste to see if salt (the soy sauce is salty) or pepper is needed. Serves 4.

Shepherd's Pie

      2 large potatoes
      Water
      ¾ to 1 lb. lean ground beef
      1 cup sliced raw carrots
      ½ large green pepper
      1 medium onion
      1 cup frozen corn
      1 can tomatoes (1 lb.)
      1 tsp. dill weed
      1 tsp. chili powder
      ½ tsp. salt
      Pepper to taste
      1 tsp. flour
      Buttermilk
      Paprika (optional)

Put potatoes on to cook in water. Sauté ground beef in a large nonstick skillet until well done. Since you want to get rid of as much fat as possible, drain off all fat and then blot cooked beef with paper towels until dry. (Do this last, of course, with the pan off the stove.) While beef is cooking, slice carrots in ⅛"-thick circles, dice green pepper in ½" cubes, and cut onion in half and slice thinly. After draining off the fat from the beef, add all vegetables and the drained tomatoes to the meat in the skillet. Season with dill weed, chili powder, salt, and pepper. Put lid on skillet and cook slowly until vegetables are tender and most of the liquid has evaporated, about 20 to 30 minutes. You may need to uncover the skillet for the last 5 to 10 minutes to evaporate the liquid. Sift or dust the flour over the mixture and place it in a casserole or deep baking dish.

Prepare mashed potatoes. Use just enough buttermilk to hold the mixture together. Spoon mashed potatoes over top of meat-and-vegetable mixture. Make a pleasing design on the top of the potatoes, using a fork. Dust with paprika or chili powder. Bake in a preheated 375° oven until potatoes are brown on tips, about 20 to 25 minutes. Serves 4.

Marinated Baked Fish, Bahamian Style

     3 lbs. fish fillets (firm flesh)
     1 whole lemon or lime
     Salt and pepper to taste
     ⅛ tsp. dried oregano
     3 cloves fresh garlic
     1 small onion, chopped
     1 small tomato, chopped
     ½ green pepper, chopped

Put the fish fillets in a glass baking dish. Squeeze the juice of the lemon or lime over them, then season with salt, pepper, and oregano. Crush garlic cloves and spread evenly over the fish. Mix together chopped onion, tomato, and green pepper and spread on the fish, covering it completely. Let the fish marinate 1 hour, or prepare it in the morning and refrigerate until evening. Bake in a preheated 350° oven until fish is just before flaking stage (fish should be opaque throughout but not flaking, because that is too dry), about 20 to 25 minutes, depending on thickness of fillets. Serves 6 to 8.

Grilled Fish Steaks

The backyard grill is as kind to a firm fish steak, such as swordfish or salmon, as it is to a T-bone. You can grill a whole fish easily, too, if you have a fish grill apparatus to hold the fish together. Fish steaks 1 to 1½″ thick are good.

First, before you light the grill, coat the grill with nonstick spray. This will help keep the fish from sticking. The grill should be very hot.

Trim fish steaks of all fat. Coat lightly with mixture of 1 part polyunsaturated oil to 1 part lemon juice. Place on grill and put lid down or cover with a tent of aluminum foil (so that you don't have to turn steak over). When fish is done, in about 5 to 10 minutes, use a spatula to lift it from the grill (it will stick a little, no doubt), sprinkle with fresh chives or dill and lemon juice and serve.

Fish with Caper Sauce

> 1 tbsp. olive oil
> 1 lb. firm fish fillets
> > Flounder, sea bass, Boston bluefish, catfish, scrod, turbot, and ocean perch are all fine.
> ½ cup flour
> ½ tsp. salt
> ½ tsp. pepper

> *Sauce*
> 1½ tbsp. soft margarine
> 1½ tbsp. red wine vinegar
> 2 tbsp. chopped parsley
> 3 tbsp. small capers

Heat olive oil in a nonstick frying pan large enough to hold all. Lightly dust fillets with flour to which you have added ½ tsp. each salt and pepper. (Shaking the fillets in a paper bag with the flour mixture works well. Fillets should be damp but not wet. Flour should coat very lightly.) Sauté fish in olive oil until done, about 5 minutes each side. This seems like very little oil in which to do this, but over moderate heat and in a nonstick pan the method works well. Just keep a close eye on the fish.

While the fish cooks, place margarine, vinegar, parsley, and capers in a small noncorrosive saucepan and heat until the mixture bubbles.

When fish is done, remove from pan to a platter, pour caper sauce over the fillets, and serve *immediately*. Serves 4.

Shrimp Curry

        1 tbsp. margarine
        1 onion, chopped
        1 tbsp. curry powder
        1½ cups chicken stock
        1½ tbsp. flour
        1 lb. raw medium shrimp, peeled and deveined

Melt margarine in a nonstick skillet over medium heat. Sauté onion until translucent, 3 to 5 minutes. Add curry powder and chicken stock and bring to a simmer. Then sift in flour, stirring continually until sauce thickens. Add peeled shrimp and cook only until shrimp turns pink, about 3 to 4 minutes. Do not overcook shrimp or it will be rubbery. Serve over rice. Serves 4.

SALADS

Three Bean Salad

        1 1-lb. can cut green beans
        1 1-lb. can cut wax beans
        1 1-lb. can kidney beans
        1 small red onion, sliced (optional)
        ⅔ cup Low-Fat and Low-Calorie Italian Dressing (recipe
          next page)

You can make this with freshly steamed beans if you like, but we think this is about the best use for canned beans. Look for the no-salt varieties.

Drain and rinse beans. Place in a large bowl with cover. Add onion if desired. Pour Italian dressing over beans and toss to cover well. Refrigerate 24 hours before serving. It's best to toss the salad a couple of times during the 24 hours, to ensure equal marinading.

Low-Fat and Low-Calorie Italian Dressing

> 1 tsp. sugar
> 1 tbsp. cornstarch
> 1 cup water
> ¼ cup red wine vinegar
> 1 tbsp. olive oil
> ½ tsp. dry mustard
> ½ tsp. dry basil
> ½ tsp. dry oregano
> ¼ tsp. garlic powder
> 8 grinds of pepper (¼ tsp.)
> ¼ tsp. salt

Mix sugar and cornstarch in a small saucepan. Add water and place over medium heat. While stirring continually to prevent lumping, cook mixture until it thickens, about 5 minutes. Take it off the heat and cool completely. Add other ingredients and mix vigorously. (Placing dressing in a jar with a lid and shaking works well.) Let mellow at least 4 hours before using. Refrigerate. Makes about 1¼ cups dressing.

You can use this salad dressing base to make other low-fat and low-calorie dressings of your choice. Just vary the herbs and spices.

Artichoke Salad

> 1 14-oz. can artichoke hearts
> ½ cup Low-Fat and Low-Calorie Italian Dressing (recipe above)
> Bibb or Boston lettuce
> Cherry tomatoes

A day before you plan to serve the salad, open and drain the can of artichoke hearts. Place hearts in a small, covered container, pour one-half of Italian dressing over, cover, and marinate in refrigerator 24 hours. If you do not use all the artichoke hearts in the salad, they will keep for a week or so refrigerated in the marinade.

To make salad, wash and break lettuce leaves into large pieces. Halve cherry tomatoes. Arrange tomatoes and artichoke hearts on bed of lettuce leaves. Use more dressing if necessary. This salad looks particularly nice if you serve it individually on salad plates. Serves up to 6.

Spinach Salad

>   ½ lb. spinach, washed and torn into large pieces
>   2 oranges, peeled and sliced (or 1 can mandarin oranges,
>   packed in juice)
>   ½ cup poppy seed dressing (recipe below)

Arrange spinach on a plate and divide orange sections equally on 4 servings of spinach. Dress with poppy seed dressing. Serves 4.

Poppy seed dressing: Place 1 tbsp. cornstarch and 1 cup water in a small saucepan and cook over medium heat, stirring constantly, until mixture thickens. Take off heat and cool. Then add 1 tbsp. honey and ¼ cup lemon juice. Stir together, then add 1 tbsp. poppy seeds. Refrigerate to store.

VEGETABLE DISHES

Ratatouille

This dish is good hot or cold. For larger quantities, double the recipe.

>   1 tbsp. olive oil
>   1 onion, chopped
>   3 to 4 cloves garlic, minced
>   1 eggplant (about 1 lb.), peeled and cubed
>   3 to 4 small zucchini squash (1 lb.), sliced
>   1 1-lb. can tomatoes
>   1 bay leaf
>   1 tsp. basil
>   ½ tsp. oregano
>   Salt and pepper to taste
>   Tomato paste (if necessary)
>   1 tbsp. lemon juice

The secret to cooking this dish with so little oil is heavy cookware and low heat. Since this takes time, you may want to make the dish a day ahead. It usually tastes even better the second day.

Heat olive oil in a heavy skillet or a saucepan (we like iron) over medium heat. Sauté onion and garlic until translucent, stirring frequently, about 3 minutes. Add eggplant, squash, tomatoes with juice, and herbs and spices. Cook slowly and stir frequently to prevent sticking. Pot should be covered. The juice from the tomatoes will prevent sticking at first and then the eggplant will exude enough liquid. If the ingredients start sticking, you have the heat too high; lower it. After 30 minutes, taste. If it's not tomatoey enough, add 1 tbsp. tomato paste. Continue simmering until eggplant and squash are well done and well blended, usually another 30 minutes. Add lemon juice. Serves 6 to 8.

Braised Red Cabbage

>1 small head red cabbage (1¼ lb.)
>1 cup water
>1 tbsp. brown sugar
>¼ cup white vinegar
>1 small tart apple, peeled and grated
>½ tsp. salt

Here, as for other dishes cooked without butter or oil, the secret is slow cooking in a heavy pot. We like an iron Dutch oven or skillet with a tight-fitting lid.

Cut cabbage in half, remove core, and slice very, very thinly across the half. Place in a pot with water, sugar, vinegar, grated apple, and salt. Bring quickly to a boil, and reduce immediately to a very slow simmer. Cover tightly so that the small amount of liquid doesn't evaporate. Stir every 15 minutes or so and check that cabbage is not scorching. If it is drying out, the heat is too high or the lid doesn't fit properly. Add a little water as needed. Cabbage is ready to eat after about 60 minutes of simmering but is even better after it simmers 1½ to 2 hours. Serves 4 to 6.

White Rice with Wild Rice and Herbs

>¼ cup wild rice
>1 cup water
>½ cup white long-grain rice
>1 cup chicken stock
>¼ tsp. onion powder
>1 tbsp. parsley
>½ tsp. salt

Rinse wild rice and place in a saucepan with 1 cup water. Cover tightly and bring to a boil, then lower immediately to a simmer. Simmer 20 minutes. Add white rice, chicken stock, onion powder, parsley, and salt. Cover, bring back to a boil, lower heat to a simmer, and simmer until all liquid is absorbed, 20 to 30 minutes. Serves 4.

Stuffed Squash

> ½ small onion, finely minced
> 2 tsp. soft margarine, melted
> 4 medium yellow squash
> 1 cup soft bread crumbs
> Salt and pepper to taste
> Paprika

Sauté onion in margarine until translucent, then set aside. Trim squash ends, cut in half, and steam until tender but not mushy. Drain. Spoon out center of squash and reserve in a small bowl. Arrange shells in a shallow baking dish. To squash centers add bread crumbs and sautéed onion. Mix together; add salt and pepper to taste. Stuffing should be stiff but should hold together. If it is too crumbly, use one egg white to bind it together or a little chicken stock. Stuff the squash shells with stuffing. Dust with paprika. Bake in a preheated 350° oven until hot and crispy, about 20 to 25 minutes. Serves 4.

Dilled Carrots

> 3 or 4 large carrots, scraped and cut into sticks
> White wine vinegar
> Dill weed, fresh or dried

Steam carrots until tender. Drain. Sprinkle with white wine vinegar and dill weed. Serves 4.

Lemony Brussels Sprouts

> 1 lb. brussels sprouts
> 1 lemon
> Sweet German mustard

Trim brussels sprouts of outer leaves, make small crosses with paring knive in stem, and steam until tender but still crunchy. In a small bowl, whisk juice of one lemon and 2 tsp. of sweet German mustard together. Drain brussels sprouts and pour dressing over them. Serves 4.

Green Beans with Pimento
> 1 lb. young green beans
> 1 pimento cut into strips or 2 tbsp. pimento strips
> ½ lemon

Trim ends of beans but leave whole. Steam until tender but still crisp. Drain. Place on a small plate or a platter and arrange pimento strips in a nice pattern over the top of beans. Squeeze lemon juice over. Serves 4.

Grilled Tomatoes
> 4 medium tomatoes
> Season-All
> Parsley, chopped

Select tomatoes that are ripe but still firm. Core but leave peel on, and cut in half horizontally. Arrange halves on a baking sheet, cut side up. Sprinkle a small amount of Season-All on each tomato and then sprinkle tomatoes with parsley. Broil 6″ from heat for about 6 minutes, or until tomatoes are cooked but not falling apart. Serves 4 to 6.

Gingery Chinese Cabbage
> 1 small head Napa cabbage or ½ larger head, about 6 cups sliced cabbage
> 2″ fresh ginger, peeled and slivered
> 1 tbsp. polyunsaturated oil
> ½ cup water or chicken stock
> 1½ tsp. white vinegar

Trim outer leaves of cabbage, cut in half, and then cut each half in very thin slices, about ⅛″ thick. Peel ginger and cut into very thin matchsticks.

Heat oil in a wok or a large nonstick skillet. Add ginger and stir-fry about 1 minute. Add all cabbage and stir-fry vigorously 1 minute. Add water or stock and continue to cook until cabbage is tender but still crisp. You may cover the pan briefly if necessary. Sprinkle vinegar over cabbage just before serving. Serves 4.

BREADS AND BREAKFAST

Muffin Mix

Mix these dry ingredients together in quantity in the following proportions and use them as a master mix for making all sorts of muffins.

> 1 cup all-purpose flour
> 1 cup whole-wheat flour
> 1½ tsp. baking soda
> 1½ tsp. baking powder
> 3 tbsp. sugar
> ¼ tsp. salt

All mixtures below should be cooked in well-greased muffin tins about 20 to 25 minutes in a preheated 400° oven. They make 10 to 12 muffins. Fill tins one-half to two-thirds full.

Wheat-germ muffins

1½ cup Muffin Mix, ½ cup wheat germ, 2 egg whites, 1 cup skim milk, ¼ cup polyunsaturated oil. Mix all ingredients together just until moist.

Oatmeal cinnamon muffins

1 cup Muffin Mix, 1 cup quick oatmeal, 2 egg whites, 1 cup skim milk, ¼ cup polyunsaturated oil, 1 tsp. cinnamon. Mix all ingredients together just until moist. Add some raisins if you like.

Graham muffins

2 cups Muffin Mix, 2 egg whites, 1 cup skim milk, ¼ cup polyunsaturated oil. Mix all ingredients together just until moist.

Fruit or nut muffins

Add up to ½ cup fruit or chopped nuts to graham muffin mixture.

Garlic Toast

This is an easy recipe to make in a hurry, to go with spaghetti or soup. Make as much or as little as you need.

Cut slices of whole-grain bread in half. Spread a very thin coating of soft margarine on each half (about ½ tsp.); dust lightly with garlic powder. Place on rack of toaster oven or large oven. Toast at medium heat until crispy and lightly browned on edges.

French Toast

For each two slices of bread, prepare the following mix: 1 egg white, 1 tbsp. skim milk, ½ tsp. sugar, ½ tsp. cinnamon. Whip vigorously with a fork.

Dip bread in mix, fry in a nonstick skillet or griddle (or pan sprayed with nonstick spray) on both sides until brown. Serve immediately with syrup, honey, or jelly.

Pancakes

You may use any pancake recipe you like, substituting two egg whites for each egg and using skim milk for whole milk. Low-fat buttermilk is also fine. We also cut the oil called for in half. If you don't have a favorite recipe, try this one. This quantity makes about 12 2½" cakes. Double or triple the recipe as required.

> ½ cup skim milk, approximately
> 2 egg whites
> 1 tbsp. safflower oil
> 1 cup all-purpose flour
> 2 tsp. baking powder
> 2 tsp. sugar
> ½ tsp. salt

Mix milk, egg whites, and oil together, then add all dry ingredients at once and stir until ingredients are moistened. Batter will be a bit lumpy. If it's too thick, thin with more skim milk. Cook on a nonstick griddle or skillet.

Banana-orange pancake sauce

Mash one banana in a small saucepan and add just enough orange juice to make the syrup the consistency you like. Sprinkle on cinnamon to taste, ¼ to ½ tsp. Heat until bubbly. Spoon over pancakes. (If this is not sweet enough for you, add a little artificial sweetener.)

DESSERTS

Baked Apples
>4 to 6 apples
>Cinnamon
>1½ tbsp. raisins for each apple

Choose crisp, tangy apples, such as Granny Smith, Stayman, or Rome. Core apples and peel a little skin from around the hole on top for looks. Sprinkle cinnamon down the core and over the top; don't be chintzy. Stuff each core with 1½ tbsp. raisins. Put apples in a glass casserole, add ½" water. Now eye them critically. Dust on a bit more cinnamon if you think you don't have enough. Then cover and bake in a preheated 375° oven until tender, about 45 minutes to 1 hour, depending on the size of the apples.

Spice Cake
>1 cup all-purpose flour
>½ tsp. baking soda
>1 tsp. baking powder
>1 tsp. cinnamon
>½ tsp. allspice
>½ tsp. nutmeg
>½ cup dark brown sugar
>2 egg whites
>½ cup skim milk
>½ cup applesauce
>¼ cup polyunsaturated oil
>
>*Glaze:*
>2 tbsp. powdered sugar
>1 tsp. lemon juice

Sift dry ingredients together. Using a mixer, blend egg whites, milk, sugar, and applesauce. Add dry ingredients gradually. Add oil. Batter should be smooth and thick. Pour into a well-greased and floured 8" or 9" square pan. Bake in a preheated 375° oven 35 to 40 minutes, or until cake springs back to touch.

Cool in pan. When cake is barely warm, mix powdered sugar and lemon juice and spread over top of cake.

Fruit Cup

Fruit cups are very versatile desserts, since they can include any fruits you like or any in season. A squeeze of lemon or lime juice or the inclusion of orange or grapefruit juice will keep cut fruit such as apples, pears, and bananas from turning brown. Here are some suggested combinations. Each makes 4 servings.

Citrus cup

Sections of 2 oranges and 1 grapefruit with 1 cup sliced fresh strawberries. A sliced banana is nice, too.

Crunchy cup

Chunk 2 red apples, 2 yellow apples, 1 pear, 1 half-cantaloupe; add 1 cup green grapes; squeeze juice of 1 lime over.

Berry cup

1 cup blueberries, 1 sliced kiwi fruit, 1 sliced peach, ½ cup sliced strawberries, 1 sliced banana, ¼ cup orange juice.

Baked Pears with Chocolate Sauce

4 pears
1 cup water
Juice of 1 lemon
Commercial chocolate hard sauce

Mix juice of lemon and water in a deep casserole with lid. Peel pears, leaving stem on. As each pear is peeled, turn it over well in the lemon water to prevent browning. Stand pears on end in water, cover casserole, and bake in a preheated 350° oven until pears are tender. Remove hot pears to serving plates and pour chocolate hard sauce carefully around top of pear. You can also heat canned pears and serve them with chocolate hard sauce. Serves 4.

Sliced Oranges with Raspberry Delight

3 large sweet oranges
1 cup ripe red or black raspberries
¼ cup orange juice

Peel oranges, making sure to cut away all the white membrane. Then slice horizontally and arrange attractively on serving plates with a twist of orange zest (the peel with all the white cut off). Heat raspberries and orange juice in a small saucepan just until raspberries begin to exude juice. Pour in equal amounts over orange slices. Serves 4.

Peach Delight

> 4 meringue shells
> 3 peaches, peeled and sliced
> ½ cup orange juice
> 1 cup black raspberries or blackberries

You may use commercial meringue shells or make them yourself from any meringue shell recipe. Peel and slice peaches and mix them with ¼ cup orange juice to prevent darkening. Heat raspberries or blackberries with ¼ cup orange juice in a small saucepan just until raspberries begin to exude juice.

Place shell on a serving plate, spoon sliced peaches into shells (divide peaches equally), and pour raspberry sauce over. Serves 4.

SNACKS

Cereal Snack Mix

> 3 cups each of two different cereals, such as Wheat Chex, Corn Chex, or Bran Chex
> ½ cup soy nuts
> 2 cups thin pretzel sticks
> 2 tbsp. Worcestershire sauce
> 2 tbsp. soft margarine
> ½ to 1 tsp. garlic or onion powder

Place cereals and soy nuts in a bowl. (Soy nuts are soy beans roasted like peanuts. You could use peanuts, but they are much higher in fat and calories, which this recipe is designed to modify.) Break pretzel sticks in half and add to cereal mixture. Melt margarine in a small saucepan. Stir in Worcestershire sauce. Sprinkle over cereal mixture while stirring mixture. You will have to work carefully here to make the sauce cover the mix, since this is relatively little sauce. So drizzle and stir; don't pour. Add garlic or onion powder to taste. Place mixture on a baking sheet or a shallow roasting pan. Bake mix in a preheated very slow oven (250°) 1 hour, stirring at least twice. Cool and enjoy. Makes about 2 quarts (8 cups) of mix. It stores nicely in a lock-seal plastic bag.

TABLE OF FOOD NUTRITIVE VALUES

How to use: You may use these tables to find the nutritive values of food called for on your daily food intake record. The foods are presented in amounts commonly eaten. If you have not eaten the exact amount, say 1 cup of vegetables, divide or multiply to get the approximate value. For instance, if you ate ½ cup of vegetables, just divide the values in half. The figures are as accurate as we can make them, but are intended for your estimations, not for more exact purposes. If you'd like even more information, consult the first two sources listed at the end of the table.

A note on the "Added Sugar" and "Fiber" categories. Very few analyses of added sugar are available. Therefore, with the exception of ready-to-eat cereals, these figures are estimations based on home recipes and derived from other data. Where we could not arrive at a useful estimate, we simply indicated that a product usually has a good bit of added sugar with a plus sign, +.

The "Fiber" column represents dietary fiber, which is composed of the indigestible part of plant foods and comes in two types—insoluble and soluble fiber (pectins and gums). Each food contains a mixture of these types, but methods of figuring dietary fiber vary. Some of our fiber figures include just insoluble fiber, others both types. The dietary fiber content for many foods is still unknown. So these figures will give you an estimate of your fiber intake, but should not be considered complete.

Cal = Calories	Carbo = Carbohydrates
g = grams	Chol = Cholesterol
Sat Fat = Saturated Fat	mg = milligrams
Poly Fat = Polyunsaturated Fat	tr = trace

Food	Amount	Weight in grams	Cal	Protein (g)	Total Fat (g)	Sat Fat (g)	Mono Fat (g)	Poly Fat (g)	Carbo (g)	Added Sugar (g)	Chol (mg)	Sodium (mg)	Fiber (g)
Alcohol—gin, vodka, rum, whiskey													
80 proof	1½ oz	42	95	0	0	0	0	0	tr		0	tr	
86 proof	1½ oz	42	105	0	0	0	0	0	tr		0	tr	
90 proof	1½ oz	42	110	0	0	0	0	0	tr		0	tr	
Alfalfa sprouts	1 cup	33	10	1	tr	tr	tr	0.1	1		0	2	1
Almonds, shelled													
Slivered, packed	1 oz	17	99	3	9	0.8	5.7	1.9	4		0	2	
Whole	1 oz	28	165	6	15	1.4	9.6	3.1	6		0	3	2
Anchovies, in oil	5 anch	20	42	6	2	0.4	0.8	0.5	0			734	
Apples													
Raw w/peel													
2¾" diam	1	138	80	tr	tr	0.1	tr	0.1	21		0	tr	4.5
3¼" diam	1	212	125	tr	1	0.1	tr	0.2	32		0	tr	5.5
Peeled, sliced	1 cup	110	65	tr	tr	0.1	tr	0.1	16		0	tr	3
Dried, sulfured	10 rings	64	155	1	tr	tr	tr	0.1	42		0	56	
Apple juice or cider, bottled or canned	1 cup	248	115	tr	tr	tr	tr	0.1	29		0	7	
Applesauce, canned													
Unsweetened	1 cup	244	105	tr	tr	tr	tr	tr	28		0	5	6
Sweetened	1 cup	255	195	tr	tr	0.1	tr	0.1	51	23	0	8	

Food	Amount	Weight in grams	Cal	Protein (g)	Total Fat (g)	Sat Fat (g)	Mono Fat (g)	Poly Fat (g)	Carbo (g)	Added Sugar (g)	Chol (mg)	Sodium (mg)	Fiber (g)
Apricots													
Raw, 12/lb	3 ap	106	50	1	tr	tr	0.2	0.1	12		0	1	
Canned, heavy syrup	3 halves	85	70	tr	tr	tr	tr	tr	18	8	0	3	
Juice pack	3 halves	84	40	1	tr	tr	tr	tr	10		0	3	
Dried (28 lge or 37 med)	1 cup	130	310	5	1	tr	0.3	0.1	80		0	13	
Apricot nectar	1 cup	251	140	1	tr	tr	0.1	tr	36		0	8	
Artichokes													
Globe, cooked	1 whole	120	55	3	tr	tr	tr	0.1	12		0	79	
Hearts	1/2 cup	84	37	2	tr	tr	tr	0.1	9		0	55	
Jerusalem, raw Sliced	1 cup	150	115	3	tr	0	tr	tr	26		0	6	
Asparagus, cooked Fresh and frozen, 1/2" at base	4 spears	60	15	2	tr	tr	tr	0.1	3		0	2	1
Canned, 1/2" at base	4 spears	80	10	1	tr	tr	tr	0.1	2		0	278	
Avocados, raw													
Calif., 2/lb	1 avocado	173	305	4	30	4.5	19.4	3.5	12		0	21	6
Fla., 1/lb	1 avocado	304	340	5	27	5.3	14.8	4.5	27		0	15	
Bacon													
Regular	3 med sl	19	110	6	9	3.3	4.5	1.1	tr		16	303	
Canadian	2 slices	46	85	11	4	1.3	1.9	0.4	1		27	711	

Bagels, plain, 3½"	1 bagel	68	200	7	2	0.3	0.5	0.7	0	38	245	
Baking powder	1 tsp	2.9	5	tr	0	0	0	0	0	1	290	
Bamboo shoots	1 cup	131	25	2	1	0.1	tr	0.2	0	4	105	3.5
Bananas, 2½"/lb	1 banana	114	105	1	1	0.2	tr	0.1	0	27	1	4
Barbecue sauce, bottled	1 tbsp	16	10	tr	tr	tr	0.1	0.1	0	2	130	
Bean sprouts, mung, Raw	1 cup	104	30	3	tr	tr	tr	0.1	0	6	6	1
Beans												
Black, dry, Cooked	1 cup	171	225	15	1	0.1	0.1	0.5	0	41	1	7
Great Northern, dry, Cooked	1 cup	180	210	14	1	0.1	0.1	0.6	0	38	13	6
Green or snap, Fresh cooked	1 cup	125	45	2	tr	0.1	tr	0.2	0	10	4	3
Green or snap, Canned	1 cup	135	25	2	tr	tr	tr	0.1	0	6	339	3
Kidney, cooked	1 cup	177	225	15	1	0.1	0.1	0.5	0	40	4	14.5
Limas, fresh, Fordhook	1 cup	170	170	10	1	0.1	tr	0.3	0	32	90	9
Limas, fresh, Baby	1 cup	180	190	12	1	0.1	tr	0.3	0	35	52	8
Limas, dry, Cooked	1 cup	190	260	16	1	0.2	0.1	0.5	0	49	4	9
Navy or pea, dry, Cooked	1 cup	190	225	15	1	0.1	0.1	0.7	0	40	13	12
Pinto, dry, Cooked	1 cup	180	265	15	1	0.1	0.1	0.5	0	49	3	10.5
Refried, canned	1 cup	290	295	18	3	0.4	0.6	1.4	0	51	1,228	

Food	Amount	Weight in grams	Cal	Protein (g)	Total Fat (g)	Sat Fat (g)	Mono Fat (g)	Poly Fat (g)	Carbo (g)	Added Sugar (g)	Chol (mg)	Sodium (mg)	Fiber (g)
Beans, baked, canned, vegetarian	1 cup	254	235	12	1	0.3	0.1	0.5	52		0	1,008	
Beef, relatively fat cuts													
Brisket, braised (33% separable fat)													
Lean and fat	3 oz	85	332	20	28	11.2	12.5	1.0	0		79	52	
Lean only	3 oz	85	205	25	11	3.9	4.9	0.3	0		79	61	
Chuck blade, braised as in pot roast (21% separable fat)													
Lean and fat	3 oz	85	330	22	26	11	11.9	1.0	0		87	53	
Lean only	3 oz	85	230	26	13	5.3	5.8	0.4	0		90	60	
Rib, whole, broiled (24% separable fat)													
Lean and fat	3 oz	85	308	18	26	10.8	11.4	0.9	0		73	52	
Lean only	3 oz	85	194	22	11	4.7	4.9	0.3	0		69	50	
Shortribs, braised (33% separable fat)													
Lean and fat	3 oz	85	400	18	36	15.1	16.1	1.3	0		80	43	
T-bone steak, broiled (19% separable fat)													
Lean and fat	3 oz	85	276	20	21	8.7	9.1	0.8	0		71	51	
Lean only	3 oz	85	182	24	9	3.5	3.5	0.3	0		68	56	
Sirloin (20% separable fat)													
Lean and fat	3 oz	85	238	23	15	6.0	6.2	0.6	0		73	52	
Lean only	3 oz	85	177	26	8	3.0	3.3	0.3	0		76	56	
Beef, relatively lean cuts													
Flank (2% separable fat)													
Lean and fat	3 oz	85	218	23	13	5.6	6.1	0.4	0		61	61	
Lean only	3 oz	85	207	22	13	5.4	5.3	0.4	0		60	61	

Round, full cut, broiled (15% separable fat)												
Lean and fat	3 oz	85	233	22	16	6.2	6.8	0.7	0	71	51	
Lean only	3 oz	85	165	24	7	2.5	2.9	0.3	0	70	54	
Round, eye of, roasted (12% separable fat)												
Lean and fat	3 oz	85	206	23	12	4.9	5.4	0.4	0	62	50	
Lean only	3 oz	85	155	25	6	2.1	2.4	0.2	0	59	52	
Tenderloin (13% separable fat)												
Lean and fat	3 oz	85	226	22	15	6.0	6.2	0.6	0	73	52	
Lean only	3 oz	85	174	24	8	3.1	3.1	0.3	0	72	54	
Beef breakfast strips	3 slices	34	153	11	12	4.9	5.7	0.5	0	40	766	
Beef, ground, cooked medium												
"Lean"	3 oz	85	227	20	16	6.1	6.8	0.6	0	66	47	
"Regular"	3 oz	85	244	20	18	7.0	7.8	0.7	0	74	51	
Beef brains, pan fried	3 oz	85	167	11	14	3.2	3.4	2.0	0	1,696	134	
Beef liver, pan-fried	3 oz	85	184	23	7	2.4	1.5	1.5	7	410	90	
Beef tongue, simmered	3 oz	85	241	19	18	7.6	8.1	0.7	tr	91	51	
Beer												
Regular	12 oz	360	150	1	0	0	0	0	13	0	18	
Light	12 oz	355	95	1	0	0	0	0	5	0	11	
Beet greens												
Cooked	1 cup	144	40	4	tr	tr	0.1	0.1	8	0	347	
Beets												
2" fresh	2 beets	100	30	1	tr	tr	tr	tr	7	0	49	1.5
Sliced	1 cup	170	55	2	tr	tr	tr	tr	11	0	83	3
Canned, sliced	1 cup	170	55	2	tr	tr	tr	0.1	12	0	466	6

Food	Amount	Weight in grams	Cal	Protein (g)	Total Fat (g)	Sat Fat (g)	Mono Fat (g)	Poly Fat (g)	Carbo (g)	Added Sugar (g)	Chol (mg)	Sodium (mg)	Fiber (g)
Biscuits, 2"													
Home recipe	1 biscuit	28	100	2	5	1.2	2.0	1.3	13		tr	195	
Refrigerated	1 biscuit	20	65	1	2	0.6	0.9	0.6	10		1	249	
Blackberries													
Raw	1 cup	144	75	1	1	0.2	0.1	0.1	18		0	tr	10.5
Blueberries													
Raw	1 cup	145	80	1	1	tr	0.1	0.3	20		0	9	4.5
Frozen, sweetened	1 cup	230	185	1	tr	tr	tr	0.1	50	30	0	2	
Bluefish, raw	3 oz	85	105	17	4	0.8	1.5	0.9	0		50	51	
Bok choy, cooked (Chinese cabbage)	1 cup	170	20	3	tr	tr	tr	0.1	3		0	58	
Bologna (8 slices in 8-oz pkg)													
Beef	2 slices	56	176	6	16	6.8	7.8	0.6	tr		36	556	
Meat	2 slices	57	180	7	16	6.1	7.6	1.4	2		31	581	
Bouillon, beef Canned, condsd	1 cup	240	15	3	1	0.3	0.2	tr	tr		tr	782	
Braunschweiger													
Slice = 1 oz	2 slices	57	205	8	18	6.2	8.5	2.1	2		89	652	
Brazil nuts	1 oz	28	185	4	19	4.6	6.5	6.8	4		0	1	
Bread crumbs, dry	1 cup	100	390	13	5	1.5	1.6	1.0	73		5	736	

Bread

Cracked wheat	1 slice	25	65	2	1	0.2	0.2	0.3	12		0	106	2
Italian	1 slice	30	85	3	tr	tr	tr	0.1	17		0	176	
Mixed grain	1 slice	25	65	2	1	0.2	0.2	0.4	12		0	106	
Oatmeal	1 slice	25	65	2	1	0.2	0.4	0.5	12		0	124	
Pita, 6½″	1 pita	65	165	6	1	0.1	0.1	0.4	33		0	339	
Pumpernickel	1 slice	32	80	3	1	0.2	0.3	0.5	16		0	177	1
Raisin	1 slice	25	65	2	1	0.2	0.3	0.4	13		0	92	tr
Rye	1 slice	25	65	2	1	0.2	0.3	0.3	12		0	175	1
White	1 slice	25	65	2	1	0.3	0.4	0.2	12		0	129	1
Whole wheat	1 slice	28	70	3	1	0.4	0.4	0.3	13		0	180	2
Broccoli													
Raw	1 spear	151	40	4	1	0.1	tr	0.3	8		0	41	
Fresh, cooked	med. spear	180	50	5	1	0.1	tr	0.2	10		0	20	7
Frozen, cooked 4½″	1 piece	30	10	1	tr	tr	tr	tr	2		0	7	1
Frozen, chopped	1 cup	185	50	6	tr	tr	tr	0.1	10		0	44	7
Brownies, frosted 1½ × 1¾	1 brownie	25	100	1	4	1.6	2.0	0.6	16	+	14	59	
Brussels sprouts Frozen, cooked	1 cup	155	65	6	1	0.1	tr	0.3	13		0	36	5
Bulgur wheat Uncooked and unsoaked	1 cup	170	600	19	3	1.2	0.3	1.2	129		0	389	

Food	Amount	Weight in grams	Cal	Protein (g)	Total Fat (g)	Sat Fat (g)	Mono Fat (g)	Poly Fat (g)	Carbo (g)	Added Sugar (g)	Chol (mg)	Sodium (mg)	Fiber (g)
Butter													
Stick, ¼ lb.	½ cup	113	810	1	92	57.1	26.4	3.4	tr		247	933 salt / 12 unsalt	
Tbsp, ⅛ stick	1 tbsp	14	100	tr	11	7.1	3.3	0.4	tr		31	16 salt / 2 unsalt	
Pat (⅓″ slice)	1 pat	5	35	tr	4	2.5	1.2	0.2	tr		11	41 salt / 1 unsalt	
Buttermilk	1 cup	245	100	8	2	1.3	0.6	0.1	12		9	257	
Cabbage, common and chinese varieties													
Raw, shredded	1 cup	70	15	1	tr	tr	tr	0.1	4		0	13	3
Cooked	1 cup	150	30	1	tr	tr	tr	0.2	7		0	29	3
Cakes, from mixes													
Angel food	1/12 cake	53	125	3	tr	tr	tr	0.1	29	25	0	269	
Devil's food													
w/frosting	1/16 cake	69	235	3	8	3.5	3.2	1.2	40	18	37	181	
	1 cupcake	35	120	2	4	1.8	1.6	0.6	20	+	19	92	
Gingerbread	2½″ sq	63	175	2	4	1.1	1.8	1.2	32	18	1	192	
Yellow													
w/frosting	1/16 cake	69	235	3	8	3.0	3.0	1.4	40	+	36	157	
Cakes, commercial													
Pound loaf	½″ slice	29	110	2	5	3.0	1.7	0.2	15	9	64	108	
White layer													
w/frosting	1/16 cake	71	260	3	9	2.1	3.8	2.6	42	+	3	176	

Candy													
Caramels	1 oz	28	115	1	3	2.2	0.3	0.1	22	+	1	64	
Chocolate													
Milk	1 oz	28	145	2	9	5.4	3.0	0.3	16	16	6	23	
Milk/almonds	1 oz	28	150	3	10	4.8	4.1	0.7	15	15	5	23	
Milk/peanuts	1 oz	28	155	4	11	4.2	3.5	1.5	13	13	5	19	
Semisweet	1 c or 6 oz	170	860	7	61	36.2	19.9	1.9	98	98	0	24	
Sweet dark	1 oz	28	150	1	10	5.9	3.3	0.3	16	16	0	5	
Fondant (mints candy corn, etc.)	1 oz	28	105	tr	tr	tr	tr	0.1	25	25	0	10	
Fudge, plain	1 oz	28	115	1	3	2.1	1.0	0.1	21	21	1	54	
Gumdrops	1 oz	28	100	tr	tr	tr	tr	0.1	25	25	0	10	
Hard	1 oz	28	110	0	0	0	0	0	28	28	0	7	
Jellybeans	1 oz	28	105	tr	tr	tr	tr	0.1	26	26	0	7	
Marshmallows	1 oz	28	90	1	0	0	0	0	23	23	0	25	
Cantaloupe, 5" diam	½ melon	267	95	2	1	0.1	0.1	0.3	22		0	24	1
Carbonated drinks													
Club Soda	12 oz	355	0	0	0	0	0	0	0	0	0	78	
Cola	12 oz	369	160	0	0	0	0	0	41	41	0	18	
Ginger ale	12 oz	366	125	0	0	0	0	0	32	32	0		
Lemon-lime	12 oz	372	155	0	0	0	0	0	46	46	0	48	
Root beer	12 oz	370	165	0	0	0	0	0	42	42	0	48	
Carrots													
Raw, 7½"	1 carrot	72	30	1	tr	tr	tr	0.1	7		0	25	2
Sliced, cooked	1 cup	156	70	2	tr	0.1	tr	0.1	16		0	103	4

Food	Amount	Weight in grams	Cal	Protein (g)	Total Fat (g)	Sat Fat (g)	Mono Fat (g)	Poly Fat (g)	Carbo (g)	Added Sugar (g)	Chol (mg)	Sodium (mg)	Fiber (g)
Carrot juice	1 cup	246	98	2	tr	0.1	tr	0.2	23		0	72	
Cashew nuts, salted, roasted	1 oz	28	165	5	14	2.7	8.1	2.3	8		0	177	
Catfish, breaded and fried	3 oz	85	194	15	11	2.8	4.8	2.8	7		69	238	
Catsup	1 tbsp	15	15	tr	tr	tr	tr	tr	4		0	156	
Cauliflower													
Raw	1 cup	100	25	2	tr	tr	tr	0.1	5		0	15	2
Cooked	1 cup	125	30	2	tr	tr	tr	0.1	6		0	15	2
Caviar, black and red	1 tbsp	16	40	4	3	tr	tr		1		94	240	
Celery	1 stalk	40	5	tr	tr	tr	tr	tr	1		0	35	0.5
Cereals, hot, cooked													
Cream of Wheat	1 cup	244	140	4	tr	0.1	tr	0.2	29		0	5	
Instant, plain	1 pkt	142	100	3	tr	tr	tr	0.1	21		0	241	
Oatmeal	1 cup	234	145	6	2	0.4	0.8	1.0	25		0	2	2
Instant, plain	1 pkt	177	105	4	2	0.3	0.6	0.7	18		0	285	
Cereals, ready to eat													
All-Bran (1/3 cup)	1 oz	28	70	4	1	0.1	0.1	0.3	21	14	0	320	9
Apple Jacks	1 oz	28	110	2	0				26	14	0	125	tr
Bran Chex	1 oz	28	90	3	0					5	0	300	5
Bran Flakes													
Kellogg's	1 oz	28	90	4	1	0.1	0.1	0.3	22	5	0	264	4
Post	1 oz	28	90	3	tr	0.1	0.1	0.2	22	5	0	260	4

Cap'n Crunch	1 oz	28	120	1	3	1.7	0.3	0.4	23	11	0	213	0.3
Cheerios	1 oz	28	110	4	2	0.3	0.6	0.7	20	1	0	307	1
Corn Chex	1 oz	28	110	2	0				25	3	0	310	tr
Corn Flakes Kellogg's	1 oz	28	110	2	tr	tr	tr	tr	24	2	0	351	tr
Corn Flakes Post	1 oz	28	110	2	tr	tr	tr	tr	24	2	0	297	tr
Crispix	1 oz	28	110	2	0					3	0	220	tr
Fiber One	1 oz	28	60	4	1	0.2	0.1	0.1	21	2	0	230	12
Froot Loops	1 oz	28	110	2	1				25	13	0	145	tr
Frosted Flakes Kellogg's	1 oz	28	110	1	tr	tr	tr	tr	26	12	0	230	tr
Fruit and Fibre, Harvest Medley	1 oz	28	90	3	1				22	4	0	190	4
Grape-Nuts (1/4 cup)	1 oz	28	100	3	tr	tr	tr	0.1	23	3	0	197	1.3
Honey Nut Cheerios	1 oz	28	105	3	1	0.1	0.3	0.3	23	10	0	257	tr
Honey Smacks	1 oz	28	105	2	1	0.1	0.1	0.2	25	16	0	75	tr
Nutri-Grain Wheat	1 oz	28	110	3	0				24	2	0	195	2
100% Natural Cereal, Quaker	1 oz	28	125	3	5	3.3	0.7	0.7	19	6	0	58	tr
Product 19	1 oz	28	110	3	tr	tr	tr	0.1	24	3	0	325	tr
Raisin Bran Kellogg's	1 oz	28	90	2	1	0.1	0.1	0.3	21	9	0	150	4
Raisin Bran Post	1 oz	28	90	2	1	0.1	0.1	0.3	21	8	0	160	4

Food	Amount	Weight in grams	Cal	Protein (g)	Total Fat (g)	Sat Fat (g)	Mono Fat (g)	Poly Fat (g)	Carbo (g)	Added Sugar (g)	Chol (mg)	Sodium (mg)	Fiber (g)
Rice Krispies	1 oz	28	110	2	tr	tr	tr	0.1	25	3	0	280	tr
Shredded													
Wheat	1 oz	28	110	3	1	0.1	0.1	0.3	23	0	0	3	3
Special K	1 oz	28	110	6	tr	tr	tr	tr	21	3	0	230	tr
Super Golden													
Crisp	1 oz	28	105	2	tr	tr	tr	0.1	26	14	0	25	tr
Total	1 oz	28	100	3	1	0.1	0.1	0.3	22	2	0	352	2
Trix	1 oz	28	110	2	tr	0.2	0.1	0.1	25	13	0	181	tr
Wheat Chex	1 oz	28	100	3	0				23	2	0	200	2
Wheaties	1 oz	28	100	3	tr	0.1	tr	0.2	23	2	0	354	1.8
Cheese, natural													
Blue	1 oz	28	100	6	8	5.3	2.2	0.2	1		21	396	
Brie	1 oz	28	95	6	8				tr		28	179	
Cheddar	1 oz	28	115	7	9	6.0	2.7	0.3	tr		30	176	
Shredded	1 cup	113	455	28	37	23.8	10.6	1.1	1		119	701	
Cream	1 oz	28	100	2	10	6.2	2.8	0.4	1		31	84	
Feta	1 oz	28	75	4	6	4.2	1.3	0.2	1		25	316	
Mozzarella													
Whole milk	1 oz	28	80	6	6	3.7	1.9	0.2	1		22	106	
Skim milk	1 oz	28	80	8	5	3.1	1.4	0.1	1		15	150	
Muenster	1 oz	28	105	7	9	5.4	2.5	0.2	tr		27	178	
Parmesan, grated	1 tbsp	5	25	2	2	1.0	0.4	tr	tr		4	93	
Port du Salut	1 oz	28	100	7	8	4.7	2.3	0.2	tr		35	152	

Provolone	1 oz	28	100	7	8	4.8	2.1	0.2	1		20	248	
Ricotta													
Whole milk	1 cup	246	430	28	32	20.4	8.9	0.9	7		124	207	
Skim milk	1 cup	246	340	28	19	12.1	5.7	0.6	13		76	307	
Swiss	1 oz	28	105	8	8	5.0	2.1	0.3	1		26	240	
Cheese, pasteurized process													
American	1 oz	28	105	6	9	5.6	2.5	0.3	tr		27	406	
Swiss	1 oz	28	95	7	7	4.5	2.0	0.2	1		24	388	
Cheesecake, 9" diam	1/12 cake	92	280	5	18	9.9	5.4	1.2	26	+	170	204	
Cherries													
Sweet, raw	10 cherries	68	50	1	1	0.1	0.2	0.2	11		0	tr	1
Sour, canned, water pack	1 cup	244	90	2	tr	0.1	0.1	0.1	22		0	17	
Chestnuts, roasted													
Shelled	1 cup	143	350	5	3	0.6	1.1	1.2	76		0	3	18.5
Chicken													
Fried w/skin, batter-dipped													
Breast	4.9 oz	140	365	35	18	4.9	7.6	4.3	13		119	385	
Drumstick	2.5 oz	72	195	16	11	3.0	4.6	2.7	6		62	194	
Fried w/skin, flour-coated													
Breast	3.5 oz	98	220	31	9	2.4	3.4	1.9	2		87	74	
Drumstick	1.7 oz	49	120	13	7	1.8	2.7	1.6	1		44	44	
Roasted, flesh only													
Breast	3 oz	86	140	27	3	0.9	1.1	0.7	0		73	64	
Drumstick	1.6 oz	44	75	12	2	0.7	0.8	0.6	0		41	42	
Stewed, light and dark, chopped (as for salad)	1 cup	140	250	38	9	2.6	3.3	2.2	0		116	98	

Food	Amount	Weight in grams	Cal	Protein (g)	Total Fat (g)	Sat Fat (g)	Mono Fat (g)	Poly Fat (g)	Carbo (g)	Added Sugar (g)	Chol (mg)	Sodium (mg)	Fiber (g)
Chicken liver, cooked	1 liver	20	30	5	1	0.4	0.3	0.2	tr		126	10	
Chicken à la king, Home recipe	1 cup	245	470	27	34	12.9	13.4	6.2	12		221	760	
Chicken chow mein, canned	1 cup	250	95	7	tr	0.1	0.1	0.8	18		8	725	
Chickpeas, cooked	1 cup	163	270	15	4	0.4	0.9	1.9	45		0	11	10
Chili w/beans, canned	1 cup	255	340	19	16	5.8	7.2	1.0	31		28	1,354	
Chocolate, baking, bitter	1 oz	28	145	3	15	9.0	4.9	0.5	8		0	1	
Chocolate syrup Thin type	2 tbsp	38	85	1	tr	0.2	0.1	0.1	22	22	0	36	
Fudge type	1 tbsp	38	125	2	5	3.1	1.7	0.2	21	22	0	42	
Clam chowder, New England, canned, condensed, prepared	1 cup	248	165	9	7	3.0	2.3	1.1	17		22	992	
Clams Canned	3 oz	85	85	13	2	0.5	0.5	0.4	2		54	102	
Raw	3 oz	85	63	11	1	0.1	0.1	0.2	2		29	47	
Cocoa Powder, no milk	¾ oz	21	75	1	1	0.3	0.2	tr	19		0	56	

Prep w/8 oz milk		265	225	9	9	5.4	2.5	0.3	30		33	176	
Powder w/milk	1 oz	28	100	3	1	0.6	0.3	tr	22		1	139	12
Coconut													
Raw, shredded	1 cup	80	285	3	27	23.8	1.1	0.3	12		0	16	
Dried, sweetened	1 cup	93	470	3	33	29.3	1.4	0.4	44		0	244	
Coffee cake, crumb, piece 2⅝" sq	1 piece	72	230	5	7	2.0	2.8	1.6	38		47	310	
Collards, frozen	1 cup	170	60	5	1	0.1	0.1	0.4	12		0	85	
Cookies													
Choc chip, 2¼"	4 cookies	42	180	2	9	2.9	3.1	2.6	28	+	5	140	
Fig bar, 1⅝" sq	1 cookie	14	53	0.5	1	0.3	0.4	0.3	11	+	7	45	
Oatmeal raisin	1 cookie	13	61	1	2.5	0.6	1.1	0.7	9	+	tr	37	
Peanut butter	1 cookie	12	61	1	3.5	1.0	1.5	0.7	7	+	6	36	
Sandwich type	1 cookie	10	49	0.5	2	0.5	0.9	0.6	7	+	0	47	
Shortbread	1 cookie	8	39	0.5	2	0.7	0.8	0.3	5	+	7	31	
Sugar, 2½"	1 cookie	12	59	0.5	3	0.6	1.3	0.9	8	+	7	65	
Vanilla wafers	10 cookies	40	185	2	7	1.8	3.0	1.8	29	+	25	150	
Corn chips	1 oz pkg	28	155	2	9	1.4	2.4	3.7	16		0	233	
Corn													
Ear 5" × 1¾"	1 ear	77	85	3	1	0.2	0.3	0.5	19		0	13	4
Kernels, canned	1 cup	210	165	5	1	0.2	0.3	0.5	41		0	571	11
Cream-style, canned	1 cup	256	185	4	1	0.2	0.3	0.5	46	often	0	730	
Cornmeal, enriched, degermed													
Dry	1 cup	138	500	11	2	0.2	0.4	0.9	108		0	1	

Food	Amount	Weight in grams	Cal	Protein (g)	Total Fat (g)	Sat Fat (g)	Mono Fat (g)	Poly Fat (g)	Carbo (g)	Added Sugar (g)	Chol (mg)	Sodium (mg)	Fiber (g)
Cottage cheese													
4% large curd	1 cup	225	235	28	10	6.4	2.9	0.3	6		34	911	
1% low-fat	1 cup	226	180	28	2	1.4	0.6	tr	8		10	840	
Nonfat	1 cup	145	125	25	1	0.4	0.2	tr	3		10	19	
Crabmeat, canned	1 cup	135	135	23	3	0.5	0.8	1.4	1		135	1,350	
Crackers													
Cheese, 1" sq	10 crkrs	10	50	1	3	0.9	1.2	0.3	6		6	112	
Cheese/peanut-butter sandwich	1 crkr	8	40	1	2	0.4	0.8	0.3	5		1	90	
Saltines	4 crkrs	12	50	1	1	0.5	0.4	0.2	9		4	165	
Snack type	1 round	3	15	tr	1	0.2	0.4	0.1	2		0	30	
Wheat, thin	4 crkrs	8	35	1	1	0.5	0.5	0.4	5		0	69	
Cranberries	½ cup	76	35	tr	tr				8		0	2	
Cranberry juice cocktail, reg	1 cup	253	145	tr	tr	tr	tr	0.1	38	+	0	10	
Cranberry sauce Canned	1 cup	277	420	1	tr	tr	0.1	0.2	108	+	0	80	
Cream													
Half & half	1 tbsp	15	20	tr	2	1.1	0.5	0.1	1		6	6	
	1 cup	242	315	7	28	17.3	8.0	1.0	10		89	98	
Light cream	1 tbsp	15	30	tr	3	1.8	0.8	0.1	1		10	6	
	1 cup	240	470	6	46	28.8	13.4	1.7	9		159	95	
Whipping, heavy	1 tbsp	15	50	tr	6	3.5	1.6	0.2	tr		21	6	
	1 cup	238	820	5	88	54.8	25.4	3.3	7		326	89	

Food	Measure												
Cream products, imitation													
Nondairy creamer													
Frozen	1 tbsp	15	20	tr	1	1.4	tr	tr	2	+	0	12	
Powdered	1 tsp	2	10	tr	1	0.7	tr	tr	1	+	0	4	
Whipped topping													
Frozen	1 cup	75	240	1	19	16.3	1.2	0.4	17	+	0	19	
	1 tbsp	4	15	tr	1	0.9	0.1	tr	1	+	0	1	
Powdered, made with whole milk	1 cup	80	150	3	10	8.5	0.7	0.2	8	+	13	121	
	1 tbsp	4	10	tr	tr	0.4	tr	tr	1	+	tr	3	
Pressurized	1 tbsp	4	10	tr	1	0.8	0.1	tr	1		0	2	
Croissants	1 reg	57	235	5	12	3.5	6.7	1.4	27		13	452	
Cucumber	6 large or 8 small slices	28	5	tr	tr	tr	tr	tr	1		0	1	tr
Currents, Eur black	1 cup	112	71	2	tr	tr	0.1	0.2	17		0	2	
Custard, baked	1 cup	265	305	14	15	6.8	5.4	0.7	29	+	278	209	6
Dandelion greens	1 cup	105	35	2	1	0.1	tr	0.3	7		0	46	
Danish pastry with fruit	1 pastry	65	235	4	13	3.9	5.2	2.9	28	+	56	233	
Dates, pitted	10 dates	83	230	2	tr	0.1	0.1	tr	61		0	2	
Doughnuts													
Cake type, 3¼"	1 donut	50	210	3	12	2.8	5.0	3.0	24	+	20	192	
Raised, 3¾"	1 donut	60	235	4	13	5.2	5.5	0.9	26	+	21	222	
Duck, roasted													
Flesh only	½ duck	221	445	52	25	9.2	8.2	3.2	0		197	144	7

Food	Amount	Weight in grams	Cal	Protein (g)	Total Fat (g)	Sat Fat (g)	Mono Fat (g)	Poly Fat (g)	Carbo (g)	Added Sugar (g)	Chol (mg)	Sodium (mg)	Fiber (g)
Eggnog (commercial)	1 cup	254	340	10	19	11.3	5.7	0.9	34	+	149	138	
Eggplant, steamed	1 cup	96	25	1	tr	tr	tr	0.1	6		0	3	2.5
Eggs													
Whole	1 egg	50	80	6	6	1.7	2.2	0.7	1		274	69	
White only	1 white	33	15	3	tr	0	0	0	tr		0	50	
Enchilada	1	230	235	20	16	7.7	6.7	0.6	24		19	4,451	
English muffin	1 plain	50	140	5	1	0.3	0.2	0.3	27		0	378	
Figs, dried	10	187	475	6	2	0.4	0.5	1.0	122		0	21	30
Filberts (hazelnuts)	1 oz	28	180	4	18	1.3	13.9	1.7	4		0	1	
Fish sticks, frozen	1 stick	28	70	6	3	0.8	1.4	0.8	4		26	53	
Fish, see particular name such as Flounder, Salmon, Trout													
Flounder													
Baked without added fat	3 oz	85	80	17	1	0.3	0.2	0.4	tr		59	111	
Flour													
White, all purpose, unsifted	1 cup	125	455	13	1	0.2	0.1	0.5	95		0	3	4
Whole wheat	1 cup	120	400	16	2	0.3	0.3	1.1	85		0	4	11.5
French toast	1 slice	65	155	6	7	1.6	2.0	1.6	17		112	257	

Fruit cocktail, canned, fruit and juice													
Heavy syrup	1 cup	255	185	1	tr	tr	tr	0.1	48	19	0	15	
Juice pack	1 cup	248	115	1	tr	tr	tr	tr	29		0	10	3
Fruit drinks or punch													
Fruit punch	6 oz	190	85	tr	0	0	0	0	22	+	0	15	
Grape	6 oz	187	100	tr	0	0	0	0	26	+	0	11	
Pineapple/ grapefruit	6 oz	187	90	tr	tr	tr	tr	tr	23	+	0	24	
Fruitcake, dark	2/3" piece	43	165	2	7	1.5	3.6	1.6	25	+	20	67	
Gelatin, dry	1 pkt	7	25	6	tr	tr	tr	tr	0		0	6	
Gelatin dessert, prepared	1/2 cup	120	70	2	0	0	0	0	17	17	0	55	
Graham crack- ers, 2 1/2" sq	2 crkrs	14	60	1	1	0.4	0.6	0.4	11	+	0	86	
Grapefruit, 3 3/4"	1/2 fruit	120	40	1	tr	tr	tr	tr	10		0	tr	1.5
Grapefruit juice	1 cup	247	95	1	tr	tr	tr	0.1	23		0	2	
Grapes	10 grapes	50	35	tr	tr	0.1	tr	0.1	9		0	1	1
Grape juice, bttl	1 cup	253	155	1	tr	0.1	tr	0.1	38		0	8	
Gravies													
Canned beef	1 cup	233	125	9	5	2.7	2.3	0.2	11		7	117	
Canned chicken	1 cup	238	190	5	14	3.4	6.1	3.6	13		5	1,373	
Mix, brown	1 cup	261	80	3	2	0.9	0.8	0.1	14		2	1,147	
Grits	1 cup	247	145	3	tr	tr	0.1	0.2	31		0	0	1
Guavas	1 fruit	90	45	1	1	0.2	0.1	0.2	11		0	2	
Haddock, cooked	3 oz	85	95	21	1	0.1	0.1	0.3	0		63	74	
Halibut, broiled	3 oz	85	140	20	6	3.3	1.6	0.7	tr		62	103	

391

Food	Amount	Weight in grams	Cal	Protein (g)	Total Fat (g)	Sat Fat (g)	Mono Fat (g)	Poly Fat (g)	Carbo (g)	Added Sugar (g)	Chol (mg)	Sodium (mg)	Fiber (g)
Ham													
Roasted,													
lean and fat	3 oz	85	205	18	14	5.1	6.7	1.5	0		53	1,009	
Roasted, lean	3 oz	85	131	21	5	1.6	2.1	0.5	0		46	1,128	
Luncheon pack—1 slice = 1 oz													
Reg cooked	2 slices	57	105	10	6	1.9	2.8	0.7	2		32	751	
Lean cooked	2 slices	57	75	11	3	0.9	1.3	0.3	1		27	815	
Herring, pickled	3 oz	85	190	17	13	4.3	4.6	3.1	0		85	850	
Hollandaise sauce													
(mix)	1 cup	259	240	5	20	11.6	5.9	0.9	14		52	1,564	
Honey	1 tbsp	21	65	tr	0	0	0	0	17	17	0	1	
Honeydew melon,													
6½"	1/10 melon	129	45	1	tr	tr	tr	0.1	12		0	13	
Hot dogs (frankfurters), 10 per lb pkg													
Beef	1 dog	45	142	5	13	5.4	6.1	0.6	tr		27	462	
Chicken	1 dog	45	115	6	9	2.5	3.8	1.8	3		45	616	
Meat	1 dog	45	145	5	13	4.8	6.2	1.2	1		23	504	
Ice cream, vanilla													
Reg (11% fat)	1 cup	133	270	5	14	8.9	4.1	0.5	32	+	59	116	
Rich (16% fat)	1 cup	148	350	4	24	4.7	6.8	0.9	32	+	88	108	
Ice milk, vanilla													
(4% fat)	1 cup	131	185	5	6	3.5	1.6	0.2	29	+	18	105	
Jams and													
preserves	1 tbsp	20	55	tr	tr	0	tr	tr	14	+	0	2	
Jellies	1 tbsp	18	50	tr	tr	tr	tr	tr	13	+	0	5	

Food	Measure												
Kale, chopped	1 cup	130	40	2	1	0.1	tr	0.3	7		0	30	tr
Kiwifruit, peeled	1 fruit	76	45	1	tr	tr	0.1	0.1	11		0	4	2
Kohlrabi, cooked and diced	1 cup	165	50	3	tr	tr	tr	0.1	11		0	35	
Lamb													
Loin chop, broiled													
Lean and fat	2.8 oz	80	235	22	16	7.3	6.4	1.0	0		78	62	
Lean only	2.8 oz	77	168	23	7	3.1	2.9	0.5	0		72	65	
Leg, roasted													
Lean and fat	3 oz	85	205	22	13	5.6	4.9	0.8	0		78	57	
Rib, roasted													
Lean and fat	3 oz	85	315	18	26	12.1	10.6	1.5	0		77	60	
Lean only	3 oz	85	195	23	11	4.8	4.5	0.8	0		75	69	
Lard	1 tbsp	13	115	0	13	5.1	5.9	1.5	0		12	0	
Leeks, cooked	1 leek	124	38	1	tr	tr	tr	0.1	10		0	13	1.5
Lemonade, fresh frozen	6 oz	185	80	tr	tr	tr	tr	tr	21	+	0	1	
Lemons, 4/lb	1 lemon	58	15	1	1	tr	tr	0.1	5		0	1	
Lemon juice	1 tbsp	15	5	tr	tr	tr	tr	tr	1		0	tr	
Lentils, dry, cooked	1 cup	200	215	16	1	0.1	0.2	0.5	38		0	26	8
Lettuce													
Iceberg, chopped	1 cup	55	5	1	tr	tr	tr	0.1	1		0	5	1
Loose-leaf	1 cup	56	10	1	tr	tr	tr	0.1	2		0	5	1
Limes (use Lemon figures)													
Liver, beef, fried	3 oz	85	185	23	7	2.5	3.6	1.3	7		410	90	
Lobster, steamed	3 oz	85	83	17	1	0.1	0.1	0.1	1		61	323	

Food	Amount	Weight in grams	Cal	Protein (g)	Total Fat (g)	Sat Fat (g)	Mono Fat (g)	Poly Fat (g)	Carbo (g)	Added Sugar (g)	Chol (mg)	Sodium (mg)	Fiber (g)
Macadamia nuts	1 oz	28	205	2	22	3.2	17.1	0.4	4		0	74	
Macaroni, cooked													
Firm stage	1 cup	130	190	7	1	0.1	0.1	0.3	39		0	1	
Macaroni & cheese													
Home recipe	1 cup	200	430	17	22	9.8	7.4	3.6	40		44	1,086	
Mackerel, cooked	3 oz	85	223	20	15	3.5	6.0	3.7	0		64	71	
Mangoes, 1½/lb	1 mango	207	135	1	1	0.1	0.2	0.1	35		0	4	3
Margarine													
Imitation (about 40% fat)													
Soft	1 tbsp	14	50	tr	5	1.1	2.2	1.9	tr		0	134	
	1 cup	227	785	1	88	17.5	35.6	31.3	1		0	2,178	
Regular (about 80% fat)													
Hard, stick	½ cup	113	810	1	91	17.9	40.5	28.7	1		0	1,066	
Hard	1 tbsp	14	75	tr	9	2.0	3.6	2.5	0		0	139	
Hard 1/3" pat	1 pat	5	25	tr	3	0.7	1.3	0.9	0		0	50	
Soft	1 cup	114	813	1	91	15.7	32.4	39.3	1		0	1,225	
	1 tbsp	14	75	tr	9	1.8	4.4	1.9	0		0	139	
Spread (about 60% fat)													
Hard, stick	½ cup	113	610	1	69	15.9	29.4	20.5	0		0	1,123	
Hard	1 tbsp	14	75	tr	9	2.0	3.6	2.5	0		0	139	
Hard 1/3" pat	1 pat	5	25	tr	3	0.7	1.3	0.9	0		0	50	
Soft	½ cup	114	613	1	69	14.6	35.6	15.7	0		0	1,128	
	1 tbsp	14	75	tr	9	1.8	4.4	1.9	0		0	139	
Mayonnaise													
Regular	1 tbsp	14	100	tr	11	1.7	3.2	5.8	tr		8	80	
Imitation	1 tbsp	15	35	tr	3	0.5	0.7	1.6	2		4	75	

Milk, fluid, no milk solids added

Whole (3.3%)	1 cup	244	150	8	8	5.1	2.4	0.3	11	33		120	
Low-fat (2%)	1 cup	244	120	8	5	2.9	1.4	0.2	12	18		122	
Low-fat (1%)	1 cup	244	100	8	3	1.6	0.7	0.1	12	10		123	
Skim, nonfat	1 cup	245	85	8	tr	0.3	0.1	tr	12	4		126	
Buttermilk	1 cup	245	100	8	2	1.3	0.6	0.1	12	9		257	
Milk, canned													
Condensed, sweetened	1 cup	306	980	24	27	16.8	7.4	1.0	166	104	+	389	
Evaporated, whole	1 cup	252	340	17	19	11.6	5.9	0.6	25	74		267	
Evaporated, skim	1 cup	255	200	19	1	0.3	0.2	tr	29	9		293	
Milk, dried, nonfat, un-mixed	1 cup	68	245	24	tr	0.3	0.1	tr	35	12		373	
Milk, chocolate, commercial													
Regular	1 cup	250	210	8	8	5.3	2.5	0.3	26	31	15	149	
Low-fat 1%	1 cup	250	160	8	3	1.5	0.8	0.1	26	7	14	152	
Miso	1 cup	276	470	29	13	1.8	2.6	7.3	65	0		8,142	8
Mixed nuts w/peanuts, salted	1 oz	28	175	5	16	2.5	9.0	3.8	6	0		185	
Molasses	2 tbsp	40	85	0	0	0	0	0	22	0	22	38	
Muffins, from commercial mix (use to estimate home recipe too)													
Blueberry	1 muffin	45	140	3	5	1.4	2.0	1.2	22	45		225	
Bran	1 muffin	45	140	3	4	1.3	1.6	1.0	24	28		385	1
Corn	1 muffin	45	145	3	6	1.7	2.3	1.4	22	42		291	4

Food	Amount	Weight in grams	Cal	Protein (g)	Total Fat (g)	Sat Fat (g)	Mono Fat (g)	Poly Fat (g)	Carbo (g)	Added Sugar (g)	Chol (mg)	Sodium (mg)	Fiber (g)
Mushrooms													
Raw, sliced	1 cup	70	20	1	tr	tr	tr	0.1	3		0	3	2
Canned, drained	1 cup	35	35	3	tr	0.1	tr	0.2	8		0	663	
Mussels, steamed	3 oz	85	147	20	4	0.7	0.9	1.0	6		48	313	
Mustard, prepared	1 tsp	5	5	tr	tr	tr	0.2	tr	tr		0	63	
Mustard greens	1 cup	140	20	3	tr	tr	0.2	0.1	3		0	22	1
Nectarines, 3/lb	1 fruit	136	65	1	1	0.1	0.2	0.3	16		0	tr	
Noodles (egg type)													
Cooked	1 cup	160	200	7	2	0.5	0.6	0.6	37		57	3	
Noodles, chow mein	1 cup	45	220	6	11	2.1	7.3	0.4	26		5	450	
Oils, salad or cooking													
Corn	1 tbsp	14	125	0	14	1.8	3.4	8.2	0		0	0	
Olive	1 tbsp	14	125	0	14	1.9	10.3	1.2	0		0	0	
Peanut	1 tbsp	14	125	0	14	2.4	6.5	4.5	0		0	0	
Safflower	1 tbsp	14	125	0	14	1.3	1.7	10.4	0		0	0	
Soybean	1 tbsp	14	125	0	14	2	3.1	7.8	0		0	0	
Soybean, hydrogenated	1 tbsp	14	125	0	14	2.1	6.0	5.3	0		0	0	

Food	Measure										
Soybean-cottonseed blend, hydrogen-											
ated	1 tbsp	14	125	0	14	2.5	4.1	6.7	0	0	0	
Sunflower	1 tbsp	14	125	0	14	1.4	2.7	9.2	0	0	0	
Okra, 3", cooked	8 pods	85	25	2	tr	tr	tr	tr	6	0	274	2.5
Olives, canned												
Green	4 med or 3 xlarge	13	15	tr	2	0.2	1.2	0.1	tr	0	312	0.5
Black (U.S.)	3 sm or 2 lrg	9	15	tr	2	0.3	1.3	0.2	tr	0	68	tr
Greek black, salt cure	2 med	5	16	tr	2	0.2	1.4	0.4	tr	0	85	tr
Onions												
Raw, chopped	1 cup	160	55	2	tr	0.1	0.1	0.2	12	0	3	1.5
Cooked	1 cup	210	60	2	tr	0.1	tr	0.1	13	0	17	2.5
Onion rings, frozen, breaded, panfried	2 rings	20	80	1	5	1.7	2.2	1.0	8	0	75	
Oranges, 2½/lb	1 orange	131	60	1	tr	tr	tr	tr	15	0	tr	2.5
Orange juice	1 cup	248	110	2	tr	0.1	0.1	0.1	26	0	2	
Oysters												
Raw, meat only	1 cup (13–19 selects)	240	160	20	4	1.4	0.5	1.4	8	120	175	
Breaded, fried	1 oyster	45	90	5	5	1.4	2.1	1.4	5	35	70	
Pancakes, 4" diam	1 pancake	27	60	2	2	0.5	0.9	0.5	8	16	160	
Papayas, ½" cubes	1 cup	140	65	1	tr	0.1	0.1	tr	17	0	9	1.5
Parsley, dried	1 tbsp	0.4	tr	tr	tr	tr	tr	tr	tr	0	2	
Parsnips, diced	1 cup	156	125	2	tr	0.1	0.2	0.1	30	0	16	5

Food	Amount	Weight in grams	Cal	Protein (g)	Total Fat (g)	Sat Fat (g)	Mono Fat (g)	Poly Fat (g)	Carbo (g)	Added Sugar (g)	Chol (mg)	Sodium (mg)	Fiber (g)
Pastrami	1 oz	28	99	5	8	3.0	4.1	0.3	1		26	348	
Peaches													
Fresh, raw, 4/lb	1 peach	87	35	1	tr	tr	tr	tr	10		0	tr	2
Canned, fruit and liquid													
Heavy syrup	1 half	81	60	tr	tr	tr	tr	tr	16	7	0	5	
Juice pack	1 half	77	35	tr	tr	tr	tr	tr	9		0	3	
Dried, uncooked	1 cup	160	380	6	1	0.1	0.4	0.6	98		0	11	
Frozen, sweetened	1 cup	250	235	2	tr	tr	0.1	0.2	60	+	0	15	
Peanuts, roasted, salted	1 oz	28	165	8	14	1.9	6.9	4.4	5		0	122	0.5
Peanut butter	1 tbsp	16	95	5	8	1.4	4.0	2.5	3		0	75	
Pears													
Fresh with skin, 2½/lb	1 pear	166	100	1	1	tr	0.1	0.2	25		0	tr	4
Canned, fruit and liquid													
Heavy syrup	1 half	79	60	tr	tr	tr	tr	tr	15	5	0	4	
Juice pack	1 half	77	40	tr	tr	tr	tr	tr	10		0	3	
Peas													
Black-eyed													
Fresh	1 cup	165	180	13	1	0.3	0.1	0.6	30		0	7	4.5
Dried, cooked	1 cup	250	190	13	1	0.2	tr	0.3	35		0	20	
Green, frozen	1 cup	160	125	8	tr	0.1	tr	0.2	23		0	139	8
Snow pea (edible pod)	1 cup	160	65	5	tr	0.1	tr	0.2	11		0	6	2.5

Food	Measure												
Split, dry, cooked	1 cup	200	230	16	1	0.1	0.1	0.3	42		0	26	
Pecans, halves	1 oz	28	190	2	19	1.5	12.0	4.7	5		0	tr	4.5
Peppers													
Hot chili	1 pepper	45	20	1	tr	tr	tr	tr	4		0	3	
Sweet, 5/lb	1 pepper	74	20	1	tr	tr	tr	0.2	4		0	2	1
Perch, ocean													
Broiled	3 oz	85	103	20	2	0.3	0.7	0.5	0			82	
Fried, breaded	1 fillet	85	185	16	11	2.6	4.6	2.8	7		66	138	
Pickles cucumber													
Dill, whole, 3¾"	1 pickle	65	5	tr	tr	tr	tr	0.1	1		0	928	
Fresh pack, ¼"	2 slices	15	10	tr	tr	tr	tr	tr	3		0	101	
Sweet gerkin, 2½"	1 pickle	15	20	tr	tr	tr	tr	tr	5		0	107	
Pickle relish, sweet	1 tbsp	15	20	tr	tr	tr	tr	tr	5		0	107	
Piecrust, 9" diam	1 shell	180	900	11	60	14.8	25.9	15.7	79		0	1,100	
Pies, piece is 1/6 of 9" diam pie													
Apple	1 piece	158	405	3	18	4.6	7.4	4.4	60	17	0	476	
Cherry	1 piece	158	410	4	18	4.7	7.7	4.6	61	33	0	480	
Creme	1 piece	152	455	3	23	15.0	4.0	1.1	59	33	8	369	
Custard	1 piece	152	330	9	17	5.6	6.7	3.2	36	17	169	436	
Lemon													
meringue	1 piece	140	355	5	14	4.3	5.7	2.9	53	35	143	395	
Pecan	1 piece	138	575	7	32	4.7	17	7.9	71	60	95	305	
Pumpkin	1 piece	152	320	6	17	6.4	6.7	3.0	37	23	109	325	

Food	Amount	Weight in grams	Cal	Protein (g)	Total Fat (g)	Sat Fat (g)	Mono Fat (g)	Poly Fat (g)	Carbo (g)	Added Sugar (g)	Chol (mg)	Sodium (mg)	Fiber (g)
Pies, fried													
Apple (or cherry)	1 pie	85	255	2	14	5.8	6.6	0.6	31	+	14	326	
Pineapple													
Fresh, diced	1 cup	155	75	1	1	tr	0.1	0.2	19		0	2	2.5
Canned, crushed or pieces													
Heavy syrup	1 cup	255	200	1	tr	tr	tr	0.1	52	13	0	3	
Juice pack	1 cup	250	150	1	tr	tr	tr	0.1	39		0	3	
Pineapple juice	1 cup	250	140	1	tr	tr	tr	0.1	34		0	3	
Pine nuts													
(piñones)	1 oz	28	160	3	17	2.7	6.5	7.3	5		0	2	
Pistachio nuts, shelled	1 oz	28	165	6	14	1.7	9.3	2.1	7		0	2	
Pizza, cheese (slice is 1/8 of 15")	1 slice	120	290	15	9	4.1	2.6	1.3	39		56	699	
Plantains	1 fruit	179	220	2	1	0.3	0.1	0.1	57		0	7	
Plums													
Fresh, 6½/lb	1 plum	66	35	1	tr	tr	0.3	0.1	9		0	tr	1.5
Canned, fruit and liquid													
Heavy syrup	3 plums	133	120	tr	tr	tr	0.1	tr	31	17	0	25	
Juice pack	3 plums	95	55	tr	tr	tr	tr	tr	14		0	1	
Popcorn, unbuttered													
Air-popped, unsalted	1 cup	8	30	1	tr	tr	0.1	0.2	6		0	tr	2.5

Oil-popped, salted 1 cup	11	55	1	3	0.5	1.4	1.2	6	0	86	
Popsicle, 3 fl oz 1 pop	95	70	0	0	0	0	0	18	0	11	
Pork, fresh, not cured											
Loin, broiled											
Lean and fat 3 oz	85	294	20	23	8.4	10.6	2.6	0	80	56	
Lean only 3 oz	85	218	24	13	4.5	5.8	1.6	0	81	64	
Loin, center rib, broiled											
Lean and fat 3 oz	85	291	21	22	8.1	10.3	2.5	0	79	52	
Lean only 3 oz	85	219	25	13	4.4	5.7	1.5	0	80	57	
Loin, center rib, pan-fried (as a chop)											
Lean and fat 3 oz	85	331	18	28	10.1	12.9	3.2	0	71	38	
Lean only 3 oz	85	219	24	13	4.8	5.8	1.6	0	69	43	
Shoulder, roasted											
Lean and fat 3 oz	85	277	19	22	7.9	10.0	2.5	0	81	58	
Lean only 3 oz	85	207	22	13	4.4	5.7	1.5	0	82	65	
Potato chips 10 chips	20	105	1	7	1.8	1.2	3.6	10	0	94	
Potatoes, cooked											
Baked, 2/lb											
With skin 1 potato	202	220	5	tr	0.1	tr	0.1	51	0	16	
Flesh only 1 potato	156	145	3	tr	tr	tr	0.1	34	0	8	
Boiled, peeled before boiling, 3/lb unpeeled 1 potato	135	115	2	tr	tr	tr	0.1	27	0	7	
French fries, frozen, strips 2"–3½"											
Heat in oven 10 strips	50	110	2	4	2.1	1.8	0.3	17	0	16	4
Fry in oil 10 strips	50	160	2	8	2.5	1.6	3.8	20	0	108	1.5
Hash browns 1 cup	156	340	5	18	7.0	8.0	2.1	44	0	53	
Mashed w/milk, no margarine 1 cup	210	160	4	1	0.7	0.3	0.1	37	4	636	

Food	Amount	Weight in grams	Cal	Protein (g)	Total Fat (g)	Sat Fat (g)	Mono Fat (g)	Poly Fat (g)	Carbo (g)	Added Sugar (g)	Chol (mg)	Sodium (mg)	Fiber (g)
Scalloped, from dry mix	1 cup	245	230	5	11	6.5	3.0	0.5	31		27	835	
Pretzels													
Stick, 2¼", long, thin	10 sticks	3	10	tr	tr	tr	tr	tr	2		0	48	
Twisted, 2¾"	1 pretzel	16	65	2	1	0.1	0.2	0.2	13		0	258	
Prunes, dried	4 xlarge or 5 large	49	115	1	tr	tr	0.2	0.1	31		0	2	8
Prune juice	1 cup	256	180	2	tr	tr	0.1	tr	45		0	10	
Puddings													
Canned													
Chocolate	5-oz can	142	205	3	11	9.5	0.5	0.1	30	+	1	285	
Vanilla	5-oz can	142	220	2	10	9.5	0.2	0.1	33	+	1	305	
Dry mix made with whole milk	½ cup	130	155	4	4	2.3	1.1	0.2	27	+	14	440	
Pumpkin													
Fresh, mashed	1 cup	245	50	2	tr	0.1	tr	tr	12		0	2	
Canned	1 cup	245	85	3	1	0.4	0.1	tr	20		0	12	
Pumpkinseed kernel	1 oz	28	155	7	13	2.5	4.0	5.9	5		0	5	
Quiche lorraine	⅛ of 8" diam	176	600	13	48	23.2	17.8	4.1	29		285	653	

Food	Measure											
Radishes	4 rad	18	5	tr	tr	tr	tr	tr	1	0	4	tr
Raisins, seedless												
Not pressed down	1 cup	145	435	5	1	0.2	tr	0.2	115	0	17	10
½-oz packet		14	40	tr	tr	tr	tr	tr	11	0	2	1
Raspberries												
Fresh	1 cup	123	60	1	1	tr	0.1	0.4	14	0	tr	9
Frozen, swtned	1 cup	250	255	2	tr	tr	tr	0.2	65	0	3	
Rhubarb, cooked with sugar	1 cup	240	280	1	tr	tr	tr	0.1	75	0	2	4.5
Rice, cooked, no added butter or margarine												
Brown	1 cup	195	230	5	1	0.3	0.3	0.4	50	0	0	
White	1 cup	205	225	4	tr	0.1	0.1	0.1	50	0	0	
Rolls, commercial												
Dinner, 2½"	1 roll	28	85	2	2	0.5	0.8	0.6	14	tr	155	
Hot dog or hamburger bun, 8 to pkg.	1 roll	40	115	3	2	0.5	0.8	0.6	1	tr	241	
Hard, 3¾"	1 roll	50	155	5	2	0.4	0.5	0.6	30	tr	313	
Submarine, 11½"	1 roll	135	400	11	8	1.8	3.0	2.2	72	tr	683	
Salad dressings, commercial, regular												
Blue cheese	1 tbsp	15	75	1	8	1.5	1.8	4.2	1	3	164	
French	1 tbsp	16	85	tr	9	1.4	4.0	3.5	1	0	188	
Italian	1 tbsp	15	80	tr	9	1.3	3.7	3.2	1	0	162	
Ranch												
Thousand Island	1 tbsp	16	60	tr	6	1.0	1.3	3.2	2	4	112	

Food	Amount	Weight in grams	Cal	Protein (g)	Total Fat (g)	Sat Fat (g)	Mono Fat (g)	Poly Fat (g)	Carbo (g)	Added Sugar (g)	Chol (mg)	Sodium (mg)	Fiber (g)
Salad dressing, commercial, low calorie													
French	1 tbsp	16	25	tr	2	0.2	0.3	1.0	2		0	306	
Italian	1 tbsp	15	10	tr	tr	tr	tr	tr	2		0	136	
Salad dressing, vinegar and oil, vinaigrette	1 tbsp	16	70	0	8	1.5	2.4	3.9	tr		0	tr	
Salami													
Beef beer	1 slice	23	76	3	7	3.0	3.2	0.3	tr		14	236	
Cooked type, 1-oz slice	2 slices	57	145	8	11	4.6	5.2	1.2	1		37	607	
Dry type, (hard) 12 slices/4 oz	2 slices	20	85	5	7	2.4	3.4	0.6	1		16	372	
Salmon													
Canned (pink)	3 oz	85	140	17	5	0.9	1.5	2.1	0		34	443	
Baked	3 oz	85	140	21	5	1.2	2.4	1.4	0		60	55	
Smoked	3 oz	85	150	18	8	2.6	3.9	0.7	0		51	1,700	
Sardines, oil pack	3 oz	85	175	29	9	2.1	3.7	2.9	0		85	425	
Sauerkraut	1 cup	236	45	2	tr	0.1	tr	0.1	10		0	1,560	
Sausages													
Brown & serve	1 link	13	50	2	5	1.7	2.2	0.5	tr		9	105	
Italian	1 link	67	217	13	17	6.1	8.0	2.2	1		52	618	
Pork link 16/lb	1 link	13	50	3	4	1.4	1.8	0.5	tr		11	168	
Patties	1 patty	27	100	5	8	2.9	3.8	1.0	tr		22	349	
Vienna	1 sausage	16	45	2	4	1.5	2.0	0.3	tr		8	152	

Scallops											
Breaded, frozen	6 scallops	90	195	15	10	2.5	4.1	2.5	10	70	298
Sesame seeds	1 tbsp	8	45	2	4	0.6	1.7	1.9	1	0	3
Sherbet	1 cup	193	270	2	4	2.4	1.1	0.1	59	14	88
Shortening, veg	1 cup	205	1,810	0	205	51.3	91.2	53.5	0	0	0
	1 tbsp	13	115	0	13	3.3	5.8	3.4	0	0	0
Shrimp											
Fresh, steamed	3 oz	85	84	18	1	0.2	0.2	0.4	0	168	190
Fried	3 oz	85	200	16	10	2.5	4.1	2.6	11		384
Snapper, broiled	3 oz	85	109	22	2	0.3	0.3	0.5	+	40	48
Sole, see Flounder											
Soups, condensed, prepared with equal volume of milk											
Cream of chicken	1 cup	248	190	7	11	4.6	4.5	1.6	15	27	1,047
Cream of mushroom	1 cup	248	205	6	14	5.1	3.0	4.6	15	20	1,076
Tomato	1 cup	248	160	6	6	2.9	1.6	1.1	22	17	932
Soups, condensed, prepared with equal volume of water											
Bean w/bacon	1 cup	253	170	8	6	1.5	2.2	1.8	23	3	951
Chicken											
noodle	1 cup	241	75	4	2	0.7	1.1	0.6	9	7	1,106
Chicken rice	1 cup	241	60	4	2	0.5	0.9	0.4	7	7	815
Minestrone	1 cup	241	80	4	3	0.6	0.7	1.1	11	2	911
Pea, green	1 cup	250	165	9	3	1.4	1.0	0.4	27	0	988
Tomato	1 cup	244	85	2	2	0.4	0.4	1.0	17	0	690
Veg beef	1 cup	244	80	6	2	0.9	0.8	0.1	10	5	1,890
Vegetarian	1 cup	241	70	2	2	0.3	0.8	0.7	12	0	822

Food	Amount	Weight in grams	Cal	Protein (g)	Total Fat (g)	Sat Fat (g)	Mono Fat (g)	Poly Fat (g)	Carbo (g)	Added Sugar (g)	Chol (mg)	Sodium (mg)	Fiber (g)
Soups, dehydrated, prepared with water, 1 pkt makes 6 fl oz													
Chicken noodle	1 pkt	188	40	2	1	0.2	0.4	0.3	6		2	957	
Onion	1 pkt	184	20	1	tr	0.1	0.2	0.1	4		0	635	
Tomato veg	1 pkt	189	40	1	1	0.3	0.2	0.1	8		0	856	
Sour cream	1 cup	230	495	7	48	30.0	13.9	1.8	10		102	123	
	1 tbsp	12	25	tr	3	1.6	0.7	0.1	1		5	6	
Soybeans, dry, cooked	1 cup	180	235	20	10	1.3	1.9	5.3	19		0	4	
Soy sauce	1 tbsp	18	10	2	0	0	0	0	2		0	1,029	
Spaghetti, al dente	1 cup	130	190	7	1	0.1	0.1	0.3	39		0	1	
Spinach													
Raw, chopped	1 cup	55	10	2	tr	tr	tr	0.1	2		0	43	1
Cooked, leaf	1 cup	190	55	6	tr	0.1	tr	0.2	10		0	163	5
Spinach soufflé	1 cup	136	220	11	18	7.1	6.8	3.1	3		184	763	
Squash, cooked													
Summer, sliced	1 cup	180	35	2	1	0.1	tr	0.2	8		0	2	3
Winter, baked	1 cup	205	80	2	1	0.3	0.1	0.5	18		0	2	2.5
Strawberries													
Fresh, whole	1 cup	149	45	1	1	tr	0.1	0.3	10		0	1	3
Frozen, sweetened	1 cup	255	245	1	tr	tr	tr	0.2	66		0	8	
Stuffing, bread, dry type	1 cup	140	500	9	31	6.1	13.3	9.6	50		0	1,254	

Sugar													
Brown, packed	1 cup	220	820	0	0	0	0	0	212	212	0	97	
Powdered, white	1 cup	100	385	0	0	0	0	0	100	100	0	2	
White, granulated	1 cup	200	770	0	0	0	0	0	199	199	0	5	
	1 tbsp	12	45	0	0	0	0	0	12	12	0	tr	
	1 pkt	6	25	0	0	0	0	0	6	6	0	tr	
Sunflower seeds	1 oz	28	160	6	14	1.5	2.7	9.3	5		0	1	3
Sweet potatoes, 2½/lb													
Baked, peeled	1 potato	114	115	2	tr	tr	tr	0.1	28		0	11	
Boiled, peeled	1 potato	151	160	2	tr	0.1	tr	0.2	37		0	20	
Candied, 2½"	1 piece	105	145	1	3	1.4	0.7	0.2	29		8	74	
Syrup (corn or maple)	2 tbsp	42	122	0	0	0	0	0	32	32	0	19	
Taco	1 taco	81	195	9	11	4.1	5.5	0.8	15		21	456	
Tahini	1 tbsp	15	90	3	8	1.1	3.0	3.5	3		0	5	
Tangerines	1 tan	84	35	1	tr	tr	tr	tr	9		0	1	1.5
Tangerine juice, canned, sweetened	1 cup	252	155	1	tr	tr	tr	0.1	41		0	15	
Tartar sauce	1 tbsp	14	75	tr	8	1.2	2.6	3.9	1		4	182	
Toaster pastries	1 pastry	54	210	2	6	1.7	3.6	0.4	38	+	0	248	
Tofu (bean curd)	2½" sq	120	85	9	5	0.7	1.0	2.9	3		0	8	0.5
Tomatoes													
Fresh, 4/lb	1 tomato	123	25	1	tr	tr	tr	0.1	5		0	10	
Canned	1 cup	240	50	2	1	0.1	0.1	0.2	10		0	391	
Tomato juice	1 cup	244	40	2	tr	tr	tr	0.1	10		0	881	
Tomato paste	1 tbsp	16	14	1	tr	tr	tr	tr	3		0	11	2.5

Food	Amount	Weight in grams	Cal	Protein (g)	Total Fat (g)	Sat Fat (g)	Mono Fat (g)	Poly Fat (g)	Carbo (g)	Added Sugar (g)	Chol (mg)	Sodium (mg)	Fiber (g)
Tomato puree	1 cup	250	105	4	tr	tr	tr	0.1	25		0	50	
Tomato sauce	1 cup	245	75	3	tr	0.1	0.1	0.2	18		0	1,482	
Tortillas, corn	1 tortilla	30	65	2	1	0.1	0.3	0.6	13		0	1	
Trout, rainbow													
Broiled	3 oz	85	129	22	4	0.7	1.1	1.3	0		62	29	
Tuna, canned													
Oil pack	3 oz	85	165	24	7	1.4	1.9	3.1	0		55	303	
Water pack	3 oz	85	135	30	1	0.3	0.2	0.3	0		48	468	
Tuna, fresh													
Tuna salad made with relish and mayonnaise	1 cup	205	375	33	19	3.3	4.9	9.2	19		80	877	
Turkey, roasted													
Light meat	3 oz	85	135	25	3	0.9	0.5	0.7	0		59	54	
Dark meat	3 oz	85	160	24	6	2.1	1.4	1.8	0		72	67	
Chopped dark and light meat	1 cup	140	240	41	7	2.3	1.4	2.0	0		106	98	
Turnip greens	1 cup	164	50	5	1	0.2	tr	0.3	8		0	25	
Turnips, diced	1 cup	156	30	1	tr	tr	tr	0.1	8		0	78	6
Veal													
Cutlet, broiled	3 oz	85	185	23	9	4.1	4.1	0.6	0		108	56	
Rib, roasted	3 oz	85	230	23	14	6.0	6.0	1.0	0		109	57	

Vegetable juice cocktail	1 cup	242	45	2	tr	tr	tr	tr	11	0	883	
Vegetables, mixed	1 cup	163	75	4	tr	0.1	tr	0.1	15	0	243	3.5
Vinegar, cider	1 tbsp	15	tr	tr	0	0	0	0	1	0	tr	tr
Waffles, 7″ diam	1 waffle	75	245	7	13	4.0	4.9	2.6	26	102	445	
Walnuts Black, chopped	1 oz	28	170	7	16	1.0	3.6	10.6	3	0	1	
English	1 oz	28	180	4	18	1.6	4.0	11.1	5	0	3	
Water chestnuts	1 cup	140	70	1	tr	tr	tr	tr	17	0	11	
Watercress	1 cup	160	52	tr	tr	tr	tr		2	0	1	
Watermelon, diced	1 cup	160	50	1	1	0.1	0.1	0.3	11	0	3	
White sauce	1 cup	250	395	10	30	9.1	11.9	7.2	24	32	888	
Wine, table	3½ oz	102	80	tr	0	0	0	0	3	5	0	tr

SOURCES

Susan E. Gebhardt and Ruth H. Matthews. *Nutritive Value of Foods.* U.S. Department of Agriculture, Human Nutrition Information Service, Home and Garden Bulletin, No. 72, 1981.

U.S. Department of Agriculture, Human Nutrition Information Service. *Composition of Foods: Raw, Processed, Prepared.* Agriculture Handbook No. 8, Volumes 1–16.

The National Cancer Institute. "Diet, Nutrition, & Cancer Prevention: The Good News." U.S. Department of Health and Human Services, NIH Publication No. 87–2878, 1986.

Gilbert A. Leveille, Mary Ellen Zabik, and Karen J. Morgan. *Nutrients in Foods.* Cambridge, Mass.: The Nutrition Guild, 1983.

"Ready to Eat Cereals." *Consumer Reports,* October 1986, pp. 628–637.

aerobic—living in air, or utilizing oxygen

aerobic dance—an organized form of rhythmic movement set to music, which meets the requirements of aerobic or cardiovascular exercise. Two major forms of aerobic dance exist: (a) high impact, which involves running in place, jumps, and leaps; and (b) a new low-impact form, which utilizes marching, lunges, and side steps to keep one foot on the ground at all times and reduce trauma to the lower joints.

aerobics—a term used to describe an activity that uses oxygen as a method of obtaining energy. Such activities are usually continuous (at least twenty minutes), rhythmical (repetitive movements), and use large muscle masses such as the legs. This form of exercise places demands on, and improves, the cardiovascular and muscular endurance systems. Such activities include running, walking, swimming, biking, etc.

aging—the process of growing older; gradual decline in physical and mental health naturally occur during this process. This term can also be used in a more technical sense to refer to the genetic biology of the aging process.

alveoli—the smallest functional part of the lung. These tiny air sacs make contact with the capillaries, the smallest part of the circulatory system, where the exchange of oxygen and carbon dioxide take place.

amino acids—the building blocks of protein, twenty amino acids have been found to exist. Of these, eleven can be created in our bodies from the food we eat, nine others must be taken in through the diet. The best, most complete source of amino acids is animal protein.

GLOSSARY

anaerobic—without oxygen; this term usually describes brief, intense activity that does not require the immediate use of oxygen. For example, you can run fifty yards while holding your breath.

angioplasty—(percutaneous transluminal coronary) an operation which enlarges a narrowed coronary artery by inserting a catheter tipped with a small balloon. The balloon is inflated at the narrowing to enlarge the inside of the vessel.

aneurysm—a thinning, stretched out blood vessel wall. This weakened area can eventually burst and lead to internal bleeding and/or death of the tissue the vessel was feeding.

arteriosclerosis—a hardening of the arteries. Occurs mainly in old age, but heredity can cause it in younger people. If we live long enough, it will occur in all of us. It is characterized by the replacement of muscle and elastic tissue in the artery with fibrous tissue and calcified plaques.

arteries—the vessels responsible for carrying blood away from the heart. Arteries are composed of three layers, a smooth inside layer, a muscular middle layer, and an outside covering.

atherosclerosis—a term used to describe damage to the inside of the arterial wall, and the subsequent buildup of fat deposits and calcification in this damaged area. These circumstances narrow the artery and cause decreased blood flow to the area which they supply.

atrophy—the wasting away of tissue. If a weight lifter were to stop lifting all together, the muscle tissue he did not require for everyday use would be broken down by the body. The body will not support that which it does not need; in a sense, if you don't use it you'll lose it.

BAL (blood alcohol level)—the concentration of alcohol in the blood after drinking. The first consistent, sizable changes in behavior occur when BAL reaches .05 percent; a level of .10 percent is legally drunk, a state in which voluntary movements are seriously impaired; at .20 percent one is "falling down" drunk; past .40 percent or .50 percent the drinker is unconscious.

blood fat profile—the analysis of the fats which can be found in the bloodstream and which contribute to your overall state of health. This profile consists of triglycerides, total cholesterol, and the transporting form of this cholesterol and fat, HDL and LDL.

blood pressure—the measure of the force of blood against the arterial walls. There are two numbers in the blood pressure reading, 120 over 80 is usually considered to be a textbook normal. The top number, the systolic, indicates the pressure of the blood in the arteries as the heart contracts. The bottom number, the diastolic, indicates the pressure in the arteries between beats, when the heart is at rest. For high blood pressure, see hypertension.

body fat—the amount of fat that a person carries within the body. It is usually expressed as a percentage of the total body weight, so that a person weighing 100 pounds and having 20 percent body fat would have 20 pounds of fat. There are two forms of fat, essential and storage. Essential fat is that amount of fat which is necessary for survival (about 3 percent in males; 12 percent in females), while storage fat is the excess fat we carry in storage form. Body fat is best determined by percentage and not by body weight.

bomb calorimeter—a hollow steel container in which food is placed for measuring its caloric content. After the container is filled with oxygen, the contents are ignited and the amount of heat given off is collected by a pool of water surrounding the calorimeter. One calorie equals the amount of energy it takes to raise one liter of water one degree celsius.

bronchioles—small tubes in the lungs which carry air to the alveoli.

bronchitis—an inflammation of the mucous membrane of the bronchial tubes which lead to the lungs. Chronic bronchitis usually consists of a cough and increased mucous secretion over a long period of time.

bypass surgery—a surgical procedure where a vessel (usually the saphenous vein from a leg) is put in place over an obstructed artery so that blood flow may be diverted away from the obstruction and continue to supply the heart.

calorie—a measurement of the energy content of food and physical work. One calorie is the amount of energy it takes to raise the temperature of one liter of water one degree Celsius. If a food contained 100 calories, then it contains enough energy to raise the temperature of 100 liters of water one degree Celsius. You will sometimes see this food calorie referred to as a kilocalorie (kcal), its more precise technical designation.

carbohydrates—a substance found in many foods, especially plants, which plays a major role in body functioning. Carbohydrates are usually termed "simple" or "complex." Simple carbohydrates are usually sugars that may contain no nutritional value (empty calories). Complex carbohydrates are found in plant products which contain vitamins and minerals for the diet.

cardiology—the study of the heart and its diseases.

cardiovascular—a term used to describe the heart, lungs, and blood transporting systems. The terms aerobic and cardiovascular are sometimes used synonymously, as the cardiovascular system transports oxygen to the working muscles.

catheter—a small, thin tube for entering into a body cavity.

cerebral hemorrhage—blood flow, usually from a burst vessel, into the brain.

chronic—long-term; most often refers to a disease that progesses slowly and proceeds for a long period of time.

cholesterol—a fatlike substance found in all animal tissue that is manufactured in many body cells, especially the liver. It is a constituent of body cells, an ingredient in certain hormones, and important for the formation of bile acids which aid digestion. Research has shown that a high level of blood cholesterol is associated with an increased risk of coronary heart disease.

circuit weight training—a form of weight training that involves a selected group of exercises performed in a sequential manner with predetermined exercise/rest periods.

cirrhosis—a progressive disease of the liver which causes damage to the liver cells.

COLD (COPD)—chronic obstructive lung (pulmonary) disease.

coronary heart disease—a term used to describe the excessive formation of atherosclerotic plaques in the coronary arteries which supply blood to the heart.

dysfunction—lack of regular function; abnormal function.

EKG—electrocardiogram; a measurement of the electrical activity of the heart.

EKG stress test—a physical exertion test usually performed on a treadmill or bicycle while the subject is hooked to an electrocardiogram. The heart's response to exercise can then be evaluated.

embolism—a floating clot in the bloodstream. This clot can lodge in a vessel, preventing blood flow. The result is death to the tissue being supplied.

embolus—a plug or stopper of clotted mass which clogs a vessel (plural: emboli).

emphysema—a lung condition characterized by destructive changes in, and a reduction in, the number of alveoli. This results in a considerable decrease in lung function.

endurance—the ability to resist fatigue. The term can be used in a weight lifting or aerobic sense.

enzyme—a chemical substance that acts like a catalyst (speeds up a reaction) in the body.

epidemiologist—a person who studies the occurence and spread of a disease in a population (a particular group of people).

exercise—a structured form of activity involving physical exertion. The term can be applied to almost any form of physical activity. Exercise is task-specific. This means you will only obtain improvement in those areas that you work; aerobics improve the cardiovascular system, weight lifting gives you strength, stretching improves flexibility, etc.

fat—a term used to describe adipose tissue, the cells which store fat. Fat is not only stored as energy but serves many other important roles, including protecting and insulating internal organs, transporting and storing the fat-soluble vitamins A, D, E, K, and depressing hunger. Dietary fats differ in their chemical structure. Saturated fats are associated with heart disease and are found in animal products. They are usually solid at room temperature. Unsaturated and polyunsaturated fats are of plant origin. They are usually liquid at room temperature.

fatty acid—a linkage of available energy substances (fats, carbohydrates, or proteins) which can be stored as fat, used as fuel, or used in a number of other bodily processes.

fitness—a state or condition of optimal performance.

free weights—barbells, dumbbells, or any other form of nonrestricted weight.

fructose—a simple sugar found in fruit.

GGT—a liver function test.

glucose—the most common sugar found in the body. It is the only fuel our brain and central nervous system use.

glycogen—the storage form of glucose in the human body. Plants store glucose as starch.

hair implant—this term may be used to designate either the injection of individual artificial hairs into the scalp (a process discovered to be dangerous and rarely performed in the United States anymore) or the use of suture implants in the scalp to secure an artificial hairpiece.

hair transplant—a surgical procedure in which small plugs of hair-growing scalp are transferred to a bald area.

HDL cholesterol—high-density lipoprotein cholesterol. Frequently called the "good" cholesterol, it may be responsible for removal of cholesterol from the body's periphery and returning it to the liver for breakdown and removal. HDL seems to be more affected by exercise than diet.

health—the absence of disease, a properly functioning organism.

heart attack—a general term used to describe a sudden affliction of the heart. Heart attacks can occur from a variety of circumstances, including lack of blood flow, sudden trauma, irregularities of the heartbeat, etc.

hernia—the protrusion of a tissue through the structure that normally contains it.

hyperplasia—an increase in the number of cells of an organ or tissue.

hypertension—high blood pressure. This condition forces the heart to pump harder and can lead to heart failure and other problems over the years. Hypertension usually carries no symptoms. Blood pressure screening should be performed on a regular basis, at least every six months.

hypertrophy—an increase in the size of a cell or tissue.

ketosis—an acidic state of the body caused by the incomplete breakdown of fats. This may be caused by a high-fat diet, an absence of carbohydrates in the diet, and/or starvation diets. This condition may lead to depression of the brain and nervous system.

GLOSSARY

LDL cholesterol—low-density lipoprotein cholesterol. Termed the "bad" cholesterol, LDL is responsible for the transport of cholesterol to the body's cells. LDLs are affected by the diet.

maximal workout range—performing an exercise movement throughout the greatest range of motion that the involved joint will allow.

metabolism—the total of all energy processes which occur in an organism. In the laboratory it can be measured by the amount of heat produced or the amount of oxygen consumed.

muscle tone—a condition in which the muscle is in a partial state of contraction. This gives it firmness and rigidity.

myocardial infarction—a lack of blood supply to the heart muscle which results in death to the tissue that was being supplied. This is one of the afflictions we generally term "heart attack."

Nautilus machine—a popular variable-resistance weight lifting machine that uses kidney-shaped pulleys to vary the weight load.

obesity—a condition of excessive body fat.

ophthalmology—the branch of medical science dealing with the structure, functions, and diseases of the eye.

overweight—weighing more than the population average for your age and height. This is usually based on insurance tables.

plaque—a small, differentiated area on a body tissue. An atherosclerotic plaque is located on the inside of an artery and looks quite different from normal arterial tissue.

power—strength multiplied by speed; strength that has the element of time involved. If two people lift a 100-pound weight and one does it in two seconds, the other in one second, then the quicker individual is said to be more powerful. Almost all athletic events require power.

preventive medicine—the practice of intervention before the onset of disease. In the medical setting this usually involves questioning the individual for current lifestyle habits, testing present health and physical condition, a review of the test results, and a counseling session to bring about improvements.

protein—a vital substance needed by the body. Almost three quarters of the dry weight of a cell is made up of protein. Protein is valuable for the roles it plays in structure, enzymes, hormones, muscles, the immune system, acid-base system, and other important functions.

skinfold test—a "pinch" test where predetermined folds of skin are measured for determining the underlying fat content. A total body fat content is then extrapolated from these figures.

stamina—the ability to endure.

strength—the application of force, usually measured by a maximal single repetition in any form of weight lifting.

stroke—a general term used to describe a lack of blood flow to the brain tissue. This results in death to the region where blood supply has been cut off.

tar—the collective particle matter in tobacco smoke.

thrombosis—the formation of a clot in a blood vessel.

thrombus—a clot in the blood vessel formed during life from the normal "ingredients" that make up blood (plural: thrombi).

"Type A" personality—a behavioral pattern typified by excess aggressiveness, time restraint, and competitive urgency.

underwater weighing—a means of determining body fat. It is considered the most accurate of body fat tests.

varicose veins—enlarged or dilated veins usually caused by malfunction of the valves in the veins which only permit blood to flow in one direction. Some known contributors to this condition are prolonged periods of standing, and pregnancy.

vascular—relating to the blood vessels, arteries, veins, capillaries.

veins—the vessels responsible for returning blood to the heart from the body's tissues.

WEIGHT LIFTING TERMS

bodybuilder—one who lifts weights for aesthetic purposes.

free weight—any form of free-moving weight. Barbells and dumbbells serve as the typical example, although anything from Heavy Hands to soup cans will qualify.

Nautilus machine—a weight lifting machine that uses a kidney-shaped cam to vary the resistance you're lifting.

Olympic lifting—the competitive form of weight lifting involving strength and technique, found in the Olympic Games. It consists of two lifts, the clean and jerk, where the weight is hoisted to the chest and then lifted overhead, and the snatch, where the weight is taken from the floor and lifted directly overhead as the lifter squats under it and then stands.

overload principle—the concept that in order for gains or progress to occur, you must stress the body in that particular area at a greater rate than what is usually encountered.

periodization (or cycle training)—this training incorporates a time table made up of specific periods of different forms of training. For example, in weight training a power lifter cannot lift maximal weights all year round or he/she will experience overtraining and eventual fatigue or injury. The training may instead revolve around six-week periods; a light weight-high repetition (20+) phase to build endurance, a medium weight-medium repetition (10–12) phase to build size and gradual strength, and heavy weights-low reps (1–6) for strength gains. This cycle can be repeated throughout the year.

power lifting—a strength competition consisting of three lifts: the bench press, the squat, and the dead lift. The bench press is performed while lying on the back and consists of lifting a weight from the chest to arm's length. The squat places the barbell on the upper back, across the shoulder blades. The lifter then squats down until the thighs are parallel with the floor and stands up. The dead lift involves simply lifting a weight off the floor until the lifter is in the standing position.

strength training—a form of weight lifting in which primary emphasis is placed on the development of strength of the individual.

Universal machine—a variable-resistance machine that uses a lever system to vary the weight.

weight lifting—any form of resistance training. The goal can be strength, endurance, tone, or muscle size.

quarters—slang term for a twenty-five-pound weight plate.

Z-bar—a crooked bar that is usually used for bicep curling. It puts the hands in a more natural position.

Introduction and Chapter 1

1.

Although conclusive evidence is not yet available, research currently in progress supports the relationship of fat distribution and a variety of disorders including diabetes, hyperlipidemia, coronary heart disease, etc. See, for example:

a) A.H. Kissebah, et al., "Relation of Body Fat Distribution to Metabolic Complications of Obesity," *Journal of Clinical Endocrinology and Metabolism*, 54:254–259, 1982.

b) B. Larsson, K. Svardsudd, L. Welin, et al., "Abdominal Adipose Tissue Distribution, Obesity, and Risk of Cardiovascular Disease and Death: Thirteen-year Follow-up of Participants in the Study of Men Born in 1913," *British Medical Journal*, 288: 1401–1404, 1984.

c) S. Fujioka, et al., "Contribution of Intra-Abdominal Fat Accumulation to the Impairment of Glucose and Lipid Metabolism in Human Obesity," *Metabolism*, 36(1):54–59, 1987.

2.

You can read more about the relationship of health and fitness in G. Legwold, "Are We Running from the Truth About the Risks and Benefits of Exercise?," *The Physician and Sportsmedicine*, 13:136–148, 1985, and P. Raber, "Aerobic Exercise in Perspective . . .," *Rx Being Well*, Nov./Dec. 1985.

3.

a) Y. Friedlander, J.D. Kark, Y. Stein, "Family History of Myocardial Infarction As an Independent Risk Factor for Coronary Heart Disease," *British Heart Journal*, 53:382–387, 1985.

b) A. Rissanen, "Premature Coronary Heart Disease: Ask About the Family," *Acta Medica Scandinavia*, 218:353–354, 1985.

c) K.-T. Khaw, E. Barrett-Conner, "Family History of Stroke As an Independent Predictor of Ischemic Heart Disease in Men and Stroke in Women," *American Journal of Epidemiology*, 123:59–66, 1986.

4.

a) K.A. Perkins, "Family History of Coronary Heart Disease: Is It an Independent Risk Factor?," *American Journal of Epidemiology*, 124(2):182–194, 1986.

b) R.M. Conroy, et al., "Is a Family History of Coronary Heart Disease an Independent Coronary Risk Factor?," *British Heart Journal*, 53:378–381, 1985.

c) K.-T. Khaw, E.B. Conner, "Family History of Heart Attack: A Modifiable Risk Factor?," *Circulation*, 74(2):239–244, 1986.

5.

A.J. Stunkard, T.T. Foch, Z. Hrubec, "Twin Study of Human Obesity," *Journal of the American Medical Association*, 256:51–54, 1986.

6.

T.B. Van Itallie, "The Overweight Patient," *Clinical Implications of Nutrition*, 1(2):1–7, 1985.

7.

F.I. Katch, W.D. McArdle, *Nutrition, Weight Control, and Exercise* (Philadelphia: Lea & Febiger, 1983), pp. 134–135.

8.

K.H. Cooper, *The Aerobics Program for Total Well-Being* (New York: Bantam, 1982), p. 221.

9.

American College of Sports Medicine, "Position Stand on the Recommended Quality and Quantity of Exercise for Maintaining Fitness in Healthy Adults," *Medicine and Science in Sports and Exercise*, 10:vii–x, 1978.

10.

For more in-depth discussion of the factors associated with increased risk of heart disease, see the following articles:

a) S.M. Fox, J.P. Naughton, W.L. Haskell, "Physical Activity and the Prevention of Coronary Heart Disease," *Annals of Clinical Research*, 3:404–432, 1971.

b) L. Wilhelmsen, H. Wedel, G. Tibblin, "Multivariate Analysis of Risk Factors for Coronary Heart Disease," *Circulation*, XLVIII:950–958, 1983.

c) W.B. Kannel, D. McGee, T. Gordon, "A General Cardiovascular Risk Profile: The Framingham Study," *American Journal of Cardiology*, 38:46–51, 1976.

d) "Lowering Blood Cholesterol to Prevent Heart Disease," *Nutrition Reviews*, 43:283–285, 1985.

e) R.A. Bruce, L.D. Fisher, K.H. Hossack, "Validation of Exercise-Enhanced Risk Assessment of Coronary Heart Disease Events: Longitudinal Changes in Incidence in Seattle Community Practise," *Journal of the American College of Cardiology*, 5:875–881, 1985.

Chapter 2

1.

The following articles give an overview of ongoing research on the relationship of activity to longevity. Your attention is particularly directed to the articles by Paffenbarger, a major researcher in the field. The Monahan article provides a good, easily accessible summary.

a) T. Monahan, "From Activity to Eternity," *The Physician and Sportsmedicine*, 14:156–164, 1986.

b) R.S. Paffenbarger, R.T. Hyde, A.L. Wing, C. Hsieh, "Physical Activity, All-Cause Mortality, and Longevity of College Alumni," *New England Journal of Medicine*, 314:605–613, 1986.

c) I. Holme, et al., "Physical Activity at Work and at Leisure in Relation to Coronary Risk Factors and Social Class," *Acta Medica Scandinavia*, 209:277–283, 1983.

d) R.S. Paffenbarger, et al., "Physical Activity as an Index of Heart Attack Risk in College Alumni," *American Journal of Epidemiology*, 8:161–175, 1978.

e) R.E. LaPorte, et al., "Physical Activity or Cardiovascular Fitness: Which Is More Important for Health?," *The Physician and Sportsmedicine*, 13:145–149, 1985.

2.

a) American College of Sports Medicine, "Position Stand on the Recommended Quantity and Quality of Exercise for Maintaining Fitness in Healthy Adults," *Medicine and Science in Sports and Exercise*, 10:vii–x, 1978.

b) S.B. Gibson, S.G. Gerberich, A.S. Leon, "Writing the Exercise Prescription: An Individualized Approach," *The Physician and Sportsmedicine*, 11:87–110, 1983.

3.

R.S. Paffenbarger, R.T. Hyde, A.L. Wing, C. Hsieh, "Physical Activity, All-Cause Mortality, and Longevity of College Alumni," *New England Journal of Medicine*, 314:605–613, 1986.

4.

W.D. McArdle, F.I. Katch, V.L. Katch, *Exercise Physiology: Energy, Nutrition, and Human Performance* (Philadelphia: Lea & Febiger, 1986), pp. 157–158.

5.

G.L. Blackburn, K. Pavlou, "Fad Reducing Diets: Separating Fads from Facts," *Contemporary Nutrition*, vol.8(7), 1983, pp. 1–2.

6.

a) E.J. Drenick, H.F. Dennin, "Energy Expenditure in Fasting Obese Men," *Journal of Laboratory and Clinical Medicine*, 81:421–430, 1973.

b) G.A. Bray, "Effect of Caloric Restriction on Energy Expenditure in Obese Patients," *Lancet*, 2:397–398, 1969.

c) A.J. Stunkard, "Anorectic Agents and Body Weight Set Point," *Life Sciences*, 30:2043–2055, 1982.

7.

R.H. Colvin, S.B. Olson, "A Descriptive Analysis of Men and Women Who Have Lost Significant Weight and Are Highly Successful at Maintaining the Loss," *Addictive Behaviors*, 8 (1983), p. 294.

8.

For a full discussion of the methods used by quacks and faddists to sell their ideas and wares, see Stephen Barrett, M.D., "Diet Facts and Fads"; and William T. Jarvis, Ph.D., and Stephen Barrett, M.D., "How Quackery Is Sold," in *The Health Robbers: How to Protect Your Money and Your Life*, edited by Stephen Barrett (Philadelphia: George F. Stickley, 1980), pp. 173–183 and 12–25, respectively.

Chapter 3

1.

Though many physicians report changes beginning as early as these time frames, remember that this may not be true for everyone. Changes may take longer to begin for some individuals. Also remember that these times represent the *beginning* of changes, not the end; change for the better continues over a much longer time if you follow the proper intake and exercise regimen. The following resources support the point made in the text and here.

a) W.R. Frontera, R.P. Adams, "Endurance Exercise: Normal Physiology and Limitations Imposed by Pathological Processes (Part 1)," *The Physician and Sportsmedicine*, 14:95–106, 1986. (cardiovascular changes)

b) P.A. Farrell, J. Barboriak, "The Time Course of Alterations in Plasma Lipid and Lipoprotein Concentrations During Eight Weeks of Endurance Training," *Atherosclerosis*, 37:231–238, 1980. (cholesterol changes)

c) A.M. Gotto, "Hypercholesterolemia: An Assessment of Screening and Diagnostic Techniques," *Modern Medicine*, 55:28–32, 1987.

d) G.H. Hartung, "Diet and Exercise in the Regulation of Plasma Lipids and Lipoproteins in Patients at Risk of Coronary Disease," *Sports Medicine*, 1:413–418, 1984. (an overview)

2.

The first two articles discuss fat-burning efficiency; articles (c) and (d) discuss the increase of pumping power, and articles (e) and (f) the increase of blood vessels.

a) P.D. Gollnick, B. Saltin, "Hypothesis: Significance of Skeletal Muscle Oxidation Enzyme Enhancement with Endurance Training," *Clinical Physiology*, 2:1–12, 1983.

b) P.D. Gollnick, "Metabolism of Substrates: Energy Substrate Metabolism During Exercise and as Modified by Training," *Federation Proceedings*, 44(2):353–357, 1985.

c) B. Ekblom, et al., "Effect of Training on Circulatory Response to Exercise," *Journal of Applied Physiology*, 24:518–528, 1968.

d) M.H. Frick, A. Konttinen, H.S. Samuli Sarajas, "Effects of Physical Training on Circulation at Rest and During Exercise," *The American Journal of Cardiology*, 12:142–147, 1963.

e) P. Anderson, J., Henriksson, "Capillary Supply of the Quadriceps Femoris Muscle of Man: Adaptive Response to Exercise," *Journal of Physiology*, 270:677–699, 1977.

f) P. Brodal, F. Ingjer, L. Hermansen, "Capillary Supply of Skeletal Muscle Fibers in Untrained and Endurance Trained Men," *Acta Physiologica Scandinavia*, suppl. 440:179(abs. 296), 1976.

3.

a) F.I. Katch, W.D. McArdle, *Nutrition, Weight Control, and Exercise*, (Philadelphia: Lea & Febiger, 1983), pp. 162–164.

b) K.D. Brownell, A.J. Stunkard, "Physical Activity in the Development and Control of Obesity," in *Obesity*, edited by A.J. Stunkard (Philadelphia: W.B. Saunders Co., 1980), pp. 300–324.

c) J.W. Kennitz, "Body Weight Set Point Theory," *Contemporary Nutrition*, 10(2): 1985.

4.

In "Diet Facts and Fads," in *The Health Robbers: How to Protect Your Money and Your Life* (Philadelphia: George F. Stickly, 1980), pp. 174–176, Dr. Stephen Barrett discusses how fasting was developed by Dr. George L. Blackburn as a strictly controlled, medically supervised last resort and how (as Dr. Blackburn had feared) the concept was seized upon by the popular press and radically distorted, misleading the public.

5.

G.A. Bray, et al., "Obesity: A Serious Symptom," *Annals of Internal Medicine*, 77(5):779–795, 1972.

6.

For an excellent discussion of most available methods and the importance of body composition for different people, see J.H. Wilmore, "Body Composition in Sport and Exercise: Directions for Future Research," *Medicine and Science in Sports and Exercise*, 15:21–31, 1983.

7.

A.S. Jackson, M.L. Pollock, "Practical Assessment of Body Composition," *The Physician and Sportsmedicine*, 13:76–90, 1985.

8.

a) F.I. Katch, B. Keller, R. Solomon, "Validity of BIA for Estimating Body Fat in Cardiac and Pulmonary Patients, and Black and White Men and Women Matched for Age and Body Fat," *Medicine and Science in Sports and Exercise*, 18(2):S80, 1986.

b) H.L. Nash, "Body Fat Measurement: Weighing the Pros and Cons of Electrical Impedance," *The Physician and Sportsmedicine*, 13:124–128, 1985.

9.

a) American Heart Association, *Heart Facts 1983*, (Dallas: American Heart Association, 1982).

b) American Heart Association, *Risk Factors and Coronary Disease: A Statement for Physicians 1980* (Dallas: American Heart Association, 1980).

c) J.T. Lampman, et al., "Effect of Exercise Training on Glucose Tolerance, in Vivo Insulin Sensitivity, Lipid and Lipoprotein Concentrations in

Middle-Aged Men with Mild Hypertriglyceridemia," *Metabolism*, 34:205–211, 1985.

10.

a) W.B. Kannel, D. McGee, and T. Gordon, "A General Cardiovascular Risk Profile: The Framingham Study," *American Journal of Cardiology*, 38:46–51, 1980.

b) J.S. Raichlen, et al., "Importance of Risk Factors in the Angiographic Progression of Coronary Artery Disease," *American Journal of Cardiology*, 57:66–70, 1986.

11.

H.A. Solomon, *The Exercise Myth* (San Diego: Harcourt Brace Jovanovich, 1984), p. 37.

12.

If you'd like to immerse yourself in the subject, the following text for administrators is recommended: M.H. Ellestad, *Stress Testing: Principles and Practice* (Philadelphia: F.A. Davis Co., 1986).

For a shorter discussion of the same issues see the following:

a) N. Goldschlager, A. Selzer, K. Cohn, "Treadmill Stress Tests As Indicators of Presence and Severity of Coronary Heart Disease," *Annals of Internal Medicine*, 85:277–286, 1976.

b) J.B. Barlow, "The False Positive Exercise Electrocardiogram: Value of Time Course Patterns in Assessment of Depressed ST Segments and Inverted T Waves," *American Heart Journal*, 110:1328–1336, 1985.

c) A.F. Calvert, "True Sensitivity of Cardiac Exercise Testing," *The Medical Journal of Australia*, 140:131–135, 1984.

d) L.M. Prisant, L.O. Watkins, A.A. Carr, "Exercise Stress Testing," *Southern Medical Journal*, 722(12):1551–1556, 1984.

13.

a) V.F. Froelicher, *Exercise Testing and Training* (New York: Le Jacq Publishing Inc., 1983).

b) M.H. Sketch, "Significant Sex Differences in the Correlation of Electrocardiographic Exercise Testing and Coronary Arteriograms," *American Journal of Cardiology*, 36:169–173, 1975.

14.

a) American College of Sports Medicine, *Guidelines for Exercise Testing and Prescription* (Philadelphia: Lea & Febiger, 1986), pp. 1–8.

b) American Heart Association, *The Exercise Standards Book*, 1979; see pp. 31–39. You may find the same information in *Circulation*, 59:421A, 1979.

15.

Unpublished data from the Cooper Clinic.

16.

P.L. McHenry, "Risks of Graded Exercise Testing," *The American Journal of Cardiology*, 39:935–937, 1977.

17.

For further discussion of the type risks see, M.H. Ellestad, *Stress Testing: Principles and Practice* (Philadelphia: F.A. Davis Co.), 1986, pp. 119–126. In addition, B.F. Walker, "Cardiac Emergency—Sudden Death in Midlife," *Cardiovascular Medicine*, Jan.:55–59, 1985, found that most people who died during exercise suffered from over 50 percent blockage of the coronary arteries.

18.

a) P. Gunby, "Future Seems Promising for Coronary Angioplasty," *Journal of the American Medical Association*, 251(3):302, 1984.

19.

a) See the section on "hypertension" in American Heart Association, *Heart Book: A Guide to and Treatment of Cardiovascular Disease* (New York: E.P. Dutton), 1980.

b) *The Merck Manual* 14th Ed., ed. R. Berkow (Rahway, N.J.: Merck Sharpe & Dohme Research Laboratories, 1982), p. 393.

20.

National Center for Health Statistics, *Health USA 1985*, DHHS Publication Number (PHS)86–1232, 1985, pp. 16–17.

21.

These articles offer an overview of the treatment of high blood pressure with exercise, diet, and weight loss:

a) M. McMahon, R.M. Palmer, "Exercise and Hypertension," *Medical Clinics of North America*, 69:57–70, 1985.

b) R. Fagard, "Habitual Physical Activity, Training, and Blood Pressure in Normo- and Hypertension," *International Journal of Sports Medicine*, 6:57–67, 1985.

c) J.J. Duncan, et al., "The Effects of Aerobic Exercise on Plasma Catecholamines and Blood Pressure in Patients with Mild Essential Hypertension," *Journal of the American Medical Association*, 254:2609–2613, 1985.

d) R. Stamler, et al., "Nutritional Therapy for High Blood Pressure: Final Report of a Four-Year Randomized Controlled Trial—The Hypertension Control Program," 257(11):1484–1491, 1987.

e) T.R. Anderson, P.E. Nielson, "Blood Pressure Lowering Effect of Weight Reduction," *The Scandinavian Journal of Clinical and Laboratory Investigation*, 45(suppl. 176):7–14, 1985.

22.

For a more extensive discussion of this subject see the following:

a) D.E. Hoekenga, "Can Coronary Atherosclerosis Be Halted or Reversed?," *Practical Cardiology*, 12(11):81–89, 1986.

b) C.J. Glueck, "Role of Risk Factor Management in Progression and Regression of Coronary and Femoral Artery Atherosclerosis," *American Journal of Cardiology*, 57:35G–41G, 1986.

23.

American Heart Association, *Textbook for Advanced Cardiac Life Support*, 1983, p. 25.

24.

a) S.P. Van Camp, R.A. Peterson, "Cardiovascular Complications of Outpatient Cardiac Rehabilitation Programs," *Journal of the American Medical Association*, 256:1160–1163, 1986.

For further reading see:

b) L.W. Gibbons, et al., "The Acute Cardiac Risk of Strenuous Exercise," *Journal of the American Medical Association*, 244:1799–1801, 1980.

c) D.S. Siscovick, W.S. Weiss, R.H. Fletcher, et al., "The Incidence of Primary Arrest During Vigorous Exercise," *New England Journal of Medicine*, 311:874–7, 1984.

25.

a) K.H. Cooper, et al., "Physical Fitness vs. Selected Coronary Risk Factors: A Cross Sectional Study," *Journal of the American Medical Association*, 12:166–169, 1976.

b) H. Blackburn, "Concepts and Controversies About Prevention of CHD," *Postgraduate Medical Journal*, 52:464–469, 1976.

26.

a) R.S. Paffenbarger, et al., "Physical Activity, All-Cause Mortality, and Longevity of College Alumni," *The New England Journal of Medicine*, 314:605–613, 1986.

27.

The first article gives an overview of the issue. If you are interested in a more technical discussion, any one of the books [(b)–(f)] will offer this.

a) "The Physician and Sportsmedicine, Exercise and the Cardiovascular System," *The Physician and Sportsmedicine*, 7(9):54–74, 1979.

b) P. Astrand, K. Rodahl, *Textbook of Work Physiology* (New York: McGraw-Hill Book Co., 1977).

c) W.D. McArdle, F.I. Katch, V.L. Katch, *Exercise Physiology: Energy, Nutrition, and Human Performance* (Philadelphia: Lea & Febiger, 1986).

d) G.A. Brooks, T.D. Fahey, *Exercise Physiology: Human Bioenergetics and Its Applications* (John Wiley & Sons: New York, 1984).

e) M.L. Pollock, J.H. Wilmore, S.M. Fox, *Exercise in Health and Disease: Evaluation and Prescription for Prevention and Rehabilitation* (Philadelphia: W.B. Saunders Co., 1984).

f) P.S. Fardy, J.L. Bennett, N.L. Reitz, M.A. Williams, *Cardiac Rehabilitation: Implications for the Nurse and Other Health Professionals* (St. Louis: C.V. Mosby Co., 1980).

Chapter 4

1.

This figure is based on data found in American Heart Association, *Risk*

Factors and Coronary Disease: A Statement for Physicians, 1980. Readers may also find this statement printed in *Circulation*, 62(1980):445A.

2.

Any one of these references provides an excellent discussion of what cardiovascular fitness entails:

a) P. Astrand, K. Rodahl, *Textbook of Work Physiology: Physiological Bases of Exercise* (McGraw-Hill, 1977).

b) American College of Sports Medicine, position stand on "The Recommended Quantity and Quality of Exercise for Maintaining Fitness in Healthy Adults," *Medicine and Science in Sports and Exercise*, 10:vii–x, 1978.

c) American College of Sports Medicine, *Guidelines for Exercise Testing and Prescription* (Philadelphia, Lea & Febiger, 1986).

d) P.B. Hultgren, E.J. Burke, "Issues and Methodology in the Prescription of Exercise for Healthy Adults," in *Exercise, Science, and Fitness*, ed. E.J. Burke (Ithaca, NY: Mouvement Publications, 1980).

3.

Readers desiring an in-depth look at lactic acid metabolism will find an excellent presentation in G.A. Brooks, T.D. Fahey, *Exercise Physiology: Human Bioenergetics and Its Applications* (New York: John Wiley and Sons, 1984).

4.

D. Costill, *A Scientific Approach to Distance Running* (Los Altos, CA: Tafnews Press, 1979), p. 60.

5.

a) L.R. Gettman, M.L. Pollock, "Circuit Weight Training: A Critical Review of Its Physiological Benefits," *The Physician and Sportsmedicine*, 9:45–60, 1981.

b) L.R. Gettman, P. Ward, R.D. Hagan, "A Comparison of Combined Running and Weight Training with Circuit Weight Training," *Medicine and Science in Sports and Exercise*, 14:229–234, 1982.

c) J.H. Wilmore, R.B. Parr, et al., "Physiological Alterations Consequent to Circuit Weight Training," *National Strength and Conditioning Association Journal*, 4:17, 1982.

6.

P.F. Freedson, et al., "Intra-Arterial Blood Pressure During Free Weight and Hydraulic Resistance Exercise," *Medicine and Science in Sports and Exercise*, 16:131, 1984. Since, as this article shows, blood pressure is raised during lifting, it follows that persons suffering from high blood pressure should not pursue an activity that could place them at even greater risk.

7.

M.H. Kelemen, et al., "Circuit Weight Training in Cardiac Patients," *Journal of the American College of Cardiology*, 7:384–2, 1986.

8.

a) C. Corbin, K. Fox, "Flexibility: The Forgotten Part of Fitness," *The British Journal of Physical Education*, 16(6):191–194, 1985.

Flexibility is the range of motion around a joint. Flexibility need not be lost as a consequence of strength training, if it's done properly. While lifting weights, make sure that you are lifting throughout the full range of motion that the exercise will allow, and you may even gain flexibility. Of course, the best way to improve flexibility is through stretching and flexibility exercises. The loss of flexibility with weight training is an old myth that doesn't seem to want to die.

9.

The following articles present research on the impact of weight training on the cardiovascular system and on factors related to that system's health:

a) P.A. Farrnell, M.G. Maksud, M.T. Pollock, et al., "A Comparison of Plasma Cholesterol, Triglycerides, and High Density Lipoprotein-Cholesterol in Speed Skaters, Weightlifters, and Non-Athletes," *European Journal of Applied Physiology*, 48:77–82, 1982.

b) B.F. Hurley, D.R. Seals, J.M. Hagberg, et al., "High Density Lipoprotein Cholesterol in Body Builders vs. Power Lifters: Negative Effects of Androgen Use," *Journal of the American Medical Association*, 252:507–513, 1984.

c) R.C. Hickson, et al., "Strength Training Effects on Aerobic Power and Short Term Endurance," *Medicine and Science in Sports and Exercise*, 12:336–339, 1980.

d) B.F. Hurley, et al., "Effects of High Intensity Strength Training on Cardiovascular Function," *Medicine and Science in Sports and Exercise*, 16: 483–488, 1984.

10.

National Strength and Conditioning Association, "Position Paper on Prepubescent Strength Training," *National Strength and Conditioning Association Journal*, 7(4):27–31, 1985.

Chapter 5

1.

For a more complete explanation of the causes of muscle soreness, see:

a) W.C. Byrnes, P.M. Clarkson, "Delayed Onset Muscle Soreness and Training," *Clinics in Sports Medicine*, 5(3):605–614, 1986.

b) M.F. Bobbert, A.P. Hollander, P.A. Huijing, "Factors in Delayed Onset Muscular Soreness of Man," *Medicine and Science in Sports and Exercise*, 18(1):75–81, 1986.

c) R.B. Armstrong, "Mechanisms of Exercise-Induced Delayed Onset Muscular Soreness: A Brief Review," *Medicine and Science in Sports and Exercise*, 16(6):529–538, 1984.

d) H.A. deVries, "Electromyographic Observations of the Effects of Static

Stretching Upon Muscular Distress," *Research Quarterly*, 32:468–479, 1961.

2.
You'll find a full discussion of the reasons for warming up, and some of the consequences of not doing so, in the following:
a) R.J. Barnard, et al., "Ischemic Response to Sudden Strenuous Exercise in Healthy Men," *Circulation*, XLVIII:936–942, 1973.
b) B.D. Franks, "Physical Warmup" in *Ergogenic Aids and Muscular Performance*, ed. W.P. Morgan (New York: Academic Press, 1972).
c) U. Bergh, B. Ekblom, "Physical Performance and Peak Aerobic Power at Different Body Temperatures," *Journal of Applied Physiology*, 46:885–889, 1979.
d) F.G. Shellock, W.E. Prentice, "Warming-Up and Stretching for Improved Physical Performance and Prevention of Sports Related Injuries," *Sports Medicine*, 2:267–278, 1985.

3.
D.L. Costill, B. Saltin, "Factors Limiting Gastric Emptying During Rest and Exercise," *Journal of Applied Physiology*, 37:679–683, 1974.

4.
R.H. Dressendorfer, et al., "Plasma Mineral Levels in Marathon Runners During a 20-Day Road Race," *The Physician and Sportsmedicine*, 10:113–118, 1982.

5.
For a thorough discussion of what's best to drink during exercise, see the following:
a) American College of Sports Medicine, position stand on "The Prevention of Thermal Injuries During Distance Running," Indianapolis, 1985.
b) D.L. Costill, B. Saltin, "Factors Limiting Gastric Emptying During Rest and Exercise," *Journal of Applied Physiology*, 37:679–683, 1974.
c) D.L. Costill, "Fluids for Athletic Performance: Why and What Should You Drink During Prolonged Exercise," in *Toward an Understanding of Human Performance*, ed. E.J. Burke (Ithaca N.Y.: Mouvement Publications, 1980).
d) D.L. Costill, et al., "Effects of Elevated Plasma FFA and Insulin on Muscle Glycogen Usage During Exercise," *Journal of Applied Physiology*, 43:695–699, 1977.
e) L. Levine, et al., "Fructose and Glucose Ingestion and Muscle Glycogen Use During Submaximal Exercise," *Journal of Applied Physiology*, 55:1767–1771, 1983.

6.
Two preliminary studies are:
a) E.F. Coyle, et al., "Muscle Glycogen Utilization During Prolonged Strenuous Exercise When Fed Carbohydrate," *Journal of Applied Physiology*, 6(1):165–172, 1986.

b) M. Millard, K. Cureton, C. Ray, "Effect of a Glucose-Polymer Dietary Supplement on Physiological Responses During a Simulated Triathlon," *Medicine and Science in Sports and Exercise*, 18(2):S6, 1986.

See also, Bonnie F. Liebman, "Sports Drinks Slug It Out," *Nutrition Action Health Letter*, July/Aug. 1986, p. 11.

7.

D.L. Costill, "Water and Electrolytes." In W.P. Morgan (ed.), *Ergogenic Aids and Muscular Performance*. (New York: Academic Press, 1972), pp. 293–320.

8.

a) S. Akgun, N.H. Ertel, "A Comparison of Carbohydrate Metabolism After Sucrose, Sorbitol, and Fructose Meals in Normal and Diabetic Subjects," *Diabetes Care*, 3:582–585, 1980.

b) P.A. Crapo, O.G. Kolterman, J.M. Olefsky, "Effects of Oral Fructose in Normal, Diabetic, and Impaired Glucose Tolerance Subjects," *Diabetes Care*, 3:575–582, 1980.

Chapter 6

1.

Position of the National Institute on Alcohol Abuse and Alcoholism cited in B. Liebman, "Drink for Your Health?," *Nutrition Action* (March, 1984), p. 12.

2.

Facts About Alcohol. U.S. Department of Health and Human Services, National Institute on Alcohol Abuse and Alcoholism, Publication Mc 81–1574, 1980, p. 8.

3.

For an interesting, informative discussion of how much social drinkers drink, when, and how, see Leonard Gross, *How Much Is Too Much: The Effects of Social Drinking* (New York: Random House, 1983). Mr. Gross's book provides a thorough, excellent presentation of the effects on health and behavior of social drinking and the questions surrounding the various issues.

4.

For a brief description of how alcohol is handled by the body, see *Facts About Alcohol & Alcoholism*, pp. 7–14, or "Alcohol in Perspective," *Consumer Reports*, July 1983, pp. 351–354. If you are interested in alcohol's effect at the cellular level, see Dora B. Goldstein, M.D., "Drunk and Disorderly: How Cell Membranes Are Affected by Alcohol," *Nutrition Today*, March/April 1985:4–9.

5.

a) *Facts About Alcohol & Alcoholism*, pp. 7–8.

b) "Alcohol in Perspective," p. 351–352.

6.

National Institute on Alcohol Abuse and Alcoholism, "The Fifth Special Report to Congress on Alcohol and Health," in *Alcohol Health and Research World 9* (Fall, 1984), pp. 20–21. See also, John R. Senior, M.D., "Alcoholic Hepatitis," *Alcohol Health and Research World, 10* (Winter 85/86):40–43.

7.

If you would like to read some of the studies themselves, here are several of the most often cited. Though the popular media leapt on the findings, please note the caution with which all the researchers present their findings. See also, note 9 below.

a) C.H. Hennekens, et al., "Daily Alcohol Consumption and Fatal Coronary Disease," *American Journal of Epidemiology*, 107:196–200, 1978.

b) C.H. Hennekens, et al., "Effects of Beer, Wine, and Liquor in Coronary Deaths," *Journal of the American Medical Association*, 242:1973–1974, 1979.

c) W.D. Castelli, "How Many Drinks a Day?" (editorial), *Journal of the American Medical Association*, 242:2000, 1979.

d) K. Yano, et al., "Coffee, Alcohol, and Risk of Coronary Heart Disease Among Japanese Men Living in Hawaii," *New England Journal of Medicine*, 297:405–409, 1977.

e) M.G. Marmot, G. Rose, et al., "Alcohol Mortality: A U-shaped Curve," *Lancet*, 1:580–583, 1981.

8.

"Alcohol in Perspective," p. 352.

9.

Though various of these arguments are mentioned by other sources, you will find succinct, comprehensive presentations in Bonnie Liebman, "Drink for Your Health?," *Nutrition Action*, March 1984, pp. 10–13; and in "Beer or Skittles?," *Harvard Medical School Health Letter*, 11(Jan. 1986):1–2.

10.

"Study Links Heavy Drinking to Increased Risk of Stroke," *New York Times*, Oct. 23, 1986, p. A22. Drinking thirty or more drinks a week was associated with increased risk of stroke, even with smoking and high blood pressure taken into account.

11.

a) "Medical Consequences of Alcohol," from *The Fifth Special Report to Congress on Alcohol and Health*, pp. 19–25.

b) The Spring 1986 issue (Vol. 10, no. 3) of *Alcohol Health and Research World*, a journal produced by the National Institute on Alcohol Abuse and Alcoholism, focuses on the relationship of alcohol and cancer. "Overview: Alcohol and Cancer," by D.M. Podolsky, gives an excellent summary of current research findings, pp. 3–9.

c) Esteban Mezey, M.D., "Alcohol Abuse and Digestive Diseases," *Alcohol Health and Diseases World*, 10 (Winter 85/86):6–9.

12.

"Medical Consequences of Alcohol," p. 67.

13.

a) Arthur Schatzkin, M.D., et al., "Alcohol Consumption and Breast Cancer in the Epidemiologic Follow-up Study of the First National Health and Nutrition Examination Survey," *New England Journal of Medicine*, 316:1169–1173, 1987.

b) W.C. Willet, M.D., M.J. Stampfer, M.D., et al., "Moderate Alcohol Consumption and the Risk of Breast Cancer," *New England Journal of Medicine*, 316:1174–80, 1987.

c) "Alcohol and Breast Cancer," *Harvard Medical School Health Letter*, 12 (July 1987):1–2.

14.

Though the study of the effect of alcohol on sleep is complicated by such factors as the amount of alcohol consumed, the alcohol tolerance of an individual, the sleep and drinking history of an individual, the difficulty of testing a sleeping subject, etc., there is evidence that even a single drink before bed affects Rapid Eye Movement sleep during the first half of the night in many subjects. More restlessness has also been observed in some studies. There is little research on the effect on nonalcoholics of several drinks (such as one might consume during a party).

Heavy drinking and long-term alcohol abuse are associated with sleep disturbance. For a review of the subject, see Alex D. Pokorny, M.D., "Sleep Disturbances, Alcohol and Alcoholism: A review," in R. L. Williams, M.D. and Ismet Karcan, M.D., eds., *Sleep Disorders: Diagnoses & Treatment* (New York: John Wiley & Sons, 1978), pp. 233–260.

Chapter 7

1.

If you'd like to read more about the mechanisms of muscular growth, see:

a) N.A.S. Taylor, J.G. Wilkinson, "Exercise-Induced Skeletal Muscle Growth Hypertrophy Or Hyperplasia," *Sports Medicine*, 3:190–200, 1986.

b) W.J. Gonyea, D. Sale, "Physiology of Weight-Lifting Exercise," *Archives of Physical Medicine and Rehabilitation*, 63:235–237, 1982.

c) L.G. Shaver, *Essentials of Exercise Physiology* (Minneapolis: Burgess Publishing, 1981), pp. 259–264.

d) S. Salmons, J. Henriksson, "The Adaptive Response of Skeletal Muscle to Increased Use," *Muscle and Nerve*, 4:94–105, 1981.

e) P.D. Gollnick, et al., "Muscle Enlargement and Number of Fibers in Skeletal Muscles of Rats," *Journal of Applied Physiology*, 50:936–943, 1981.

2.

a) "Roundtable: Strength Training and Conditioning for the Female Athlete," *National Strength and Conditioning Association Journal*, 7(3):10–29, 1985.

b) T. Moritani, H.A. deVries, "Neural Factors Versus Hypertrophy in the Time Course of Muscle Strength Gain," *American Journal of Physical Medicine,* 58(3):115–130, 1979.

3.

a) A.L. Goldberg, et al., "Mechanism of Work-Induced Hypertrophy of Skeletal Muscle," *Medicine and Science in Sports and Exercise,* 7:185–198, 1975.

b) R. Zak, "Nitrogen Metabolism and Mechanics of Protein Synthesis and Degradation," *Circulation* 72(suppl IV):IV-13—IV-17, 1985.

4.

a) W.J. Gonyea, D. Sale, "Physiology of Weight-Lifting Exercise, *Archives of Physical Medicine and Rehabilitation,* 63:235–237, 1982.

b) E.F. Coyle, et al., "Specificity of Power Improvements Through Slow and Fast Isokinetic Training," *Journal of Applied Physiology,* 51:1437–1442, 1981.

5.

The following position papers reflect the collective reasoning on steroids by two of the largest and most respected professional organizations in their fields.

a) American College of Sports Medicine, "The Use Of Anabolic-Androgenic Steroids in Sports," *American College of Sports Medicine Position Stands and Opinion Statements* (Indianapolis: 3rd Ed. 1985).

b) National Strength and Conditioning Association, "Position Statement: Use and Abuse of Anabolic Steroids," *The National Strength and Conditioning Association Journal,* 7:27, 1985.

6.

See E.L. Smith, "Exercise for Prevention of Osteoporosis: A Review," *The Physician and Sportsmedicine,* 10(3):74, 1982. Although there is evidence that stress placed on a bone will increase its mineral content, and though studies are underway on the possible effect of weight lifting on osteoporosis, the experts advise that there is as yet no conclusive scientific evidence that weight lifting will *reverse* the effects of osteoporosis. Since there is evidence that weightbearing activities such as walking or aerobic dance increase bone mass (see note 8 below), there is a good probability that lifting will be shown to be useful, particularly as a preventive measure. See note 7.

7.

Although studies are not yet complete, exercise physiologists speculate that since activities such as walking, jogging, or aerobic dance increase bone mass on the weightbearing bones, then weight lifting, which can place beneficial stress on other areas, *may* prove helpful in preventing or retarding bone mass. However, no one should rush into a program without consulting his or her physician. Remember, safety must always be a prime consideration. Using low weights and many repetitions is safer, and the exercise more closely resembles those weightbearing activities which have been shown to be helpful.

8.

The following articles discuss the kinds of benefits weightbearing exercise offers.

a) E.L. Smith, "Exercise for Prevention of Osteoporosis: A Review," *The Physician and Sportsmedicine*, 10(3):72–83, 1982.

b) C.E. Goodman, "Osteoporosis: Protective Measures of Nutrition and Exercise," *Geriatrics*, 40:59–70, 1985.

c) P.L. Fitzgerald, "Exercise for the Elderly," *Medical Clinics of North America*, 69:189–196, 1985.

d) R.J. Stillman, et al., "Physical Activity and Bone Mineral Content in Women Aged 30 to 85 Years," *Medicine and Science in Sports and Exercise*, 18:576–580, 1986.

9.

a) A.D. Martin, C.S. Houston, "Osteoporosis, Calcium and Physical Activity," *Canadian Medical Association Journal*, 136:587–593, 1987.

b) C.W. Callaway, "Dietary Effects on Osteoporosis," *Journal of the American Medical Association*, 257(12):1652, 1987.

c) A.C. Santora, "Role of Nutrition and Exercise in Osteoporosis," *The American Journal of Medicine*, 82(suppl. 1B):73–79, 1987.

d) D. Muram, D. Massouda, "Osteoporosis," *Southern Medical Journal*, 80(2):219–222, 1987.

10.

a) T.E. Auble, L. Schwartz, R.J. Robertson, "Aerobic Requirements for Moving Handweights Through Various Ranges of Motion While Walking," *The Physician and Sportsmedicine*, 15(6):133–140, 1987.

b) J.E. Zarandona, "Physiological Responses to Hand Carried Weights," *The Physician and Sportsmedicine*, 14:113–120, 1986.

11.

a) C.R. Kyle, "Athletic Clothing," *Scientific American*, March:104–110, 1986.

b) C.R. Kyle, V.J. Caiozzo, "The Effect of Athletic Clothing Aerodynamics upon Running Speed," *Medicine and Science in Sports and Exercise*, 18:509–515, 1986.

12.

a) P.O. Astrand, "Human Physical Fitness with Special Reference to Sex and Age," *Physiological Review*, 36:307–335, 1956.

Chapter 8

1.

Kenneth H. Cooper, M.D., Ph.D., *Running Without Fear: How to Reduce the Risk of Heart Attack and Sudden Death During Aerobic Exercise* (New York: M. Evans and Company, Inc., 1985).

NOTES

2.

V.F. Froelicher, "Exercise Testing-Screening: Positive Tests in Asymptomatic Patients. Estimation of Severity of Coronary Heart Disease," cited in *The Exercise Myth*, Harold A. Solomon (San Diego: Harcourt Brace Jovanovich, 1984), pp. 37–38.

3.

You may find a good description of what cholesterol is and how the body uses it in A.C. Guyton, *Testbook of Medical Physiology*, 7th Ed. (Philadelphia: W.B. Saunders Co., 1986), pp. 825–826.

4.

Reported in Marion Burros, "Diet Guidelines Revised by Heart Association," *New York Times*, Aug. 27, 1986, p. C4.

5.

A.C. Guyton, *Textbook of Medical Physiology*, pp. 825–826.

6.

a) R. Ross, et al., "Endothelial Injury: Blood-Vessel Wall Interactions," *Annals New York Academy of Sciences*, 401:260–264, 1982.

b) S.M. Schwartz, "Disturbances in Endothelial Integrity," *Annals New York Academy of Sciences*, 401:228–233, 1982.

The physical processes in the development of atherosclerosis have not yet been conclusively determined. I have picked the explanation by Ross and colleagues because it gives a very clear picture of the total process which may be occurring, and the role the risk factors (which you can control) play in its development. Other noted authorities also excel in this area of study. The Nobel Prize was recently won by two Texas scientists (cited in reference [c]) who have devoted their work to the mechanisms of LDL cholesterol and its receptors in the body. Their work supports the idea that injury does not have to occur for the atherosclerotic plaque to develop (although injury surely helps). You may read about their work in:

c) M.S. Brown, J.L. Goldstein, "How LDL Receptors Influence Cholesterol and Atherosclerosis," *Scientific American*, 251:58–66, 1984.

7. and 8.

a) Information from the National Center for Health Statistics, U.S. Public Health Service, Department of Health and Human Services, 1980, cited in M.L. Pollack, J.H. Wilmore, S.M. Fox, *Exercise in Health and Disease* (Philadelphia: W.B. Saunders Co., 1984), pp. 3–4.

b) American Heart Association, *Heart Facts 1983*, Dallas, 1982.

9.

You may read about some of the ongoing research on drug treatment for atherosclerosis in the following:

a) H. Engelberg, "Heparin, Heparin Fractions, and the Atherosclerotic Process," *Seminars in Thrombosis and Hemostasis*, II(1):48–54, 1985.

b) D.H. Blankenhorn, "Drugs to Produce Atherosclerosis Regression," *Atherosclerosis Reviews*, 12:1–8, 1984.

c) C. Nakazima, et al., "Rules of Smooth Muscle Cell in the Atherosclerotic Model and Effects of Drugs on the Atherosclerosis," *The Japanese Journal of Pharmacology*, 39:133, 1985.

d) A.M. Gotto, "Hypercholesterolemia: Implications of Drug and Diet Therapy, *Modern Medicine*, 55:38–44, 1987.

e) A.M. Gotto, P.H. Jones, "Hyperlipidemia: Current Management Guidelines," *Drug Therapy*, May 1986, pp. 47–59.

10.

T. Corcos, et al., "Percutaneous Transluminal Coronary Angioplasty for the Treatment of Variant Angina," *Journal of the American College of Cardiology*, 5:1046–1056, 1985.

11.

There has been a lot of publicity about the benefits of fish oil lately; a good summary of research findings can be found in reference (a). For more technical information in the area, see references (b), (c) and (d). The remaining references discuss the effect of fiber on cholesterol and other blood factors.

a) J. Dusheck, "Fish, Fatty Acids and Physiology," *Science News*, 128:252–254, 1985.

b) W.S. Harris, W.E. Conner, M.P. McMurry, "The Comparative Reductions of the Plasma Lipids and Lipoproteins by Dietary Polyunsaturated Fats: Salmon Oil Versus Vegetable Oils," *Metabolism*, 32:179–184 1983.

c) J.Z. Mortensen, et al., "The Effect of N-6 and N-3 Polyunsaturated Fatty Acids on Hemostasis, Blood Lipids and Blood Pressure," *Thromb Heamostas* (Stuttgart), 50:543–546, 1983.

d) J.E. Kinsella, "Dietary Fish Oils," *Nutrition Today*, Nov./Dec. 1986, pp. 7–14.

e) "Dietary Fiber, Exercise and Selected Blood Lipid Constituents," *Nutrition Reviews*, 38:207–209, 1980.

f) J.W. Anderson, et al., "Hypocholesterolemic Effects of Oat-Bran or Bean Intake for Hyphercholesterolemic Men," *American Journal of Clinical Nutrition*, 40:1146–55, 1984.

12.

Here's only a sample of the research which supports this statement.

a) R.J. McCunney, "The Role of Fitness in Preventing Heart Disease," *Cardiovascular Reviews & Reports*, 6:776–781, 1985.

b) S.M. Grundy, "Dietary Intervention—Diet and Hypercholesterolemia," *Cardiovascular Medicine*, Jan. 1985, pp. 39–52.

c) K.H. Cooper, "Physical Training Programs for Mass Scale Use: Effects on Cardiovascular Disease–Facts and Theories," *Annals of Clinical Research*, 14 (suppl. 34):25–32, 1982.

d) R.D. Hagan, M.G. Smith, L.R. Gettman, "High Density Lipoprotein Cholesterol in Relation to Food Consumption and Running Distance," *Preventive Medicine*, 12:287–295, 1983.

e) Z.V. Tran, et al., "The Effects of Exercise on Blood Lipids and Lipo-proteins: a Meta-analysis of Studies," *Medicine and Science in Sports and Exercise*, 15:393–402, 1983.

f) P.D. Wood, W.L. Haskell, "The Effect of Exercise on Plasma High Density Lipoproteins," *Lipids*, 14:417–425, 1979.

g) P.A. Farrell, J. Barboriak, "The Time Course of Alterations in Plasma Lipid and Lipoprotein Concentrations During Eight Weeks of Endurance Training," *Atherosclerosis*, 37:231–238, 1980.

13.

a) P.A. Wolfe, "Risk Factors for Stroke," *Stroke*, 16:359–360, 1985.

b) P. Mustacchi, "Risk Factors in Stroke," *The Western Journal of Medicine*, 143:186–192, 1985.

14.

See the discussion in note 1, Chapter 3.

15.

M. Friendman, R.H. Rosenman, *Type A Behavior and Your Heart* (Greenwich, Conn.: Fawcett Publications Inc., 1974).

16.

J.S. Greenberg, *Comprehensive Stress Management* (Dubuque, Iowa: Wm. C. Brown Co., 1983). This book covers in depth the psychological aspects of handling stress.

17.

a) A.M. Gotto, "Treatment of Hyperlipidemia," *American Journal of Cardiology*, 57:11G–16G, 1986.

b) I. Hjermann, et al., "Effect of Diet and Smoking Intervention on the Incidence of Coronary Heart Disease," *Lancet*, 2(8259):1303–1310, 1981.

c) Lipid Research Clinic Program, "The Lipid Research Clinic Primary Prevention Trial Results. I. Reduction in Incidence of Coronary Heart Disease. II. The Relationship of Reduction in Incidence of Coronary Heart Disease to Cholesterol Lowering," *Journal of the American Medical Association*, 251:351–374, 1984.

Chapter 9

1.

If you are still a doubter, the following studies will convince you of the futility of spot reduction.

a) M. Noland, J.T. Kearney, "Anthropometric and Densitometric Responses of Women to Specific and General Exercise," *The Research Quarterly*, 49:322–328, 1978.

b) F.I. Katch, et al., "Effects of Sit-Up Exercise Training on Adipose Cell Size and Adiposity," *Research Quarterly for Exercise and Sport*, 55:242–247, 1984.

c) G. Gwinup, R. Chelvam, T. Steinberg, "Thickness of Subcutaneous Fat and Activity of Underlying Muscles," *Annals of Internal Medicine*, 74:408–411, 1971.

2.

Quoted in Richard Trubo, "Fad Diets: Unqualified Hunger for Miracles," *Medical World News*, Aug. 11, 1986, p. 46. Also, see Chapter 3, note 6.

3.

Quoted in Trubo, p. 46.

Chapter 10

1.

The old figures for cholesterol in shellfish included cholesterol and other sterols (chemical compounds resembling fat). Now we know that there is a distinction between the two, and that actual levels of cholesterol in shellfish are much lower than originally thought, so the cautions against eating shellfish have been dropped.

2.

Since many of the risk factors for stroke can be modified through proper eating habits, then it stands to reason that reducing your risk factors can reduce your chances of a stroke. Recommended reading: *Stroke: A Guide for the Family* (Dallas: American Heart Association, 1981).

3.

For an overview of the facts and controversies about vitamin supplementation see the following:

a) "Vitamin Supplements," in E.M. Hamilton, E.N. Whitney, *Nutrition: Concepts and Controversies* (St. Paul: West Publishing Co., 1982), pp. 45–49.

b) "Some Facts and Myths of Vitamins," *FDA Consumer*, HHS publication No. (FDA) 79-2117.

c) D.A. Roe, J. Levinson, "Vitamin Facts & Fallacies," *Rx Being Well*, March/April 1985.

d) "The Vitamin Pushers," *Consumer Reports*, March 1986, pp. 170–175.

e) "Vitamin Preparations as Dietary Supplements and as Therapeutic Agents," *Journal of the American Medical Association*, 257(14):1929–1936, 1987.

f) E.J. van der Beek, "Vitamins for Endurance Training: Food for Running or Faddish Claims?," *Sports Medicine*, 2:175–197, 1985.

g) Joint Nutrition Monitoring Evaluation Committee Report—May 1986: Nutritional Status of U.S. Population. *Nutrition Today*, 21(3): 23–29, 1986.

4.

"Nutrition: Food Nutrient Interactions," *Journal of Dentistry for Children*, May–June, 1985, p. 206.

5.

Many food faddists hoping to make a quick buck often argue the opposite.

But this opinion that people eating a varied and balanced diet from the four food groups don't need vitamin supplementation reflects the overwhelming and scientifically established opinion of trained professionals in the field of nutrition. For a fuller discussion, see:

a) E.M. Hamilton, E.N. Whitney, *Nutrition: Concepts and Controversies* (St. Paul: West Publishing Co., 1982).

b) F.I. Katch, W.D. McArdle, *Nutrition, Weight Control, and Exercise* (Philadelphia: Lea & Febiger, 1983).

c) "American Dietetic Association Statement: Nutrition and Physical Fitness," *Journal of the American Dietetic Association*, 76:437–443, 1980.

6.

"Vitamin Supplements," *The Medical Letter*, 27:66–68, 1985.

7.

a) F.R. Sinatra, "Food Faddism in Pediatrics," *Journal of the American College of Nutrition*, 3:169–175, 1984.

b) "Toxic Effects of Vitamin Overdosage," *Medical Letter*, 26:73–74, 1984.

c) R.M. Issenman, et al., "Children's Multiple Vitamins, Overuse Leads to Overdose," *Canadian Medical Association Journal*, 12032:781–784, 1985.

d) D. Rudman, P.J. Williams, "Megadose Vitamins: Use and Abuse," *New England Journal of Medicine*, 309(8):488–489, 1983.

e) "Toxic Effects of Vitamin Overdosage," *Medical Letter on Drugs and Therapeutics*, 26(667):73–74, 1984.

8.

a) R.M. Hanning, S.H. Zlotkin, "Unconventional Eating Practises and Their Health Implications," *Pediatric Clinics of North America*, 32(2):429–445, 1985.

b) V. Herbert, "Facts and Fictions about Megavitamin Therapy," *Journal of the Florida Medical Association*, 66:475–481, 1979.

9.

You can find tables of comparison for these and other foods in E.M. Hamilton, E.N. Whitney, *Nutrition: Concepts and Controversies*, pp. 573–609. Other good nutrition textbooks also have tables; ask your librarian for help.

10.

S. Palmer, S. Berkow, "Nutrition Education in American Medical Schools," *Nutrition Today*, 21(1):4–15, 1986.

11.

The Health Robbers, Second Ed., S. Barrett, M.D., ed. (Philadelphia: George F. Stickley Co., 1986). See also the National Council Against Health Fraud's position paper on chiropractic for a concise statement of the issues.

12.

a) Food and Nutrition Board, *Committee on Recommended Allowances, Recommended Daily Allowances*, 9th ed. (Washington, D.C.: National Academy of Sciences, 1980).

b) Food and Nutrition Board Statement, "Recommended Dietary Allowances: Scientific Issues and Process for the Future," *Journal of Nutrition Education*, 18(2):82, 1986.

13.

a) D.L. Elliot, L. Goldberg, "Nutrition and Exercise," *Medical Clinics of North America*, 69(1):71–82, 1985.

b) V. Aronson, "Protein and Miscellaneous Ergogenic Aids," *The Physician and Sportsmedicine*, 14:199–202, 1986.

14.

For a clear description of the process, see:

a) W.D. McArdle, F.I. Katch, V.L. Katch, *Exercise Physiology: Energy, Nutrition, and Human Performance*, (Philadelphia: Lea & Febiger, 1986), p. 8.

b) A.C. Guyton, *Textbook of Medical Physiology*, 7th ed. (Philadelphia: W.B. Saunders Co., 1986), pp. 816–817.

15.

a) "Dietary Fiber," *Harvard Medical School Health Letter*, 11(10):1–4, 1986.

b) R.M. Kay, "Dietary Fiber," *Journal of Lipid Research*, 23:221–236, 1982.

c) D. Kritchevsky, "The Role of Dietary Fiber in Health and Disease," *Journal of Environmental Pathology, Toxicology and Oncology*, 6:273–284, 1986.

16.

a) J.W. Anderson, et al., "Hypocholesterolemic Effects of Oat-bran or Bean Intake for Hypercholesterolemic Men," *American Journal of Clinical Nutrition*, 40:1146–1155, 1984.

b) T.A. Miettinen, "Dietary Fiber and Lipids," *American Journal of Clinical Nutrition*, 45:1237–1242, 1987.

17.

a) G.R. Newell, "Cancer Prevention: Update for Physicians, Four Years Later," *The Cancer Bulletin*, 37(3):103–107, 1985.

b) M.H. Floch, et al., "Practical Aspects of Implementing Increased Dietary Fiber Intake," *Nutrition Today*, 21(6):27–30, 1986.

18.

a) F.C. Luft, M.H. Weinberger, "Sodium Intake and Essential Hypertension," *Hypertension*, 4(supp III):III-14–III-19, 1982.

b) H.P. Dustin, et al., "Excessive Sodium Retention as a Characteristic of Salt-Sensitive Hypertension," *American Journal of Medical Sciences*, 292(2):67–74, 1986.

19. and 20.

a) M. Jacobson, B.F. Liebman, "Dietary Sodium and the Risk of Hypertension," *New England Journal of Medicine*, 303(14):817–818.

21.

a) P.C. Pozinak, "The Carcinogenicity of Caffeine and Coffee: A Review," *Journal of the American Dietetic Association*, 85:1127–1133, 1985.

b) T.L. Whitsett, C.V. Manion, "Cardiovascular Effects of Coffee and Caffeine," *American Journal of Cardiology*, 53:918–922, 1984.

c) D.S. Thelle, E. Arnesen, O.H. Forde, "The Tromso Heart Study: Does Coffee Raise Serum Cholesterol?," *New England Journal of Medicine*, 308:1454–1457, 1983.

d) M.F. Jacobsen, B.F. Leibman, "Caffeine and Benign Breast Disease," *Journal of the American Medical Association*, 255(11):1438–1439, 1986.

Chapter 11

1.

This list of physiological factors affected by age was derived primarily from resources (c) and (d). Additional supporting data is found in the other two.

a) H.A. deVries, "Tips on Prescribing Exercise Regimens for Your Older Patient," *Geriatrics*, 35:75–81, 1979.

b) P.L. Fitzgerald, "Exercise for the Elderly," *Medical Clinics of North America*, 69:189–196, 1985.

c) G.A. Brooks, T.D. Fahey, *Exercise Physiology: Human Bioenergetics and Its Applications* (New York: John Wiley and Sons, 1984), pp. 683–700.

d) W.D. McArdle, F.I. Katch, V.L. Katch, *Exercise Physiology: Energy, Nutrition, and Human Performance*, 2nd ed. (Philadelphia: Lea & Febiger, 1986), pp. 563–570.

2.

a) J.A. Wessel, W.B. Van Huff, "The Influence of Physical Activity and Age on Exercise Adaptation of Women Aged 20–69 Years," *The American Journal of Sports Medicine*, 9:173–180, 1969.

b) Sharon Begley, "Why Do We Grow Old?," *Newsweek*, June 16, 1986, p. 61.

3.

a) P. Lemon, K.E. Yarasheski, D.G. Dolny, "The Importance of Protein for Athletes," *Sports Medicine*, 1:474–484, 1984.

b) I. Gontzea, R. Sutzescu, S. Dumitrache, "The Influence of Adaptation to Physical Effort on Nitrogen Balance in Man," *Nutrition Reports International*, 11:231–236, 1975.

4.

American Dietetic Association Statement, "Nutrition and Physical Fitness," *Journal of the American Dietetic Association*, 76:437–443, 1980.

5.

The following two articles discuss different points of view on the supplementation of iron:

a) W.H. Crosby, "Yin, Yang and Iron," *Nutrition Today*, 21(4)14–16, 1986.

b) J.L. Beard, "Iron Fortification—Rationale and Effects," *Nutrition Today*, 21(4): 17–20, 1986.

6.

A.C. Guyton, *Textbook of Medical Physiology*, 7th ed. (Philadelphia: W.B. Saunders Co., 1986), p. 670.

7.

D.C. Cumming, et al., "Reproductive Hormone Increases in Response to Acute Exercise in Men," *Medicine and Science in Sports and Exercise*, 18:369–373, 1986.

Chapter 12

1.

a) H.A. deVries with Dianne Hales, *Fitness After Fifty* (New York: Scribner & Sons, 1982).

b) H.A. deVries, "Tips on Prescribing Exercise Regimens for Your Older Patient," *Geriatrics*, 35:75–81, 1979.

Chapter 13

1.

H. Kraus, *Clinical Treatment of Back and Neck Pain* (New York: McGraw-Hill, 1970).

2.

A. Melleby, *The Y's Way to a Healthy Back* (Piscataway, N.J.: New Century Publishers, 1982).

3.

a) G. Timothy Johnson, M.D., and Stephen E. Goldfinger, M.D., eds. *The Harvard Medical School Health Letter Book* (Cambridge, Mass: Harvard University Press, 1981), p. 43.

b) T. Gerard Aldhizer, M.D., Thomas M. Krop, M.D., and Joseph Dunn, *The Doctor's Book on Hair Loss* (Englewood Cliffs, N.J.: Prentice Hall, 1983), pp. 55, 65, 80–88.

4.

You'll find an interesting presentation of the types of hair quackery in *The Doctor's Book on Hair Loss*, pp. 80–88, and in Herbert S. Feinberg, M.D., *All About Hair: Avoiding the Ripoffs, Making It Better, Replacing It If It Is Gone* (New York: Simon & Schuster, 1979), pp. 3–29.

5.

If you'd like to read more about hair weaving, you can do so in *All About Hair*, pp. 108–111. An interview with a cosmetologist who performs hair weaving is offered in John Mayhew, *Hair Techniques And Alternatives to Baldness*, (Owerri: Trado-Medic Books, 1983).

6. and 7.

For a good discussion of the pros and cons of these suture implants, see *All About Hair*, pp. 113–114, or *The Doctor's Book on Hair Loss*, pp. 103–105.

8.

If you are contemplating a hair transplant, you may want to read about it in several sources. The following books have clear, illustrated discussions and are available in many libraries.

a) *The Doctor's Book on Hair Loss*, pp. 109–122.

b) *All About Hair*, pp. 117–166.

c) James J. Reardon, M.D., and Judi McMahon, *Plastic Surgery for Men: The Complete Illustrated Guide* (New York: Everest House, 1981), pp. 67–85.

d) Dr. Walter P. Unger & Sidney Katz, *The Intelligent Man's Guide to Transplants and Other Methods of Hair Replacement* (Chicago: Contemporary Books, Inc., 1979).

9.

Anastasia Toufexis, "Some Bald Facts About Minoxidil," *Time*, July 14, 1986, p. 43.

10.

"Going Bald? 'Miracles' May Be Costly—and Risky," *Business Week*, July 28, 1986 p. X.

11.

Toufexis, *Time*, p. 43.

12.

"Dental Implants," an interview with Dr. Paul Schnitman, head of the Department of Implant Dentistry at the Harvard School of Dental Medicine, in *The Harvard Medical School Health Letter*, 11 (Oct. 1986):5–8.

13.

Marilyn Linton, The new price of a smile, *MacLeans*, Jan. 28, 1985, p. 48.

14.

a) Marshal F. Goldsmith, "*Caveat Emptor* tops the eyechart for radial keratotomy candidates," *Journal of the American Medical Association*, 254 (Dec. 27, 1985):3,401–3,403.

b) Maureen K. Lundergan, M.D., George L. White, Jr., M.S.P.H., and Richard T. Murdock, "What Patients Should Know About Radial Keratotomy," *American Family Physicians*, 33 (May 1986):169–172.

c) "The Nearsighted Operation," *The Health Letter* 27 (Jan. 1986):2–3.

d) "Radial Keratotomy: an Unkind Cut?," *Science News*, 128 (Oct. 12, 1985):229.

15.

For an excellent summary of the issues and events in the case, see Colin Norman, "Clinical Trial Stirs Legal Battles," *Science*, 227 (March 15, 1985):1,316–1,318. See also Karen Freifeld, "Myopic Haste?," *Forbes* (May 6, 1985):95–98.

16. and 17.

"Follow-up and Feedback: Surgery for Nearsightedness," *Harvard Medical School Health Letter*, 10 (Oct. 1985):8.

Chapter 14

1.

"Vitamin Supplements," in Eva May Nunnelley Hamilton and Eleanor Noss Whitney, *Nutrition, Concepts and Controversies*, 2nd Edition, (St. Paul: West Publishing Company, 1982), pp. 45–49, includes an excellent discussion of this and other points.

For a longer look at the issues related to vitamins and "natural" foods, see Victor Herbert, M.D., J.D., and Stephen Barrett, M.D., *Vitamins and "Health" foods: The Great American Hustle* (Philadelphia: George F. Stickley Company, 1982).

2.

W.H.B. Denner, "Colourings and Preservatives in Food," *Human Nutrition: Applied Nutrition* 38A:435–449, 1984.

3.

a) James DeBrosse, "Some Patients Lose Only Money: Some Pay with Their Lives," *St. Petersburg Times*, Sunday, July 29, 1984.

b) James DeBrosse, "FDA Has Strict Rules on Health Product Claims," *St. Petersburg Times*, July 30, 1984.

c) James DeBrosse, "FDA, Industry Dispute Value of Herb Use," and "Herbalife Rally," in *St. Petersburg Times*, July 31, 1984.

The above articles are part of a series written by James DeBrosse, who holds master's degrees in public health as well as journalism. The FDA Press Office and many FDAers encouraged the series, publication of which was delayed because of threats of prepublication suits against the *Times*. Readers who wish to read the whole series will find it reprinted in the *Health* volumes of the *Social Issues Resources Series* (*SIRS*) in most libraries.

d) William T. Jarvis, Ph.D. and Stephen Barrett, M.D., "How Quackery Is Sold," in *The Health Robbers*. Stephen Barrett, M.D. ed., Second Ed. (Philadelphia: George F. Stickly Company, 1980), pp. 12–25.

e) William T. Jarvis, "Food Faddism, Cultism, and Quackery," *Annual Review of Nutrition*, 3:35–52, 1983.

4.

William Jarvis, quoted in "Quick Hits," in *50 Plus*, July 1986, p. 12. Also in personal phone interview.

5.

Quoted in James DeBrosse, "Some People Lose Only Money . . ."

6.

a) Eva May Nunnelley Hamilton and Eleanor Noss Whitney, *Nutrition, Concepts and Controversies*, p. 19.

b) Michael A. Dubick, "Dietary Supplements and Health Aids—A Critical Evaluation, Part 3—Natural and Miscellaneous Products," *Journal of Nutrition Education*, 15(1983): 123–129.

7.

a) "Cytotoxic Testing Advertised As Money Maker," *National Council Against Health Fraud Newsletter,* 8 (March/April 1985):3.

b) "Cytotoxic Testing," *Nutrition and the M.D.* 11(1985):1.

c) "Pennsylvania Prohibits Cytotoxic Testing for Food Allergies," *National Council Against Health Fraud Newsletter,* 8(Nov./Dec. 1985): 1.

d) "Hair Analysis," *Harvard Medical School Health Letter,* 11(June 1986), p. 8.

e) S. Barrett, "Commercial Hair Analysis: Science or Scam?," *Journal of the American Medical Association* 254:1041, 1985.

8.

a) Dubick, p. 125.

b) Judith Willis, "About Body Wraps, Pills and Other Magic Wands," *FDA Consumer,* Nov. 1982, pp. 18–19.

9.

a) "What's This Glucomman?," *FDA Consumer,* Feb. 1984, p. 31.

b) Willis, p. 19.

10.

a) Stephen Barrett, M.D., "Diet Facts and Fads," in *The Health Robbers,* p. 181.

b) Willis, p. 19.

11.

Leo Tolstoy, *War and Peace,* trans. Ann Dunnigan (New York: New American Library), p. 790.

Chapter 15

1.

The Health Consequences of Smoking: Chronic Obstructive Lung Disease, report of the surgeon general. U.S. Department of Health and Human Services, DHHS Publication No. (PHS) 84-50205, 1984, p. 417. The urban dweller breathes in an average of two milligrams of particulate matter from the air per day; the smoker of two packs of cigarettes a day at twenty milligrams tar, about 800 mg.

2.

As reported in "Number of Adult Smokers Down by 7 Percent Since 1976, Study Shows," The Miami Herald, Oct. 19, 1986, p. 12A.

3. and 4.

a) *The Health Consequences of Smoking: Chronic Obstructive Lung Disease,* p. 417.

b) *The Health Consequences of Smoking: Cardiovascular Disease,* report of the surgeon general. U.S. Department of Health and Human Services, DHHS Publication No. (PHS) 84-50204, 1984, pp. 206–208.

5.

You can find this information in many places, but a very clear description may be found in Doctors Myra B. Shayevitz and Berton R. Shayevitz, *Living Well with Emphysema and Bronchitis* (New York: Doubleday, 1985), which is available in many public libraries. For a much more technical discussion, see Chapter 5, "Mechanisms by Which Cigarette Smoke Alters the Structure and Function of the Lung," in *The Health Consequences of Smoking: Chronic Obstructive Lung Disease*, pp. 251–328.

6.

For a review of the research on the various ways in which smoke damages the lung, see "Cigarette Smoke Toxicology," in *The Health Consequences of Smoking: Chronic Obstructive Lung Disease*, pp. 426–450.

7.

Health Consequences of Smoking: Chronic Obstructive Lung Disease, p. viii.

8.

National Center for Health Statistics, *Health USA 1985*, DHHS Publication No. (PHS) 86-1232, Dec. 1985, p. 16.

9.

a) *Health USA 1985*, p. 16.

b) *The Health Consequences of Smoking and Women*, a report of the surgeon general. U.S. Department of Health and Human Services, Public Health Service, 1980.

10.

The figure was given to us in a phone interview with the office. Earlier printed sources put the figure at 340,000, but at least one authority, Dr. Elizabeth Whelan, writing as executive director of the American Council on Science and Health, put the estimate of premature deaths associated with smoking at 400,000 ("Big Business vs. Public Health: The Cigarette Dilemma," *USA Today* [magazine], May 1984, p. 62).

11.

U.S. Department of Health and Human Services, Public Health Services, Office on Smoking and Health, *A Physician Talks About Smoking: A Slide Presentation* (Title document No. A14700), p. 27.

12.

a) *A Physician Talks About Smoking*, p. 7.

b) See also, *The Health Consequences of Smoking: Cancer*, a report of the Surgeon General, U.S. Department of Health and Human Services, DHHS Publication No. (PHS) 82-50179, 1982.

c) *Smoking, Tobacco, & Health: A Fact Book*, U.S. Department of Health and Human Services. DHHS Publication No. (PHS) 80-50150.

13.

a) Whelan, "Big Business vs. Public Health: The Cigarette Dilemma," p. 63.

b) *The Health Consequences of Smoking: Cancer*, pp. vi–vii, 5–8.

14.

Facts About Smoking and Your Heart, U.S. Department of Health and Human Services. This pamphlet is excerpted from the text of Dr. Koop's

Nov. 17, 1983, press conference announcing the release of the 1983 *Report on the Health Consequences of Smoking: Cardiovascular Disease.* For further information consult this volume, pp. iii–vii.
15.
Facts About Smoking and Your Heart.
16.
The following articles will give you an overview of the relationship of smoking and heart disease.
a) David W. Kaufman, Constituents of Cigarette Smoke and Cardiovascular Disease, in *The Cigarette Underworld*, ed. Alan Blum, M.D., a publication of the Medical Society of New York (Secaucus, N.J.: Lyle Stuart, Inc., 1985), p. 27.
b) Lloyd W. Klein, M.D., "Effects of Cigarette Smoking on Systemic and Coronary Hemodynamics," in *The Cigarette Underworld*, pp. 24–26.
c) See also, *Health Consequences of Smoking: Cardiovascular Disease*, pp. 209–219 for a discussion of the effects of nicotine, and pp. 219–224 for those of carbon dioxide.
17.
a) "Older People and Smoking," *From the Surgeon General*, a newsletter published by U.S. Department of Health and Human Services, Public Health Service, 1986.
b) Robert Lee Holtz, "It's Never Too Late to Stop Smoking," *Atlanta Constitution*, June 4, 1985, p. 4A.
18.
David Kaufman, "Constituents of Cigarette Smoke and Cardiovascular Disease," *The Cigarette Underworld*, p. 27.
19.
T.F. Pechacek, A.R. Folsom, R. de Gaudermaris, et al., "Smoke Exposure in Pipe and Cigar Smokers Serum Thiocyanite Measures," *Journal of American Medical Association*, 254:3330–3332, 1985.
20.
Jack Henningfield of the Addiction Research Center of the National Institute of Drug Abuse, quoted in Diane E. Edwards, "Nicotine: A Drug of Choice," *Science News*, 129 (Jan. 18, 1986):44.
21.
For a further description of the addictive qualities of nicotine see:
a) Edwards, "Nicotine: A Drug of Choice," pp. 44–45.
b) William Pollin, M.D., "Why People Smoke Cigarettes," a statement developed from testimony before Congress by the director of the National Institute on Drug Abuse, March 16, 1982. PHS Publication No. (PHS) 83-50195.
22.
I have drawn these types from the National Institute of Health pamphlet,

"Why Do You Smoke?," NIH Publication No. 84-1822, 1984. It includes a short self test.
23.
The U.S. Office on Smoking and Health has free materials to help you quit; write and ask them.
24.
"What RPH's [Registered Pharmacists] Should Know Re New Smoking Cessation Drug," *American Druggist*, March 1984, pp. 108–110.
25.
"Gum to Help You Stop Smoking," *Consumer Reports*, Aug., 1984, pp. 434–435.

Chapter 16

1.
M. Duda, "The Medical Risks and Benefits of Sauna, Steambath, and Whirlpool Use," *The Physician and Sportsmedicine*, 15(5):170–182, 1987.
2.
B. Stamford, "Massage for Athletes," *The Physician and Sportsmedicine*, 13:178, 1985.
3.
For a complete guide to biofeedback applications, see G.E. Schwartz and J. Beatty, eds., *Biofeedback: Theory and Research* (New York: Academic Press, 1977).

Chapter 19

1.
You may obtain the complete *Rockport Fitness Walking Test*, which includes a fitness walking program, from the Rockport Walking Institute, P.O. Box 480, Marlboro, Mass. 01752. The cost was $1.00 as of this printing.
2.
This test, adapted from the *Rockport Fitness Walking Test*, may be found in "Walking: A Program for Life," *Berkeley Wellness Letter*, Feb. 1987, p. 6.
3.
K. H. Cooper, *The Aerobics Program for Total Well-Being* (New York: Bantam Books, 1982), pp. 271–272. Dr. Cooper's book is highly recommended for anyone who wants to know more about aerobics and all the possible activities.

Chapter 20

1.
Jack H. Wilmore, *Training for Sport and Activity: The Physiological Basis of the Conditioning Process*, 2nd edition (Boston: Allyn and Bacon, Inc., 1982), p. 241.

2. and 3.

T. Kavanagh, "Guidelines for Cold Weather Exercise," *Journal of Cardiac Rehabilitation*, 3:70–73, 1983.

4.

You may read more about Hulda Crook's achievements in the *Los Angeles Times*, August 11 to 14, 1986, and earlier in Jim Russell, "The Backpacking Octogenarian," *Aging*, Oct.–Nov. 1984, pp. 22–25.

5.

H.A. deVries, "Physiological Effects of an Exercise Training Regimen upon Men Aged 52 to 88." *The Journal of Gerontology*, 25:325–336, 1970.

6.

H.A. deVries, "Tips on Prescribing Exercise Regimens for Your Older Patients," *Geriatrics*, 34:75–81, 1979.

7.

President's Council on Physical Fitness, *Aqua Dynamics: Physical Conditioning Through Water Exercises* (Washington, D.C.: U.S. Government Printing Office [1985]), p. 3.

8.

If you'd like to read more about fitness swimming, see J. Katz and N.P. Bruning, *Swimming for Total Fitness* (New York: Dolphin Books, Doubleday & Company, Inc., 1981).

Chapter 23

1.

A.E. Thomas, D.A. McKay, and M.B. Cutlip, "A Nomograph Method for Assessing Bodyweight," *The American Journal of Clinical Nutrition*, 29:302–304, 1976.

While the Body Mass Index is a handy tool for estimating desirable weight, it is not intended to provide a complete assessment since it does not take into account such factors as distribution of body fat and health risk factors. Such factors must be taken into account for the most accurate picture.

2.

From the American Diabetes Association and the American Dietetic Association, *A Guide for Professionals: The Effective Application of "Exchange Lists for Meal Planning,"* 1977, in American Dietetic Association, *Handbook of Clinical Diabetes* (New Haven: Yale University Press, 1981), p. F17.

3.

a) U.S. Department of Agriculture and U.S. Department of Health and Human Services, "Nutrition and Your Health: Dietary Guidelines for Americans," Home and Garden Bulletin, N. 232, 2nd edition, 1985.

b) "Dietary Guidelines for Healthy Americans: A Statement for Physicians and Health Professionals by the Nutrition Committee, American Heart Association," *Circulation* 74 (Dec.):1465A–1467A, 1986.

c) U.S. Department of Health and Human Services, National Cancer Institute, "Diet, Nutrition, and Cancer Prevention: The Good News," NIH Publication No. 87-2878, 1986.

4. and 5.

American Heart Association, "Dietary Guidelines," p. 1466A.

6.

Chris Lecos, "New Regulation to Help Sodium-Conscious Consumers," *FDA Consumer*, May 1986, p. 17.

7.

Adapted from the chart in U.S. Department of Agriculture, *Food*, Home and Garden Bulletin, No. 228, 1979. See also Jean A.T. Pennington, "Considerations for a New Food Guide" in I.S. Scarpa, H.C. Kiefer, Rita Tatum, eds., *Sourcebook on Food and Nutrition*, 3rd edition (Chicago: Marquis Academic Media, 1982), pp. 16–18.

8.

Jane Brody, *Jane Brody's Nutrition Book*, (New York: Bantam Books, 1987), p. 515. If you want to know more about labels, Ms. Brody's book has an excellent and extensive chapter.

9.

If you'd like to read more about how to achieve these dietary goals, the Human Nutrition Information Service of the Department of Agriculture has published a series of booklets, one for each guideline. They are Home and Market Bulletins, Numbers 232-1 through 232-7. The titles are (1) "Eat a Variety of Foods"; (2) "Maintain Desirable Weight"; (3) "Avoid Too Much Fat, Saturated Fat, and Cholesterol"; (4) "Eat Foods with Adequate Starch and Fiber"; (5) "Avoid Too Much Sugar"; (6) "Avoid Too Much Sodium"; and (7) "If You Drink Alcoholic Beverages, Do So in Moderation."

10.

"Fish Oil Pills: Jumping the Gun," *Berkeley Wellness Letter*, Feb. 1987, p. 1.

11.

"Avoid Too Much Sodium," Home and Market Bulletin 232-6, p. 4.

12.

"Avoid Too Much Sodium," p. 5.

RESOURCE ORGANIZATIONS

National Council Against
Health Fraud
P.O. Box 1276
Loma Linda, CA 92354
*You may receive a bimonthly
newsletter at $15 per year.*

Lehigh Valley Committee
Against Health Fraud
P.O. Box 1602
Allentown, PA 18105
*Information on consumer health,
quackery, and health frauds.*

U.S. Department of Agriculture
Food and Nutrition Information Center
10301 Baltimore Blvd.
Beltsville, MD 20705
*Provides information on nutri-
tion and diet.*

Food and Drug Administration
5600 Fishers Lane
Rockville, MD 20857

The American Dietetic Association
430 North Michigan Ave.
Chicago, IL 60611

American Heart Association
7320 Greenville Ave.
Dallas, TX 75231

American Medical Association
535 North Dearborn St.
Chicago, IL 60610

American Cancer Society
777 Third Ave.
New York, NY 10017

American Lung Association
1740 Broadway
New York, NY 10019

Office on Smoking and Health
U.S. Department of Health,
Education, and Welfare
5600 Fishers Lane
Park Building, Room 110
Rockville, MD 20857

The National Strength and
Conditioning Association
Journal
P.O. Box 81410
Lincoln, NE 68501
*A great place to get a compre-
hensive view on weight training;
used by many strength coaches.*

I N D E X